Into Thin Air

INTO THIN AIR

A History of Aviation Medicine

in the RAF

by

T.M. GIBSON and
M.H. HARRISON

Foreword by
Air Marshal Sir David Atkinson KBE, QHP, RAF

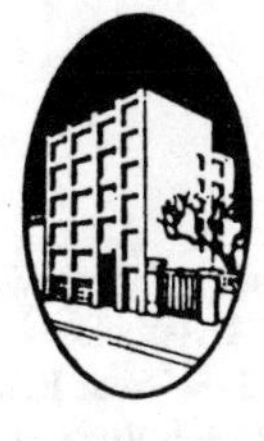

ROBERT HALE · LONDON

First published in Great Britain 1984

ISBN 0 7090 1290 X

Robert Hale Limited
Clerkenwell House
Clerkenwell Green
London EC1R 0HT

Photoset in North Wales by
Derek Doyle & Associates, Mold, Clwyd
Printed in Great Britain by
St Edmundsbury Press, Bury St Edmunds, Suffolk
Bound by Woolnough Bookbinding Limited

To the memory of Air Marshal Sir Harold Whittingham,
the inspiration for many who have gone before and, perhaps
through this book, the inspiration for many yet to come.

Contents

Illustrations

Acknowledgements

The illustrations in this book are Crown copyright with the exception of the following: National Portrait Gallery, 1; Royal Society of Medicine, 3; Imperial War Museum, 4, 6, 10; Professor Sir Bryan Matthews, 7; Australian War Memorial, 37; Wing Commander K. Bazarnik, 38; Martin Baker Aircraft Company, 41; Audio Visual Centre, University of Newcastle, 46; JRNMS, 57

List of Abbreviations

AEA	Aircrew Equipment Assembly
AEG	Aircrew Equipment Group
AFC	Air Force Cross
AMTC	Aviation Medicine Training Centre
AR	Aircrew Respirator
ATDR	Automatic Thermal Data Recorder
AVS	Air Ventilated Suit
BOAC	British Overseas Airways Corporation
CAA	Civil Aviation Authority
CAM	Catapult Armed Merchant Ship
CB	Companion of the Order of the Bath
CBE	Commander of the Order of the British Empire
CDE	Chemical Defence Establishment
CinC	Commander-in-Chief
CME	Central Medical Establishment
DFC	Distinguished Flying Cross
DGMS	Director General of Medical Services
DHR	Director of Health and Research
DMS	Director of Medical Services (title used until the 1940s)
DPMO	Deputy Principal Medical Officer
EHC	Electrically Heated Clothing
ESA	European Space Administration
FPMO	Flying Personnel Medical Officer
FPRC	Flying Personnel Research Committee
FRCP	Fellow of the Royal College of Physicians
FRCS	Fellow of the Royal College of Surgeons
FRS	Fellow of the Royal Society

HMS	His/Her Majesty's Ship
IAM	Institute of Aviation Medicine
KHP	Honorary Physician to the King
KHS	Honorary Surgeon to the King
LCS	Liquid Conditioned Suit
L/min	Litres per minute
MA	Master of Arts
MAP	Ministry of Aircraft Production
MC	Military Cross
MD	Doctor of Medicine
ME	Mechanical Engineering Department of the RAE
mm Hg	Millimetres of mercury
MSFU	Merchant Ship Fighter Unit
MOD	Ministry of Defence
MOD(PE)	Ministry of Defence (Procurement Executive)
MOP	Medical Officer Pilot
MOS	Ministry of Supply
MP	Member of Parliament
MRC	Medical Research Committee (until 1920; Council from 1920)
NASA	National Aeronautics and Space Administration
NBC	Nuclear, Biological, Chemical
OBE	Officer of the Order of the British Empire
OBOGS	On-Board Oxygen Generating System
OM	Order of Merit
PMO	Principal Medical Officer
PRU	Photographic Reconnaissance Unit
RAAF	Royal Australian Air Force
RAC	Royal Armoured Corps
RAE	Royal Aircraft Establishment
RAF	Royal Air Force
RAMC	Royal Army Medical Corps
RCAF	Royal Canadian Air Force
RNAS	Royal Naval Air Service
RFC	Royal Flying Corps
ScD	Doctor of Science

SDFD	Spatial Disorientation Familiarization Device
SMA	Sensori-Motor Apparatus
UK	United Kingdom of Great Britain and Northern Ireland
USA	United States of America
USAF	United States Air Force
VIP	Very Important Person

Foreword

by Air Marshal Sir David Atkinson KBE, QHP, RAF

We in the Royal Air Force, because of our comparatively short history, are perhaps less aware than we ought to be of the need to record events before they fade too far from memory. It is therefore all the more encouraging that these two young authors have taken this opportunity to tell the story of aviation medicine in the Royal Air Force. Such an account is, of course, virtually the story of the development of the Royal Air Force Institute of Aviation Medicine at Farnborough, Hampshire. The authors, appropriately one a serving officer, the other a civilian, write from the IAM, where they have been fortunate to have access to collected records and research papers dating from the establishment of the Institute's predecessor, the RAF Physiological Laboratory. They have, moreover, taken full advantage of the astounding memories of some of those most closely involved in the aviation medicine scene during World War II; men like Professor Sir Bryan Matthews and that founder member and doyen of the RAF Medical Branch, to whose memory this book is dedicated, the late Air Marshal Sir Harold Whittingham.

The reader will see that the problems of aviation psychology, as well as physiology, which arose in the Second World War have been covered. Whilst some of the advances which psychological research brought may have arrived too late to be of decisive value in that conflict, there is no doubt that the work has been of inestimable value in the jet age which followed and which has led to an enormous increase in aircrew workload.

The authors have demonstrated that medical scientists have made vital contributions to safety in aviation, both military and civil, and the book has added to the understanding of the role of the doctor in an air force. It is unquestioningly accepted by his non-medical colleagues that he provides general practitioner and hospital services as well as medical cover for the flying programme. It is not so frequently understood that the doctor is often the first to see the results of human frailty or error and of failure of machine or equipment. Gibson and Harrison have demonstrated this in a most convincing fashion and shown that medicine can predict and contribute to the solution of practical aviation problems. In so doing they have also pointed to the outstanding courage shown by experimenters over the years at the IAM.

This is a story that needed telling, and whilst they would not expect me to agree with all their views, there is not much with which I would quarrel. They are to be congratulated for the qualities they have admired in so many of their predecessors at the Institute – enthusiasm, initiative and tenacity of purpose. The authors have expressed a wish to transfer the income from their share of the royalties on the sale of this book to the Trust which commemorates the life and work of Air Vice-Marshal W.K. Stewart CB, CBE, AFC, a former Commandant of the Royal Air Force Institute of Aviation Medicine. As Chairman of the Stewart Memorial Trust, I thank them for this most generous gesture and, unashamedly, wish the book every success.

Authors' Preface

As aircraft have become increasingly sophisticated, human tolerances have more and more set the limits to which the aircraft can be used. Aviation medicine evolved in order to match the performance of the man to that of the machine. Only one accurate account of the history of aviation medicine has been published (*The Dangerous Sky*, by D.H. Robinson), but that was concerned mainly with American advances. Here in Britain, we have led the world in some areas of aviation medicine and still do in others.

The history of British military aviation medicine is very much the story of one scientific research establishment – the Royal Air Force Institute of Aviation Medicine (IAM). Although this Institute was actually a fairly late arrival on the aviation scene, its ancestry can be traced back to the end of the First World War. Because the IAM is a military establishment, whose function is to advise the RAF, our story has a strongly military bias. Moreover, the 'medicine' in 'aviation medicine' is not medicine as generally understood by the layman. Aviation medicine is essentially preventive – not curative or clinical; it aims to help the man withstand the stresses of flight. Accordingly our history is concerned with physiology, ergonomics, protective clothing, psychology and engineering. While this may sound a formidable list, our task is made slightly easier by the fact that the problems have remained largely the same from the earliest days of flight to the present day. Only the solutions have changed.

The history has been written for the layman who is interested in flying, to show him an aspect of aviation that he may not have hitherto considered. Medical jargon is avoided and is simply explained when it is necessary. The aim has been to produce a history that is at the same time definitive and yet easily readable. The approach has been to treat events chronologically, although, from World War II onwards, to deal separately with the historical development of various different aspects of aviation medicine.

As the present Head of the RAF Institute of Aviation Medicine, Air Commodore Peter Howard, has observed, the compilation of a history of aviation medicine in the United Kingdom has been often discussed and sometimes started. Perhaps it was never finished because the would-be historians belatedly appreciated the enormity of their task. Certainly being confronted with filing cabinet after filing cabinet full of archival material – reports, memoranda, committee papers, books and files – was a daunting experience for us. For this, in a literal sense, was 'that great dust-heap called "history" '. But, to quote Carlyle, 'The history of the world is but the biography of great men', and we have indeed been fortunate in having access to some of the great men of British aviation medicine. With their help, we tried to blow away the dust and tell, for the first time, a story not just of British scientific achievement and success but of personal courage, dedication and self-sacrifice of Service and civilian personnel alike.

First and foremost amongst these great men is Sir Harold Whittingham, to whose memory this book is affectionately dedicated, for without him there might never have been an IAM. He and Lady Whittingham gave us every assistance and encouragement, for which we thank them. Help, hospitality and anecdotes have also been liberally dispensed by Sir Bryan Matthews, Surgeon Vice-Admiral Sir John Rawlins, Air Vice-Marshal T.C. Macdonald, Air Vice-Marshal H.L. Roxburgh, Dr and Mrs John Gilson, the late Group Captain H.P. Ruffell-Smith and Mr B. Kervell. We are also very grateful to Mr O. Blunt, Mr N. Burn, Mr B. Limbrey, Mr R. Needham and finally Wing Commander R.H. Winfield's widow, Mrs H.D. Ridgeon, for allowing us to borrow her late husband's papers. It would be invidious to attempt to single out individuals at the Institute for acknowledgement – so many have been of service, but mention must be made of the staff in the typing pool, the photographic section and Dr Byford and his computer staff, all of whom have made our task so much easier. We are particularly grateful to our Commandant, Air Commodore Howard, for allowing us the time and facilities to compose this history, and to Air Commodore R.A. Probert and Air Marshal Sir David Atkinson for advice and guidance. Finally, we wish to record our indebtedness to our wives and families for their forbearance of the neglect they have experienced during the time this book has been in preparation.

'To understand science, one must know its history.'

Auguste Comte

'You cannot be a good human physiologist unless you regard your body, and that of your colleagues, ... as something to be used and, if need be, used up.'

J.B.S. Haldane

The views expressed in this book are those of the authors alone and should not be interpreted in any way as representing the opinion of the Ministry of Defence.

1 First Awakenings

The morning of 17 December 1903 dawned cold at Kitty Hawk, North Carolina, and along the beach a blustery wind whipped the sand hard across the dunes. An unlikely setting, perhaps, for the realization of a dream as old as Man himself. But that is exactly what was about to happen. At just after 10.30 Orville Wright climbed aboard a flimsy-looking, spruce-framed biplane. There was a roar from a 12 h.p. engine, and two large propellers at the back started to spin. Brother Wilbur let go of the rope, and within seconds the machine was in the air. It did not go very high, nor very far, but it was enough. Thanks to two bicycle manufacturers from Ohio, the world would never be quite the same again.

Just over sixty years later, a span of time short enough for at least a few of those out at Cape Kennedy on that July morning to remember the momentous event way back in 1903, the count-down was in progress for the realization of another dream. Beneath a blue sky and hot sun, Apollo Eleven was ready to take the first men to the surface of the moon.

During those intervening six and a half decades, the fragile aircraft of the early years of the century, all struts, wire and aeroplane dope, had given way to streamlined metal machines, devoid even of propellers. Altitude, originally measured in hundreds of feet, can now be measured in miles. Speed, at least for aircraft like Concorde and for jet fighters, is measured in terms of the speed of sound, rather than miles per hour. Yet, although aircraft have changed almost beyond recognition since Flier 1 staggered off the beach at Kitty Hawk, those who fly them have not. This seemingly self-evident observation has important consequences. It means that man's performance in the air is limited not so much by his machine as by himself. Just a few years after the events at Kitty Hawk, it was being recognized, at least by some, that there was a need to match the man to his machine. In response to this recognition a new science emerged – aviation medicine.

To be strictly accurate, there had really been a speciality of aviation medicine for many years before 1903. Several hundred years ago physicians were aware of the sickness and debilitation associated with mountain travel, and in the nineteenth century the increasingly high altitudes to which balloons were ascending brought to the attention of the medical world the twin hazards of altitude/hypoxia (that is, a lack of oxygen) and cold. It was only with the classic experiments of Paul Bert, described in his 1878 monograph *La Pression Barométrique*, that it became generally recognized that the effects of altitude were caused not by a lack of oxygen but by the diminished partial pressure of oxygen associated with the reduced barometric pressure.

In Britain during the nineteenth century, ballooning was no less popular than elsewhere in Europe – the only difference was that the British scientific contributions in this field were virtually nil. The military potential of balloons had been appreciated very early on – at least by the French. In 1794 they actually formed an Aeronautical Company, and tethered balloons were used for observation purposes that year in the Battle of Fleurus, fought against the Austrians. Balloons were used in the American Civil War and also during the siege of Paris in the Franco-Prussian War for the conveyance of dispatches – and people – out of the beleaguered city. Balloons were first used by the British Army in the Bechuanaland Expedition of 1884, and then again in the Boer War. A Balloon School had been established at Woolwich in 1878 for the instruction of Royal Engineers in military aeronautics. Near to the school, at Chatham, was a factory for making balloons, and in 1890 both were moved to Aldershot so that balloons could be used during army exercises. In 1905 the factory was moved again, this time to South Farnborough, where it would eventually become the present Royal Aircraft Establishment. Despite the achievements of the Wright Brothers in America, however, the emphasis in this country remained with balloons until 1909; the War Office saw little of military value in the aeroplane![1]

This attitude was changed by the then Secretary of State for War, Lord Haldane. He had a strong belief in the future of the aeroplane, based, no doubt, not just upon events across the Atlantic but also on an awareness of the tremendous advances being made by the French, who from 1909 to 1914 led the aviation world. Additionally, in 1908 the first entirely British aircraft had taken to the air at Farnborough, when 'Colonel' Samuel F. Cody covered a distance of about 460 yards in 'British Army Aeroplane Number 1'. Haldane overcame the War Office obduracy by the simple expedient of bypassing it! An advisory committee on aeronautics was set up which reported directly to Prime Minister Asquith.[2] In 1910 a Mr O'Gorman was made head of the Balloon Factory, which was soon renamed the Aircraft Factory. It became the Royal Aircraft Factory in 1912 and gained its present name, the Royal Aircraft Establishment, in 1918.

Military aviation in Britain achieved a belated recognition in 1911 with the formation of an Air Battalion (which superseded the Balloon School), to be followed by the Royal Flying Corps (RFC) with two wings, one naval and the other military. The Corps was based at the Central Flying School at Upavon, on the Salisbury Plain, and from the start was dominated by the Army. So very quickly the two wings grew apart and by the outbreak of war were virtually separate organizations. This was despite the fact that the Command Paper creating the RFC had stipulated that 'the British aeronautical service was to be regarded as one.'[3] The first medical officer attached to the Central Flying School was Captain E.G.R. Lithgow, who several years later was to be involved in the medical selection of flying officers. To the naval wing – or the Royal Naval Air Service (RNAS) as it became in 1914 – was attached Staff Surgeon H.V. Wells, who was to contribute much on matters of safety in the air. Both doctors proved keen aviators, being the first medical men in the UK to learn to fly.

In fact, until the outbreak of World War I there was relatively little interest in aviation medicine, either in Europe or in America. A few medical articles did appear, mainly from the French and the Italians, and in 1911 the Englishman F.I. Wilbur published an article in *Flight* magazine entitled 'Aviation and Common Sense'. This contained a colourful account of some of the physiological problems reputed to beset the aviator – including haemorrhaging from fingernails and lips and loosening of the femur in its socket! Most of the symptoms he described relate specifically to hypoxia, and so Wilbur's suggestion that recourse should be made to inhalation from bags of oxygen was eminently sensible. Rather more questionable were his recommendations that laxatives should be taken prior to flight 'to excite the circulatory organs' and that perhaps bleeding would relieve feelings of 'congestion' and 'lividity'. He pointed out that in the Andes animals were sometimes given relief from 'congestion of blood in the capillaries' by cutting a piece from the ears or by making a slit in the nostril!

Rather more practical suggestions would follow from the studies of H.V. Wells which he began in 1913; indeed, Wells was undoubtedly the first person in Britain to apply rigorous scientific and medical principles to aviation and to the aviator. He was, however, pre-empted into print by J.E. Alder, who in 1914 published his 'Notes on the Medical Aspect of Aviation' in Hamel and Turner's book *Flying*. The significance of Alder's contribution lay with his emphasis on the importance of the medical examination for the would-be aviator. That apart, he concentrated mainly on the physiology of altitude rather than on the physiology of flying, and wrongly ascribed airsickness to lack of oxygen. From a practical point of view, however, the two papers published by Wells, one in 1915 and one and 1916, were of far greater consequence.[4] They were concerned with accidents and flight safety and considered in some detail the advantages and disadvantages afforded by the recently introduced seat-belts and flying helmets. Also, like Alder, Wells drew attention to the physical requirements military pilots should be asked to fulfil.

The work of Alder and Wells and of others such as Lithgow and Surgeon-Lieutenant H.G. Anderson,[5] although immensely valuable, lacked any formal authority. There was no organization within the UK specifically concerned with the medical problems of flying. By way of contrast, in Germany it had been recognized as early as 1910 that special qualifications were needed to be a successful aviator, and consequently the German selection procedures were considerably more advanced than those of their adversaries at the outbreak of war. C.B. Heald, a medical officer who served with the RFC in France during World War I, in an unpublished account of the origins of the Air Force Medical Service[6] draws attention to the disquieting official attitude towards aviation medicine in Britain at that time, which was one of total indifference. This he found surprising in view of the internationally recognized contributions made to medicine by the balloonists and to respiratory physiology by the Englishmen J.S. Haldane (brother of the Secretary of State of War) and J.G. Priestley. However, with regard to ballooning (as opposed to pure physiology), it had consistently been the French, and later the Germans, who had taken the lead. So it should come as no surprise that these countries should be the first in Europe to recognize the military potential of the aeroplane. Necessarily accompanying this recognition was the realization that the success or failure of any aerial enterprise depended in no small part on the 'fitness' of those required to fly the aeroplane. Despite Heald's assertions to the contrary, there were in fact several notable contributions to aviation medicine from France and Germany, and also from the Italians, immediately before the outbreak of war and during the first few years of the war. Most of these were concerned with the effects of flying on blood-pressure, with the causes and prevention of airsickness and with the establishment of minimum physical standards of aviators.

It was to be 1918 before Britain had a medical air service comparable with that of Germany (established in 1915) and France (1917). Nevertheless, the early years of the war were a watershed in British military thinking, at least in terms of the military application of the aeroplane. Once it became accepted that the aeroplane *was* important, then, as a logical corollary, the aviator also became important. The Royal Air Force Medical Service, inaugurated in 1918, was really conceived in 1916, largely as a result of one man's singlemindedness and farsightedness; that man was Major-General (subsequently Lieutenant-General) Sir David Henderson. That he succeeded was due primarily to the fact that by 1916 the aeroplane had become an accepted part of military strategy.

At the outbreak of war the RFC had 179 aircraft, and the RNAS, as it would shortly become, had 91. During the first two years of the war the RFC's aircraft were used mainly for locating enemy batteries and for directing, or 'spotting', artillery fire at the enemy – a singularly hazardous occupation, as the aircraft was generally fired on by both sides! The RNAS's aircraft were used for home defence (particularly against airships), for observation of enemy shipping and for attacks on enemy installations. By 1915 air combat and ground strafing were becoming commonplace, and the casualty rate had begun to rise dramatically, increasing the demand for pilots. Even in pre-war days the methods of teaching had been very hit-and-miss. Now training was so accelerated that even basic escape and evasion manoeuvres could not be taught, and pilots with only a few hours' solo experience were sent to the Front, where the superiority of the enemy was often more a function of his adversaries' inexperience than of any inferiority of allied aircraft. The lesson was learned the hard way, but it was learned. Late in 1917, at Gosport in Hampshire, a new flying school was established, where Captain R. Smith-Barry, using aircraft fitted with dual controls, taught his pupils every conceivable type of manoeuvre that might aid in bewildering and defeating the army. Described by Trenchard as 'the man who taught the world to fly', Smith-Barry owed his success, in no small measure, to a truly revolutionary communication system devised by one of his fellow instructors at the school, a Major Parker. Until then one of the most intractable problems facing flying instructors had been that of communicating with their pupils. Parker devised a system of paired flexile tubes, to be known thereafter as Gosport Tubes, which connected earphones in the instructor's and pilot's helmets to mouthpieces mounted at the opposite ends of the tubes.

Another important step had been taken the previous year with the establishment of a Special Medical Board of the RFC. This Board, which was to be concerned with the medical selection of flying officers, and also with the invalidating and rehabilitation of the injured, was the beginning of the 'formal authority' that was to give aviation medicine credibility; it marked the genesis of British aviation medicine.

According to C.B. Heald, it was Sir David Henderson, the General Officer Commanding RFC in the Field, who in 1916 recommended to the Air Board at the War Office that a Special RFC Medical Board should be formed – this to be concerned with the medical 'vetting' of prospective pilots. There seems little doubt that Henderson forced through his recommendations despite considerable opposition from established opinion in the Army Medical Service, which generally took the view that there were *no* special medical problems to flying. Henderson, a tall, gentle, yet extremely purposeful man, seems to have been one of the more enlightened, forward-thinking army officers of his time. A veteran of the Sudan and the South African Wars, he first became interested in aviation in 1908, following the demonstration flights given in Europe by Wilbur Wright. He learned to fly in 1911 – at the age of forty-eight – and the following year played a key role in the creation of a unified flying service – the RFC. At the outbreak of war he was the Director General of the Military Aeronautics Directorate but was soon made General Officer Commanding the RFC, a post he held until October 1917. In 1918 he would briefly become Vice-President of the newly formed Air Council. He died in 1921 at the age of fifty-nine.

Henderson's arguments were undoubtedly given additional force by the mounting casualty rate in the RFC at that time, which was causing much concern. The climate of opinion would therefore have been favourably disposed towards any suggestions which might lead to a reduction in these losses. Henderson's case would have been based on the reports he was continually receiving from medical officers attached to RFC units at the Front, showing that many of those recruited and trained as pilots and observers were often not really medically 'fit' for flying duties. Today it is well known that certain medical conditions, both chronic and acute, which may be fairly innocuous on the ground, can cause considerable distress under conditions of cold, hypoxia and reduced atmospheric pressure; the common cold is a good example. But in 1916 these lessons were still being learned, and with flying training being so inadequate at that time, learning the lessons also meant adding unnecessarily to casualty lists.

It was from the attempts of the Board to distinguish between candidates who would make successful aviators and those who would not that the need for scientifically designed testing procedures became apparent. The Secretary of the Medical Research Committee (MRC; it became the Medical Research Council in 1920), Sir Walter Morley-Fletcher, was approached by Charles Heald for advice on this matter, and as a result a member of that Committee, Dr Martin Flack, was attached to the Board as 'an adviser on research connected with the physiological aspects of flying'. Flack, an accomplished physiologist, was to prove an invaluable acquisition not just for the Special RFC Medical Board but subsequently for the RAF too. As a medical student working at the London Hospital under the distinguished anatomist Sir Arthur Keith, he had discovered the sino-auricular node, the tissue in the heart responsible for the initiation of contraction. Just before the outbreak of war he had become assistant to Sir Leonard Hill, a physiologist of international repute, with whom he worked first at the London Hospital and then in the Department of Applied Physiology of the Medical Research Committee. In later years Air Marshal Sir Harold Whittingham would remember Flack as 'stoutish, with no military bearing'. This, however, certainly did not prevent Flack from being commissioned as a Captain, RAMC, immediately upon his detachment from the Department.

From the start the Army Medical Service was sceptical about the new selection procedures adopted by the Board. However, as time progressed, the accumulating statistical evidence conclusively showed that far more of the entrants who passed through the Special Medical Board were ultimately successful than of those who passed through the Army Selection Boards.[7] Since each failed aviator cost the country an estimated £2,000, the work of the RFC Board quickly became highly regarded – so much so that in the autumn of 1917 it was enlarged and moved from its slightly incongruous location in the Hotel Cecil in the Strand to new headquarters at Mount Vernon in Hampstead, London. But by this time events of much greater significance were taking place, events which would lead to the formation of the Royal Air Force Medical Service.

Whether there would have been an independent Air Medical Service had the RFC and the RNAS not been amalgamated is unclear – although it would seem unlikely. What is clear is that, once the decision had been made to combine the two air forces, then it was taken for granted that the new Service would need to have its own separate medical service. Consequently, just how the decision came about to join the two air forces together is a matter of some relevance to a history of British aviation medicine.

Two factors were of crucial importance. First, relationships between the RFC and the RNAS grew increasingly acrimonious as the war progressed. Despite the Command Paper stipulation referred to earlier, relationships between the two services were never good, and as the war continued were made even more difficult by competing demands for men and machines – so much so that by 1916 there was little consultation, and even less co-operation, between the RFC under the War Office and the RNAS under the Admiralty. The situation became so bad that a Joint War Air Committee was set up under Lord Derby to provide recommendations as to how the two air services could be drawn closer together. Unfortunately the committee had no executive powers, and it accomplished virtually nothing. It survived only a few months, but in his letter of resignation Lord Derby pointed out that the only logical solution was to combine the RFC and the RNAS. This impasse was not to last long, however, for a few months later the German Air Force launched its bombing offensive against southern England. Against the Gothas flying at 80 m.p.h. and at 15,000 feet, the British air forces proved singularly ineffective. Indeed, so ineffective were they and so indignant both public and government opinion, that in July of that year the War Cabinet appointed a committee consisting of the Prime Minister (Lloyd George) and Lieutenant General J.C. Smuts to examine defence arrangements against air raids, air organization generally and the direction of aerial operations. The first of these issues is of little concern here, but it was the report of General Smuts on the second that was to have such profound consequences. This report concluded with eight recommendations. The three most pertinent of these were that an Air Ministry should be instituted as a matter of urgency, that an Air Staff should be created and that the RFC and RNAS should be absorbed into a new, independent Air Service.[8] These recommendations were accepted, the appropriate legislation prepared, passed and enacted, and on 1 April 1918 the Royal Air Force (known irreverently to the other Services for some years as the 'Royal April Fool'!) was born. Unfortunately, however, by this time plans for the new Air Force Medical Service had already run into trouble. The main problem was that the medical branches of the other two services thought that they, and not the RAF, should run it.

Once it had been agreed that there was to be an independent Air Force, Sir David Henderson had asked C.B. Heald to draw up proposals for the conditions of service and method of administration of the Medical Branch. Charles Heald, a large, powerful, well-built man, had been attached to Sir David's staff during his convalescence following an air crash in France in 1916, when he survived a fractured neck. He was to go on to be a medical consultant to the RAF in the Second World War and remained active in medicine until shortly before his death in 1974 at the age of ninety-one. In 1917, however, Heald quickly discovered that any departure from the existing rules and regulations of the Navy and Army Medical Services provoked immediate opposition from those services. His task proved too difficult and onerous for 'a mere Captain R.A.M.C.', and a Flying Services Medical Advisory Committee was therefore set up, under the chairmanship of Sir William Watson-Cheyne, to give 'form and authority' to Heald's proposals. This Committee unreservedly supported the need for a separate medical service, saying that aviation presented new 'physiological and pathological problems which require special study and which can only be dealt with satisfactorily by a specially trained body of men'. The Committee's proposals for the new Medical Service were given unqualified approval by the Air Board but encountered powerful opposition from both the War Office and the Admiralty. Much ill-tempered wrangling and a reconstitution of the Cheyne Committee followed, until eventually a compromise was reached. The compromise received little support from Watson-Cheyne himself and even less support from the Air Board, which made a strong protest to the Treasury in February 1918. All efforts were in vain, however; the obduracy, and even active obstruction, of the other two services prevented a completely independent Air Medical Service from emerging until after the war.

Under the agreement a Medical Administrative Committee, under the control of the Directors General of the Army and Navy

Medical Services, was set up. The compromise agreement also meant that the medical officers serving in the field with the RFC and the RNAS remained 'on loan' from their parent services. This situation lasted only until 18 April 1918, however, when a Weekly Order from the newly formed Air Ministry decreed that all medical officers within the RAF (then eighteen days old!) were to become the responsibility of the Air Force Medical Department.

Indeed, the Committee itself was to have neither a long nor a particularly happy life. In many ways its existence, and also, therefore, the opposition of the Navy and Army Medical Services, was rendered irrelevant once the Air Force (Constitution) Act received the Royal Assent. For then the RAF existed as an independent service with control of its own organization. Needless to say, inter-service rivalries quickly made themselves apparent on the Committee, and to maintain the peace the War Office was obliged to bring in an 'outsider' to act as Chairman. Major-General Sir Matthew H. Fell, a distinguished veteran of the South African War and a born leader of men, proved an admirable choice, quickly earning the goodwill of his colleagues. So successful was he that, when the Committee was discharged in November 1918, he became the first Director of Medical Services of the RAF, in the rank of acting Air Commodore.

One of his first actions was to select fifty medical officers, most of whom had already seen service with the RFC or the RNAS, to fill essential administrative and professional posts. Over the next three years he firmly established the basic principles upon which the RAF Medical Service is still, to this day, based. Perhaps the most important of these was that specialist medical officers should be allowed to practise their specialities unless they voluntarily elected to be transferred to administrative or other duties. This particular dictum would have significant consequences for the future Institute of Aviation Medicine. Matthew Fell can justly be regarded as the Father of the RAF Medical Service. He went on to become the Director General of the Army Medical Services in 1926 (the only person ever to be a DMS of two services), an appointment he held until his retirement in 1929. He died in 1959 at the age of eighty-six.

2 All You Need is 'Hands'

Just what the prevailing attitude towards the aviator was during the war years is well illustrated by a paper in *The Lancet* of September 1918. This described the typical aviator's character as possessing 'resolution, initiative, presence of mind, sense of humour, judgement'; he was 'alert, cheerful, optimistic, happy-go-lucky, generally a good fellow, and frequently lacking in imagination'. Almost invariably a sportsman, for amusement he likes the theatres, music ('chiefly ragtime'!) and dancing, and 'it appears necessary for the well-being of the average pilot that he should indulge in a really riotous evening at least once or twice a month.' One of the most important characteristics of the successful aviator was his 'hands'. The meaning of this was explained by analogy with horse-riding. Apparently the authors of the paper had never known a man 'who has consistently been in the first flight in the hunting field make anything but a good pilot.'[1]

The paper is quoted at some length because it shows just how archaic and unscientific prevailing attitudes towards flying were in Britain at that time – and remember this was over twelve years after the very first aeroplane flight. Indeed, as late as 1930 a wing commander, writing in the *RAF Quarterly*, advocated riding as an aid to efficiency in the RAF. He claimed that equitation developed 'an eye for the country' and an appreciation of 'communication' and 'hands'.[2] The creation of the Special RFC Medical Board was, therefore, an event of some significance, and during its brief existence it did much to dispel attitudes such as these – although obviously not enough to prevent the ill-informed opinions of some people from being made public. In fact, much of the credit for the medical research conducted at this time lies not with the RFC Board but with the Medical Research Committee. Although they did not, as their 1920 publication *The Medical Problems of Flying*[3] suggests, actually initiate much, if any, research, they did, to quote C.B. Heald again, 'respond generously to requests and appeals for help'. And help was certainly needed. In 1918 aircraft were flying twice as fast and eight times higher than in 1914. Cold had been a serious problem from the beginning, even when altitudes rarely exceeded 3,000 feet. In 1916 altitudes of 20,000 feet were attainable in theory (although rarely in practice), at which air temperatures were commonly below minus 20°C – and the aircraft still had open cockpits! Taking wind-chill into account, the dangers of frostbite were very real. Equally dangerous at these high altitudes, and certainly more insidious, were the effects of hypoxia.

The practical significance of other problems was also becoming more widely appreciated. Reference has already been made to the totally inadequate medical examination and selection procedures applied to prospective aviators. Then there was the question of safety – should safety-belts be worn or protective helmets or even parachutes! It was also being recognized that the stress of operational flying in wartime was exacting its own psychological toll. There were the problems of how to overcome fatigue and loss of confidence. So it is not really surprising that 1917 proved to be the year in which both aviation medicine and aviation physiology, to quote C.B. Heald, 'made the most memorable forward strides'.[4]

It was shortly after Heald had sought advice from the Secretary of the MRC on the possibility of devising special pre-selection tests for pilots that the Committee formally offered its services to the Air Board. Whether this offer was made as a result of the meeting between Heald and Sir Walter Morley-Fletcher or whether the Committee had already decided that it was time to formalize the association with the Air Services, which had been building up unofficially during 1916, is not clear. Perhaps Heald was the catalyst; certainly events moved quickly thereafter. Early in 1917 the Air Board Research Committee (Medical) was formed (soon after renamed the Air Medical Investigation Committee), the members of which included commissioned officers in the RAMC attached to the RFC and eminent scientists from the world of physiology and medicine. The main task of the Committee was to co-ordinate the scientific work already being done for and by the RFC and the RNAS. In addition, specific research projects were given financial and other assistance, and a research team was set up. The MRC also loaned to the War Office a hospital building which they had recently acquired at Hampstead for the proposed National Institute for Medical Research. This was used as a hospital for flying officers, and it also housed a new Physiological Laboratory under Martin Flack, the MRC secondment to the RFC Medical Board. Twenty-eight years later, this laboratory would become the RAF Institute of Aviation Medicine at Farnborough.

The problems to which the research team devoted most of its attention were those of aircrew protection and aircrew selection. The most urgent of the former were those of protecting the airmen against the elements – the cold, wind and rain – and against his aircraft when it crashed. It was not, however, to the solution of these that physiology made its most significant contribution but to that of providing protection against the effects of hypoxia.

Contemporary medical writers devoted much attention to the physiology of hypoxia and to methods of alleviating the symptoms of hypoxia. Yet its importance is easily exaggerated, for throughout the war the great majority of aircraft rarely flew much over 10,000 feet, and many of the pilots and observers almost certainly never saw an oxygen mask. On the other hand, as the war progressed, the important advantage which altitude conferred in aerial combat became more generally appreciated, and there seems little doubt that there was a tendency to fly higher and higher. However, Major J.L. Birley, the medical officer in charge of Field Headquarters RFC, considered that 20,000 feet was the absolute ceiling for combat and that most action occurred below 15,000 feet. The greatest altitudes were attained by the reconnaissance aircraft and by the bombers, but even then only for relatively short periods of time.[5]

Why, therefore, was so much attention devoted to this problem? No clear-cut answer can be given, but several observations are possible relevant. First, the deaths of the Frenchmen Sivel and Crocé-Spinelli, during their balloon ascent to 28,200 feet in April 1875, had proved to the world that hypoxia could be a killer. Twenty years later, during an ascent to 30,000 feet, Berson and Gross had both lost consciousness, despite the fact that they were (presumably very ineffectively) using oxygen. These events must surely have impressed upon the nascent flying services that lack of oxygen at altitude was a problem not to be lightly dismissed. A second point is that the Englishmen J.S. Haldane and J.G. Priestley were internationally recognized authorities on altitude physiology. The armed services had, therefore, an immediately accessible source of expert opinion on the physiological consequences of hypoxia. Thirdly, as the war progressed, it became apparent that many of the medical problems which beset the aviator could be attributed to effects of oxygen deficiency, and in March 1917 Birley had submitted a memorandum to that effect to the War Office. For example, the fatigue which was always present after long flights tended to be more severe the higher the altitude. There were also many cases reported of erratic and irrational behaviour at altitude. Both Birley and Flack cited examples where observers failed to change photographic plates between photographs or were unable to recognize the countryside over which they were flying – even if it was their own! There were cases of pilots failing to engage the enemy and even waving cheerily to them! Landings made after sustained flights at altitude were often well below par and sometimes downright dangerous. Afterwards the pilot would be unsteady on his feet and would usually be extremely short-tempered and complain of a severe headache which could last for many hours. Birley was of the opinion that it was the repeated flights at these high altitudes which produced the frequently observed rapid deterioration in mental and physical well-being. Flack and Heald considered that some deterioration also occurred as a result of flights at relatively low altitudes and that performance could be improved by breathing oxygen. This view was based upon experiments conducted by them in 1917 at Brooklands Airfield; a dozen or so pilots and observers flew short sorties of thirty minutes' duration at low altitudes with and without supplementary oxygen. According to Heald, these were the first experiments in aviation medicine to be carried out specifically for a fighting service. It was, almost certainly, the first field trial.

Field trials, however, have their disadvantages; they are usually expensive to mount, and, more importantly, highly trained aircrew can rarely be spared from operational duties just to take part in scientific experiments. So attempts were made to develop laboratory apparatus for evaluating the effects of 'oxygen want'. Of course, decompression chambers were the ideal solution, but at that time there was only one in the UK suitable for carrying out experiments using human subjects. This was at Siebe Gorman & Co's works in London, where it had been installed in 1912. It was made available for use by the flying services throughout the war. Then in 1917 Lieutenant Colonel Dreyer RFC (afterwards Professor Dreyer) devised a simple apparatus which allowed the pressure of inspired oxygen to be changed at any desired rate, thus simulating the falling pressure of increasing altitude but without the effects of a decreased atmospheric pressure. Flack subsequently devised an even simpler apparatus – rebreathing into a five-litre bag from which the expired carbon dioxide was continuously removed by an absorbent cartridge. By analysing the oxygen content of the bag at points when adverse symptoms were first noted, it was possible to estimate the approximate height at which such symptoms might be expected to develop.

Both the Dreyer and the Flack apparatus were used by Lieutenant-Colonel Corbett RAMC and Lieutenant-Colonel Bazett RAMC in an investigation of the cardiovascular and respiratory reactions of flying personnel to diminished oxygen pressure. This remarkable study was carried out during 1917 in two of the British Expeditionary Force's General Hospitals in France. They showed that, at altitudes of 18,000 feet and above, the usual reaction to hypoxia was an increase of the heart rate and a slowing but deepening of the respiration. Deviations from this normal response generally indicated a poor tolerance to lack of oxygen.

In a subsequent study Bazett showed that a large lung volume and slow respiration rate were characteristic features of those best able to tolerate hypoxia. Corroboration of these observations was provided by Dr Grace Briscoe, who had been working independently at the Physiological Laboratory at Hampstead. She noted that pilots who had become unfit for flying-duties generally had an abnormally rapid and shallow type of respiration, and also that unfit pilots and observers had a higher metabolic rate (as indicated by the amount of oxygen consumed per minute) than their fit colleagues. The significance of Corbett, Bazett and Briscoe's findings was that they showed that some individuals were less sensitive to the adverse effects of hypoxia than others. Since presumably these relatively insensitive people would make better aviators, then would it not be possible to devise tests which would allow them to be identified at the selection boards? It was precisely to this question that Martin Flack addressed himself in April 1917 after his attachment to the RFC Medical Board.

The tests he devised became known as the 'Flack Tests' and were used, although with some modifications, in the selection of airmen until the Second World War. Their usefulness ended only when techniques for the administration of oxygen became so improved that a tolerance of hypoxia was really unnecessary. Flack's approach to the problem of distinguishing normal and abnormal responses to the hypoxia of altitude was very similar to that of Corbett, Bazett and Briscoe. He compared the respiratory responses of fit pilots with those of pilots suffering from the stress of service flying, and on the basis of his findings recommended four specific tests which could be applied to prospective aviators:

1. The measurement of the maximum volume of air which could be expired. This volume was reduced in cases of flying fatigue.
2. The measurement of breath-holding capacity. This, Flack maintained, gave some indication of resistance to hypoxia. (In fact, the breaking-point in breath-holding is determined not so much by the falling oxygen content of the blood as by the effect of the increasing carbon-dioxide content.)
3. The measurement of expiratory force (by blowing a mercury column up a U-tube as high as possible.)
4. Sustaining a forty-millimetre column of mercury in the U-tube, with the breath held, for as long as possible.

Tests 3 and 4 were intended to provide a measure of impaired expiratory force and of resistance to respiratory fatigue. The pulse would also be taken during these two tests, an abnormally large rise being considered unsatisfactory. For all the tests, criteria determining what was 'normal' and what was 'abnormal' had been established on the basis of the many hundreds of comparative measurements on fit and unfit pilots and observers. The approach was thus entirely empirical; contemporary physiology and psychology were far too little advanced for it to be anything else. Perhaps it was because the tests were born of experience that they were so effective in identifying candidates with poor respiratory responses to hypoxia – although whether those rejected candidates would still have made good aviators remains something of a moot point. The evidence from studies carried out much later, during the Second World War, was to cast considerable doubt on the value of many of the 'special tests' used for predicting future flying potential.

Despite all the evidence pointing to its value, there was a very great reluctance amongst pilots and observers to use oxygen – a reluctance attributed by Staff Surgeon Sheldon Dudley to 'unreasonable prejudice'.[6] Dudley, however, was almost certainly committing a grave injustice here, for, whilst there may have been a few who considered it 'soft' to use oxygen, generally the objection was not to the oxygen but to the apparatus used to administer it – either a pipe-stem mouthpiece or a face mask. The first face mask had been invented by the Viennese physiologist Hermann von

Schrötter in about 1900, and over the succeeding years many different types, of all shapes and sizes and made of different materials, had been produced; all shared one common feature – unpopularity. At least part of the problem was psychological; to paraphrase Birley, 'No pilot relished the prospect of seeking out and destroying the enemy with a mask over his face and nose.' There were, however, other, more practical difficulties. For example, the moist expired air would freeze on the mask, obstructing valves and tubing and preventing the flow of oxygen. The masks were uncomfortable, and the dry oxygen passing over the face caused drying of the mouth and nose which led to irritation and sores. For these reasons pipe-stem mouthpieces continued to be used throughout the war. Yet they were not without their problems either. It was fatiguing to grip the pipe stem with the teeth; it required considerable concentration to breathe entirely through the mouth; and if you breathed through your nose, or breathing rate increased, then the inspired oxygen became diluted with air.

Whichever system was used, the oxygen was generally supplied continuously to the aircrew, which meant that the gas supplied during the period of expiration was wasted – amounting to some two-thirds of the total delivered. Haldane, in 1917, did design an apparatus which overcame this particular problem, although it was intended not for aviators but for treating the victims of poisonous gas attacks. An oxygen cylinder supplied a constant flow of oxygen through a reducing valve and regulator to a collecting bag and face mask. During expiration the bag acted as a reservoir, filling with oxygen whilst the expired air passed out of the mask through a rubber flap-valve. During inspiration the negative pressure within the mask closed the valve and caused oxygen to be sucked in from the collecting bag. Thus oxygen, despite being supplied continuously, was used far more economically since it was not wasted during the expiratory phase of respiration.

An apparatus very similar to Haldane's was manufactured by Siebe Gorman for use by aviators. The only difference was the position (and size) of the collecting bag, which was described by Siebe Gorman as an 'oxygen economiser flexible bag'. It does not, however, appear to have been very successful. Birley refers to the 'complexity and vulnerability of the expiratory valve and collecting bag' and to complaints that the system took up 'much valuable space'. By 'vulnerability' he meant that the valve froze and the bag tended to blow off![7] This, however, is far from the end of the story, since the concept was to be resurrected at the start of the next war – as the highly successful Oxygen Economiser.

The problem of the space taken up by oxygen apparatus, alluded to by Birley, was an important one. The later balloonists had used bags to contain the oxygen, but as well as being bulky, bags failed to provide a constant stream of gas. Von Schrötter was the first to propose the use of steel cylinders for storing the oxygen – either as gas or liquid. The disadvantage of cylinders is that they are heavy, and for the aircraft of the period this could mean a considerable reduction in the effective payload or in the speed or altitude ceiling attainable – a recurring problem of aviation. For this reason, towards the end of the war the Germans used liquid oxygen, which reduced the size of the cylinder required by half compared with that needed for compressed gas. The disadvantage of liquid gas at that time was the difficulty of producing it and particularly of storing it, since there was a continuous and considerable loss by evaporation. Throughout the war the British used gaseous oxygen, although Siebe Gorman did manufacture some liquid oxygen systems which were used in aircraft for a short time after the war.

Whether the oxygen is in gaseous or liquid form, some device for controlling its rate of delivery is necessary; that device is the oxygen regulator. Liquid and gaseous oxygen require different types of regulator, and that the Germans were able to use liquid oxygen so successfully was due largely to a system for controlling the rate of evaporation of the gas – a system with which the Allies appear not to have been familiar. The system did have one disadvantage, however; less oxygen was evaporated as altitude increased, due to the fall in temperature.

In Britain oxygen regulators were manufactured by Siebe Gorman. The simplest of these merely had three settings which had to be adjusted manually at certain altitudes to increase the flow of gas. However, apart from having to deliver the right amount of oxygen, it quickly became apparent that regulators needed to provide some indication of how much gas was left in the supply cylinder and also some confirmation of the fact that the oxygen was flowing at the appropriate rate. So regulators became more complicated; pressure gauges were incorporated, and sometimes flow meters. The most famous oxygen regulator of the war was one invented by Dreyer while he was serving in France. This was an aneroid device which automatically increased the amount of oxygen delivered as altitude increased.

From personal records which have survived, and from correspondence and articles in the aviation journals of the time, it is abundantly clear that the overriding concern of the airmen during World War I, apart from simply surviving, was how to keep warm. Nor was this problem limited to the colder months of the year; even on the warmest days of summer the forward motion of the aircraft created a gale which blew straight into the face of the pilot. And, of course, as altitude increased, so the air temperature dropped and the gale became an icy, bone-chilling blast. Even so, there were always some who scorned virtually any sort of protective clothing or safety device. These were the pilots who would endure the most extreme discomfort just to remain free of encumbrances which might impair their ability to see, and outmanoeuvre, the enemy.

To help keep the cold at bay, the World War I aviator had a very considerable selection of different types of flying clothing to choose from.[8] The word 'choose' is used quite deliberately, for, until 1917, there was no official policy regarding what constituted the most appropriate flying clothing assembly. Consequently it was possible to see almost every conceivable variation on the general theme of 'keeping warm'. There *was* an issue of flying clothing made to airmen by the RFC and the RNAS – just a knee-length leather coat, which was usually worn with thigh-length sheepskin 'fug-boots'. Totally inadequate alone, the coat was generally supplemented by clothing purchased by the airmen, out of their own pockets, from commercial suppliers. These suppliers had started out by designing and producing protective clothing for the early motorists, and certainly to begin with there was little difference between the clothing assembly of the motorist and that of the aviator.

There was, then, no attempt being made to develop a really effective flying clothing assembly. On a trial-and-error basis airmen tried all types of fabric and combinations of fabric – silks, wool, leather etc – and all were found to be in some measure unsatisfactory. For example, fur, which was beautifully warm when dry, quickly became matted when wet and lost most of its insulating properties. No clothing seemed to be totally windproof – the cold air always managed to get through the flying coats, however tightly they were buttoned. A continual problem was cold air coming up through the bottom of the coat, freezing the feet, legs and thighs, despite the fug-boots.

The situation did not improve until 1917. That it did so then was due to a fortuitous observation made by a young RNAS pilot, Sidney

Cotton. Being on one occasion obliged to fly his aircraft wearing not his usual flying clothing but just his old ground overall, he was surprised to note that on returning to base he was actually still quite warm. On reflection, he attributed this to the fact that the overalls not only covered virtually his entire body but were also liberally besmeared with aircraft oil and grease, so providing effective windproofing. The overalls thus acted as an airtight bag, keeping the body heat in. This deduction was to lead to the development of the most famous flying suit ever – the Sidcot Suit (named after Cotton, i.e., SIDney COTton) which, although extensively modified over the years, was to see service with the RAF until the early 1940s.

In fact there was little new in the basic concept of a one-piece coverall. The famous French pioneer Blériot had flown in a boiler suit, and single-piece flying suits had been available commercially for years. What was new was that Cotton had stumbled on a very effective way of improving the weather-proofing of clothing; since no single fabric was sufficiently effective alone, why not combine several layers of different fabric? This is exactly what the firm of Robinson and Cleaver did, to whom Cotton took his idea. The suit they eventually produced bore little resemblance to his oil-spattered overall. It was a triple-layer (later to increase to seven layers) garment, having an internal lining of fur, an intermediate layer of silk (for windproofing) and an outer layer of a new ventile fabric, gabardine, which combined wind- and water-proofing; the result was the first truly weather-proof flying coverall. By the end of the year it was being produced by Robinson and Cleaver as the first official service aircrew coverall.

A second breakthrough in the fight against cold came in 1917 with the introduction of electrically heated clothing (EHC) by the RNAS. Although heated waistcoats, socks and gloves were available, it was the latter which were particularly useful, allowing exposed metal surfaces, such as guns or cameras, to be touched, with much reduced risk of receiving cold burns. Electrically heated clothing did have its problems, however, not least of which was obtaining a suitable supply of electrical power; generators mounted on the airframe were common, but then the power generated varied with the speed of the aircraft. An even greater problem, and one which was to bedevil designers and manufacturers for many years thereafter (indeed, was to result ultimately in the virtual abandonment of the idea of EHC by the RAF), was that the heating wires frequently broke, leading to short-circuits and painful burns. Since the feet and particularly the hands were most subject to flexing, it was in the socks and gloves that these short-circuits mainly occurred – i.e. just where electrical heating was most needed. Even today the problem of protecting the hands and feet from the cold, whilst at the same time retaining mobility and tactility, remains a difficult one to resolve.

Cold, rain and wind were not the only environmental hazards with which the early aviator had to contend. The engines of the 'tractor' style aircraft, apart from adding to the din, also had the discomforting habit of spraying the entire cockpit with oil. Even the sun could cause difficulties; at dawn and dusk, when flying eastwards and westwards respectively, the dazzling light coming from low on the horizon could be blinding. Some form of protection to the eyes and ears in particular, and the head in general, was therefore absolutely vital. However, these same problems, although admittedly rather less severe in their impact, had confronted the first motorists. And so, by the outbreak of war, the aviator had available to him as wide a selection of headgear as he had other items of flying clothing – and just as little guidance as to which was best. Just to take goggles as an example; these were available in all manner of shapes and sizes, some with tinted (chlorophyll) glass to reduce glare, some with splinter-proof (Triplex) glass and even some with wipers attached for removing rain and oil. Earplugs were used to protect against the noise, although gradually flying caps and helmets, which had been available well before 1914, became increasingly effective, and preferred, for sound attenuation. The caps were generally soft and fur-lined, serving principally for cold protection, whilst the harder leather helmets strongly advocated for safety reasons by the flying medical officers (men such as Wells, Anderson and Dudley) served also for head protection against impact. Beneath cap or helmet one or more balaclavas might be worn, both for additional warmth and to protect the exposed face, particularly the nose and cheeks, from frostbite.

Just as, until the Sidcot Suit, there had been a clear need for a completely weatherproof flying suit, so by late 1917 there was an obvious requirement for a new flying helmet which incorporated the most recent technological advances. Specifically, these advances were in communication and in aircraft performance. The Gosport Tube system introduced during 1917 and the increasing application of the radio-telephone and wireless telegraphy for ground-to-air and air-to-air communication, all needed earphones and microphones. The ever-increasing altitude attainable by the new aircraft was leading to the increasing use of oxygen equipment. The logical solution was an integrated helmet assembly, incorporating communication and oxygen-supply systems. And, for once, logic prevailed – probably because this was also the time of the major reorganization of the flying services resulting from the Smuts report. Just a few months before hostilities ceased, the very first official issue RAF flying helmet, the Mk 1, appeared. Essentially a leather, fur-lined flying cap, it had attachments for a detachable oxygen mask with mounted microphone and pockets at the side for earphones. It was to remain in service until the early 1930s.

The final year of the war also saw attention, somewhat belatedly, being given to the question of flight safety. Thus the Mk 1 flying helmet was designed to provide impact protection. The RNAS was looking into problems of sea survival, and the first immersion suits were available shortly after the war. The Davidson life-saving dress appeared in 1917; with inflatable flotation bags, this was a great advance on the cumbersome cork life-jackets. Seat-belts, at first rigid but then elasticized, with quick-release fasteners, had been introduced (but not necessarily used) into Avro aircraft before the war. Then in 1917 Oliver Sutton devised a much superior restraint system, which was to remain in service almost to the end of the next war. This had shoulder and waist straps, which came together to hold the pilot firmly in his seat, even when flying inverted. Completely neglected, however, was the one item of safety equipment which might have saved hundreds, if not thousands, of lives – the parachute. This was particularly surprising when it is realized that parachutes had already been around for well over one hundred years, that they were issued throughout the war to the occupants of observation balloons and that by the end of the war the Germans were using them, with considerable success, in many of their aircraft. Admittedly these were crude and cumbersome things, being of the 'static' or 'attached' type, depending on a line attached to the balloon or aircraft to open the parachute after bailing out (the free-fall parachute, opened manually, was not invented until after the war). Yet, throughout the war, the official attitude seemed to be that parachutes would cause aircraft to be abandoned unnecessarily! It was even denied by some that the parachute was a worthwhile life-saving device![9]

In addition to its work on the effects and prevention of hypoxia, the MRC, with the RFC Medical Board, devoted considerable attention to the problem of disorientation. All aviators quickly became aware that their senses could provide a completely misleading impression of the attitude of their aircraft in flight. However, provided there was a clear field of vision and a specific visual reference point, it was easy for a pilot to orientate himself correctly. But without adequate visual cues, such as when flying on dark, cloudy nights devoid of moon or stars, or when flying through fog, smoke or cloud, a pilot could become lost within minutes, even seconds. Blind flying was to remain an exceptionally dangerous occupation until the invention of the artificial horizon by the American Elmer Sperry in 1928.

In the absence of visual cues, disorientation occurs because the information provided by other sense organs is either inadequate or erroneous. This information is provided mainly by the sense organ concerned with the maintenance of the correct orientation of the body in space, the vestibular apparatus of the inner ear. Contemporary medical opinion during the later months of the war appears to have been inclined to the view that this disorientation was a product of an abnormally functioning or over-sensitive vestibular apparatus and that consequently it should be possible to minimize problems of disorientation in the air by selecting only those individuals who had a good sense of 'balance and stability' (this being one of the reasons that good horsemen, and particularly cavalry officers, were assumed to make the best pilots). Therefore, in 1917, whilst Flack was working on his altitude tests, A.H. Cheatle was tasked with devising some tests for measuring the balance and stability of candidates presenting themselves to the RFC Medical Board for flying duties. The tests he developed were intended to measure not just vestibular function but also 'muscle sense' and nervous stability. The latter was judged from the candidate's medical history, by tremor of the hands and in particular by an inability to balance a rod on a flat board with eyes open. Muscle sense was evaluated in terms of how a candidate balanced the rod on the board with his eyes closed and by his capacity to stand on one foot for fifteen seconds with eyes closed. Finally, as a test of vestibular function, the candidate had to walk along a line heel-to-toe and then turn completely around on one foot so as to face the opposite direction.

These tests were widely applied from mid 1917 onwards and for some years after the end of the war. However, by early 1919 sufficient data had been accumulated for a scientific evaluation to be made of their efficacy. This evaluation was carried out by Professor

Head, a member of the Air Medical Investigation Committee – and his findings were not encouraging. He considered that rod-balancing and line-walking were not tests of 'muscle sense' or 'vestibular stability' and provided no indication of ability to fly – only of the existence of some functional abnormality. The only cast-iron indicator of a poor sense of balance and stability in the air was hand tremor, and that, of course, should not have needed a special test to be detected! According to Birley, interest in the internal ear, and its possible role in disorientation, overshadowed the far more important practical problem of so-called 'pressure vertigo' which often accompanied rapid ascents to altitude. This could be powerful and sudden in onset and, although often lasting only ten to fifteen seconds, could produce, in addition to dizziness, a blurring of vision and severe nausea. It is now known to be caused by pressure changes in the middle ear.

On descent from altitude another serious problem can arise if the rising pressure in the outer ear pushes the ear-drum inwards, so causing intense pain. There were many instances of damaged ear-drums during the war, and some aviators actually gave up flying as a result.[10] The cause was usually blocked or partially blocked Eustachian tubes (the tubes which connect each middle ear to the throat and which serve normally to maintain the middle ears at near the ambient pressure). In many people compression of the throat tissue by a rising external pressure caused the Eustachian tubes to become blocked. However, this is severely aggravated by even mild infections of the upper respiratory tract, such as colds, which cause additional mucous congestion. Ascent to altitude is only very rarely a problem, since the falling ambient pressure and rising middle ear pressure tend to keep the Eustachian tubes open, thereby allowing the expanding gas to escape. But during descent, so great could be the discomfort that Birley considered that airmen should not fly if they were unable to clear their Eustachian tubes by such actions as swallowing, chewing or expiring forcefully against a closed glottis.

When assessing the suitability of candidates for flying duties, all the Military and Naval Selection Boards laid great emphasis on a very high standard of medical, physical, and psychological fitness. What distinguished the Special RFC Medical Board from these other Boards was the use it made of the special tests devised by Board members such as Flack and Cheatle. It is important to remember, however, that those were not the only special tests developed and used at this time. Almost perfect vision was mandatory for all prospective aviators, and great emphasis was laid upon perfect colour vision because of the importance of picking out the colour or markings of hostile machines, recognizing signal lights and judging the nature of landing-grounds. The most important contribution to the setting of appropriate visual standards for pilots during the war was made by Dr Edward C. Clements. In 1917, whilst working part-time for an RFC flying training station near Lincoln, he discovered that trainee pilots who were having difficulty landing their aircraft had defective binocular vision – a condition he termed heterophoria – and were consequently unable to judge distance accurately. Furthermore, in many cases he was able to correct this defect by a course of eye exercises. He presented his findings to the Special RFC Medical Board, which was sufficiently impressed to have Clements commissioned and transferred to the Medical Flight at Stanmore Aerodrome, London. This Medical Flight had been established in July of that year for the purpose of testing and evaluating clothing and equipment developed for aircrew. For the remainder of the war all trainee pilots who regularly made faulty landings were referred to Clements for treatment. After the war he joined Flack at Hampstead.

Hearing received rather less attention, which is not surprising when it is remembered that, until the advent of the Gosport Tube (page 28), verbal communication was almost impossible above the roar of the aircraft engines and the howling of the wind. In theory 'normal' hearing was required, as tested by a forced whisper at a distance of twenty feet. Attempts were also made to test a candidate's 'nerves', i.e. his emotional response to a disturbing stress. The effect of, for example, a revolver shot or a magnesium flare on respiratory rhythm, skin blood flow and tremor would be measured. In the best type of candidate (with good 'nerves'), the effects recorded would be of short duration, whilst in unsuitable candidates the respiratory rhythm remained increased for some time, and there would be a reduction in skin blood flow and marked tremor. Unfortunately, later evaluation of such tests of 'nerves' showed them to have been virtually useless for predicting nervous instability.

Attempts were also made to predict flying aptitude by measuring the time taken to respond to visual, auditory and tactile stimuli, although these were to make little headway either during or for many years after the war. Reaction-time tests had been pioneered by the French but tended to be over-simplistic, requiring little of the co-ordinated limb movement so necessary when flying an aircraft. It was for this reason that an ingenious apparatus, designed in 1918 by Lieutenant L.E. Stamm RAMC for measuring reaction time, was never used in the routine examination of candidates. Nevertheless, Stamm was on the right lines, for his Reaction Time Apparatus can be regarded as the forerunner of many such attempts to simulate at least some of the normal responses required of the aviator, and which would eventually evolve into the computer-controlled flight simulators of today. A more elaborate reaction-testing device was developed a few years later by two Flight Lieutenants, G.H. Reid and H.L. Burton. Known as the Reid Reaction Tester, it was claimed by its inventors to provide a reliable measure of an individual's co-ordinating ability, and hence of whether he could learn to fly.[11] It could also be used to follow the progress of flying training and to teach the rudiments of flying. Unfortunately it also appears to have suffered the same fate as Stamm's apparatus, as there is no record of its being used in the manner proposed by Reid and Burton.

When the war came to an end in November 1918, so, very nearly, did aviation medicine in Britain. Within a mere 14 months the RAF reduced its operational strength from 188 squadrons, with 291,000 men, to 12 squadrons and 31,500 men. Although an account of the medical research conducted during the war was published by the MRC in the form of a series of special reports, little appeared either in the scientific journals of the time or in the popular Press. Consequently, during the 1920s aviation medicine returned to the backwaters from whence it had so recently emerged, and the names of many of those who had contributed so much were forgotten. Only Flack remained to provide a semblance of continuity.

Yet the achievement had been remarkable. Quite obviously the decisive event had been the establishment of an independent Royal Air Force, and with it a Royal Air Force Medical Branch. However, without that creation of Sir David Henderson, the Special RFC Medical Board, it is unlikely that there would have been such a fertile and productive period of research as that conducted in the eighteen months between early 1917 and the end of the war. That Sir David was so successful was due, in no small measure, to the valuable, factual information provided by medical officers working with the RFC squadrons in France and elsewhere – officers like F.R.G. Lithgow, H.G. Anderson, C.B. Heald and especially J.L. Birley. Whilst living and working with the airmen, through virtually all of the war (he was twice mentioned in despatches), and making many flights as an observer, Birley applied himself to a study of all the many medical, psychological and physiological problems which beset the wartime aviator, and particularly the problems of fatigue and mental illness induced by the stress of war. He also made important contributions to Sir Henry Head's investigations of disorientation in flight. In fact, the role Birley played was very similar to that of the Flying Personnel Medical Officer of the next war. Demobilized in 1918, he was made Consultant Physician to the RAF, a position he held until his death, at the age of forty-nine, in 1934. Perhaps his greatest achievement was his presentation of the Goulstonian Lectures to the Royal College of Physicians in 1920. These must still rank as one of the best attempts ever made to describe the physiological, psychological and physical reactions of the normal individual to the stress and strain of flying. Although the lectures were published (in *The Lancet*), he was not a prolific writer, and this may explain why his work has been largely forgotten; which is a great pity, for he must certainly rank alongside Matthew Fell as one of the founding fathers of British aviation medicine.

3 Ever Higher, Ever Faster

Although virtually no aviation medicine research was undertaken in the years immediately following the end of the war, under the guidance of Air Commodore Fell a considerable reorganization of the newly created RAF Medical Branch did take place. In May 1919 the RAF lost its hospital at Hampstead when the MRC requested that the buildings be returned to them, but a new hospital was opened at Halton. Also, the MRC invited the RAF to keep its Physiology Laboratory at Hampstead as a part of the National Institute for Medical Research. This invitation was accepted, and the Physiology Laboratory was joined shortly after by the Medical Selection Board, the successor to the Special RFC Medical Board. The complete unit was named the Central Medical Establishment (CME) and was placed in the charge of Wing Commander (as he had by now become) Martin Flack. Unfortunately the heavy teaching and administrative commitments of the post, coupled with his poor health (he suffered from a recurrent illness which he called 'flu' but which was, in fact, far more serious), meant that Flack had little time available for research. Nevertheless, with his two assistants, Dr Grace Briscoe and Squadron Leader 'Handsome' Harry (later Air Commodore) Hewat, some investigations were undertaken. Among the more important of these was the testing of the responses of pilots to conditions of reduced temperature and pressure in an environmental chamber, the prevention of head injuries by padding the cockpit coaming, a study of the deafness resulting from noise in flight, the provision of adequate ventilation for the enclosed aircraft cockpits that began to appear shortly after the war, and the optimum layout of dashboards for greater ease in reading instruments.

In 1927 the Physiological Laboratory moved, with the Central Medical Establishment, from Hampstead to even smaller accommodation at Clement's Inn, just off the Strand. The size of the accommodation and the dearth of facilities gave rise to several amusing misunderstandings with foreign visitors, who refused to believe that the research effort was so miniscule and therefore convinced themselves that the British were actually hiding a large amount of secret work.

When Group Captain Flack died in 1931, at the early age of forty-nine, E.C. Clements was promoted to Group Captain and took over command of the CME, while Flack's work at the Physiological Laboratory became the responsibility of Squadron Leader Gerald Struan Marshall who, over the next few years, was to be involved with helping the RAF in its pursuit of the world high-altitude record. This pursuit of records, not just altitude but also speed and distance, was deliberate service policy at that time. For, if military aviation was still in the doldrums during the early 1930s, civil aviation most definitely was not. The imagination of the public had been captured by the race to see how far, how fast and how high aeroplanes could go. These questions became issues of national prestige, from which Britain could not stand aloof. They also led directly to the re-birth of aviation medicine in the UK.

In 1932 Mr C.F. Uwins, Chief Test Pilot of the Bristol Aeroplane Company, reached 43,976 feet in an open-cockpit Vickers Vesper biplane, so becoming the first Englishman to hold the world altitude record for heavier-than-air craft. He did so using the standard RAF oxygen apparatus made by Siebe Gorman & Co Ltd but modified to allow pure oxygen to be breathed. The flow of oxygen had to be manually set on the regulator for different altitudes, and any extra volume of gas for breathing in came as a 'top-up' from cabin air. The system had several shortcomings, the most serious of which was that half the oxygen supplied was wasted, since it flowed continuously. Apparently Haldane's idea for an 'economizer' system, and Siebe Gorman's oxygen economizer flexible bag system, had come to nought.

Before Uwins made his flight, he had sought the advice of Struan Marshall at the Physiological Laboratory, who arranged for him to experience hypoxia in the decompression chamber at the RAE. Unfortunately the occasion was to prove embarrassing for Marshall and for Mr Taylor of the RAE, both of whom accompanied Uwins on this his first experience of hypoxia in a decompression chamber. For everything that could go wrong seemed to go wrong. Taylor fainted and then, when recovering consciousness, tried to remove his oxygen mask. While Marshall was trying to restrain Taylor, he himself passed out. He recovered a short time later to see Uwins standing at the other end of the chamber, about twenty feet away, wondering what he could do to help but tethered to his own oxygen supply by the short oxygen-delivery hose.[1] The episode did, however, illustrate admirably another serious shortcoming of the RAF oxygen system: the continuous flow could not cater for changes in the requirement for oxygen following an increase in physical activity.

And the lesson was certainly not lost on Struan Marshall. In July 1932 he wrote a report to the Director of Medical Services, Air Vice-Marshal John McIntyre, drawing attention to the enormous wastage of oxygen which occurs with continuous-flow oxygen regulators, particularly when trying to cater for all needs at all altitudes. He also pointed out that it would be advantageous to keep the pressure of the inspired oxygen similar to that which obtains at sea-level.[2] There are two reasons for this. First, breathing pure oxygen for prolonged periods damages the lungs, and second, delivering more oxygen to the mask than is needed is wasteful. A system was therefore needed whereby the oxygen supplied to the mask was diluted with air, preferably automatically, so doing away with the need for manual adjustment of flow. Marshall went on to suggest a possible system based on Haldane's economizer concept. Oxygen was delivered continuously to a regulator, but only intermittently to the oxygen mask, a mixture of oxygen and air being stored in a distensible bag. The air was introduced through an orifice in the regulator, being sucked in by the negative pressure created by the oxygen passing through the regulator. With enviable precognition, Marshall drew attention to two potentially serious problems of such a system, which were to cause headaches several years later at the RAF Physiological Laboratory, namely loss of flexibility of the bag with extreme cold, and freezing of valves at altitude. The report ended strongly: '... other things being equal, in a flight at over 20,000 feet, the man with the more efficient oxygen supply will win.'

Air Vice-Marshal McIntyre must have been favourably impressed, for within a matter of weeks the RAE was working on a prototype oxygen regulator to Marshall's specification. By the time it was ready for testing, however, two other regulators were made available to the RAE, one of German manufacture and the other made by Siebe Gorman. The three systems were tested in the decompression chamber at simulated altitudes up to 40,000 feet and in the air up to 33,000 feet. The first flight, with a modified version of the German regulator, was completely successful, but the second, in a Fairey Fox aircraft flown by Flight Lieutenant G. Stainforth (a very recent holder of the world air-speed record), with a Mr Watson of the RAE using the regulator, was marred by an oxygen malfunction. It seems that either Mr Watson became detached from his oxygen supply or that his inspiratory or expiratory valve froze; in any event, he lost consciousness at 28,000 feet and did not recover until he was in hospital.[3] Subsequently all three systems were found to work well, resulting in a considerable saving of oxygen compared to the existing RAF system.

Over the next few years, development work continued, with emphasis being laid on the Siebe Gorman regulators, now referred to as the Type D. All along, however, there was a problem with the face masks for use with the regulators. Since the intermittent delivery of oxygen from the regulator to the lungs depended upon the creation of a negative pressure within the mask during inspiration, the mask had to fit tightly and securely to the face; otherwise, considerable amounts of outside air would be inspired, so diluting the oxygen coming from the regulator. Since existing masks were inadequate, a new one was designed and made by the RAE. It was tested in flight for its performance in cold conditions by the wearer leaning out into the slipstream where the air temperature was minus 35°C! A major disadvantage of the design was that there was no inward relief valve in the mask (the then current RAF mask had nostril holes); the net result was that, if the oxygen supply failed or the inspiratory valve iced up, the pilot suffocated! This, coupled with the fact that, in tests, the Type D regulator performed miserably, resulted in the abandonment of the entire programme by 1938. Nevertheless, the work did lay the foundations for the very successful development of the RAF Physiological Laboratory's oxygen economizer system early in the Second World War.

In 1935 Struan Marshall was again involved in high-altitude record attempts. By this time the altitudes being reached were such that no oxygen regulator, however good, would supply enough oxygen. As Hermann von Schrötter had perceptively pointed out at the turn of the century, at altitudes much above 40,000 feet flight would become increasingly hazardous without a pressurized supply of oxygen. The reason for this is that at 40,000 feet when breathing 100 per cent oxygen, the oxygen tension in the lungs is only some 55 to 60 millimetres of mercury (mm Hg), compared to a tension of about 100 mm Hg when breathing air at sea-level. The resulting diffusion gradient between the lung tissue and the blood is barely sufficient to maintain a sufficient oxygen pressure in the blood to meet the oxygen demands of the body – and particularly of the brain. Mental function, therefore, starts to be impaired under these conditions, although still only slightly – about the same as it is when breathing air at 10,000 feet. The critical altitude at which the oxygen tension in the lungs falls below the sea-level equivalent, even though pure oxygen only is breathed, is 33,000 feet. Above this altitude, the oxygen tension can only be maintained at the sea-level value by providing a supply of oxygen under pressure. This 'pressure breathing' is today generally regarded as being mandatory when flying at altitudes above 43,000 feet and is strongly recommended above 40,000 feet. Hence, during the mid and late 1930s, pressure breathing was essential if altitudes much above that attained by Uwins were to be reached; this was the purpose of the pressure suit.

The original idea for a pressure suit had come from J.S. Haldane many years before. In his book *Respiration*, published in 1920, he said, '... if it were required to go much above 40,000 feet, to a barometric pressure below 130 mm, Hg, it would be necessary to enclose the airman in an airtight dress, somewhat similar to a self-contained diving dress, but capable of resisting perfectly safely an internal pressure of about 130 mm Hg. This dress could be so arranged that even in a complete vacuum the contained oxygen would still have a pressure of 130 mm Hg. There would then be no physiological limit to the height obtainable.'[4] Haldane's idea was not taken up until 1933, when an American balloonist, Mark Ridge, wrote to him asking if he could use the 'diving-dress' method in an altitude-record attempt. Ridge's letter was given to Mr R. (later Sir Robert) Davis of the Siebe Gorman Company who undertook to make the dress. This was easily done since it was actually just a modification of a self-contained diving-suit already manufactured by the company. The resulting high-altitude suit was extensively tested in the firm's own high-altitude and low-temperature chambers and, in its final form, provided perfect protection at a simulated altitude of 90,000 feet – equivalent to a barometric pressure of 20 mm Hg.[5]

In the event, Ridge never used the suit because he could not obtain the necessary financial support for his record attempt. All the effort was not wasted, however, for the Air Ministry had become interested. Which was why, in 1935, Struan Marshall found himself back at the RAE, this time working with Professor Haldane and Mr Davis on the full pressure suit which had been intended for Mark Ridge. The suit, which was made of a rubberized fabric, was in two parts, securely joined together by a flexible steel band around the waist, whilst the helmet, also made of rubberized fabric, incorporated a large, double-layered, curved visor. A closed-circuit breathing-system with a chemical absorber for expired carbon dioxide was fitted to the helmet, and the suit was inflated with oxygen to a maximum pressure of 2½ pounds per square inch. It was tested at Farnborough on volunteers to an altitude of 80,000 feet, and then it was used first by Squadron Leader F.D.R. Swain, who reached 49,957 feet in 1936, and by Flight Lieutenant M.J. Adam, who reached 53,937 feet the next year.

However, full pressure suits would never be popular, mainly for reasons which had been put forward by Marshall himself two years earlier. In a lecture to the Royal Aeronautical Society[6] he had pointed out that pressure suits would necessarily be unwieldy and would therefore interfere with the pilot's freedom of movement. There would also be some rebreathing of expired air, and the normal resistance to breathing would be reversed – so the wearer would have to work hard to breathe out. One problem that Marshall did not anticipate was the severe misting of the visor experienced at altitude by Swain and Adam. Another was that, being highly insulating, the suit quickly became uncomfortably hot and the occupant exceedingly sweaty. On the other hand, the discomforts of pressure breathing alluded to by Marshall were less serious than anticipated, being somewhat alleviated by the counterpressure applied over the body surface.

In that same lecture to the Royal Aeronautical Society in 1933, Struan Marshall addressed himself to the problem of 'blacking out' under the stress of increased gravitational force, or increased 'g'. The phenomenon was already fairly well known. Visual disturbances occurring during the execution of tight turns had been described by some pilots during World War I, and the increased g-forces acting on the aircraft structure during such manoeuvres, and others such as pulling up from steep dives, were of major concern to the designers and engineers of the day. However, it was only with the great air races of the 1920s and 1930s, when pilots had to make tight turns round pylons on the courses, that the physiological effects of increased g became more widely known.

Increased g, in the form of centrifugal force, will be familiar to anyone who has had occasion to be whirled and twirled at the fairground. For the pilot of an aircraft, however, the consequences of this increased g can be serious. If he is executing an inward turn (i.e. his head is directed towards the centre of the turn), then he is pulled hard down into his seat – he feels heavier. Also pulled downwards is his blood, which tends to pool in his lower limbs. The pressure of the blood in the head is reduced and, if it falls too far, may not be able to overcome the intrinsic pressure of the eyeball. If blood flow through the eyeball is diminished, visual disturbances occur, classically a dimming and tunnelling of the vision ('grey-out') preceding a total loss of vision ('black-out'). Consciousness, and hence mental function, is retained for a short while, but eventually unconsciousness supervenes if the increased g is sustained. If this 'positive' g is increased high enough for long enough, death can ensue. The effects of g are reversible (as long as permanent damage has not been sustained as a result of too long an exposure to too high a level of g), vision returning as the g-level diminishes. In an outward turn (i.e. the pilot's head is directed away from the centre of the turn), the blood moves in the opposite direction, into the head; this is known as negative g. Blood accumulates in the brain and eyes, and a red haze ('red-out') obscures the vision. Exposure to too high a level of negative g can result in brain haemorrhages. Generally a pilot's tolerance to positive g is between two and three times his tolerance to negative g. At the time Marshall delivered his lecture in 1933, little work on problems of increased g had been carried out by the RAF. However, reports from pilots taking part in air races had indicated that blacking out could occur after about one second at $3\frac{1}{2}$ to 4g, but that forces of 6 to 7g had been experienced without mishap.

The RAF interest in problems of increased g had been aroused by its involvement, from 1927 onwards, in the air races for the Schneider Trophy, for which a special High Speed Flight had been set up. Although for seaplanes only, the Schneider Trophy was the blue-riband event of the racing calendar. First held in 1913, by the mid 1920s it had become completely dominated by the French, Italians and Americans, who at that time were threatening to take permanent possession of the trophy by winning three consecutive races. Continuing poor performance by the British team after their last victory in 1922 had led, in 1927, to the RAF being given full responsibility for the British effort. Great emphasis was now laid on training the team pilots, all of whom were RAF officers. In particular, many hours were spent practising tight, high-speed turns around the pylons located at the turning-points of the course, and it would probably have been during this training that the phenomena of grey-out and black-out were first regularly encountered. Group Captain Flack had been approached for advice and had devised an elastic belt that was intended to overcome the adverse effects of the increased g. The belt was, however, not liked by the team pilots as it tended to slip down under increased g and also restricted movement in the cramped cockpit.[7] They found that g-tolerance could be better improved by tensing their muscles, especially their abdominal muscles. However, they had to be careful to continue breathing, for they found that, if they held their breath and strained to increase muscle tension whilst pulling g, they lost consciousness. The pilots also noticed that training and experience appeared to increase the level of g at which symptoms first appeared. They found that black-out did not seem to occur below $4\frac{1}{2}$g and also that they were able to stay blacked-out for as long as twenty seconds in a descending turn without losing consciousness and whilst still retaining the 'feel' (and hence control) of the aeroplane.[8]

In 1931 Struan Marshall inherited from Flack the problem of how to provide protection against the effects of increased g. Marshall believed that blacking out was due to 'anaemia of the eye' caused by pooling of blood in the lower blood-vessels, particularly the relatively unsupported vessels of the abdomen. To counteract the problem, he suggested bracing the muscles of the abdomen either by careful training or by a pneumatic corset. Struan Marshall's idea, first put forward in 1933,[9] was for an air scoop, on the surface of the aircraft, which was to be forced out into the airstream by the g-force acting against a weight on a spring. The scoop would then ram air into an inflatable belt worn by the pilot. As the g-force lessened, the scoop would be returned to its resting position by the spring, and the belt would deflate. However, it was the opinion of the pilots in the High Speed Flight, and of Flight Lieutenant Stainforth in particular, that such a system would be disconcerting to the pilot, especially if the corset suddenly inflated in the middle of the pilot's turn. Another suggestion put forward at this time was by a Lieutenant Commander C.N. Colson RN, who noted that flying in the prone position would, theoretically, provide maximum protection against blacking out; more was to come of this idea later. For the time being, however, the High Speed Flight team decided that g protection was unnecessary; instead, the team evolved a technique for rounding the pylons without making such tight turns, whilst still keeping the airspeed up.

In fact, little work on blacking out was done in the next few years, since the RAF High Command, in their wisdom, did not expect aerobatics to be a prominent feature in any future war; they thought that dogfights would be a thing of the past since modern aeroplanes would be a mile apart within five seconds of passing each other.[10] Certainly no further work was carried out on Struan Marshall's idea of an air scoop. The next occasion that serious consideration was given to problems of increased g was in 1938, when Flight Lieutenant J.B. Wallace submitted an MD thesis on the subject to the University of Glasgow. Wallace constructed a simple g-meter for use in flight and was able to define grey-out limits and levels of g at which blacking out occurred. He experimented with several belts, including a pad that already had air contained in it. He was able to achieve a diminution in the fatigue experienced by the pilots after an aerobatic flight (i.e., the fatigue provoked by repeated exposures to high g) and a slight raising of the grey-out and black-out thresholds of some pilots. Wallace also tried the effect of breathing a hundred per cent oxygen on black-out threshold, but with no beneficial results. He concluded that correctly tailored and fitted belts would help aircrew, although he had some reservations: '... all service pilots are burdened with too many encumbrances already, and to enforce the use of an abdominal belt would merely add to their troubles.' Little did he know of what the future had in store for the poor pilots!

4 Birth of 'The Lab'

In May 1937 Wing Commander (later Air Marshal Sir Philip) Livingston visited Germany to view the aviation medicine research facilities of the Luftwaffe. Livingston, a tall, athletic Canadian, was the RAF Consultant in Ophthalmology, a position he had been appointed to following Clements' retirement in 1934. On arriving in Germany, he was received with courtesy and openness and was given a comprehensive tour of the various centres. He found all the establishments to be elaborately equipped and staffed with scientists of high calibre. Thoroughly alarmed, Livingston returned to London and submitted a report to the DMS, Air Vice-Marshal Sir Alfred Iredell, comparing Britain's backwardness in aviation medicine and her paucity of research facilities with Germany's advanced knowledge, experience and resources.[1] Iredell, in turn, referred the matter to the Air Council for their consideration. However, the result, as in 1934 when the Air Defence of Great Britain Command had pressed for better research facilities in aviation medicine for the RAF, was disappointing. Apart from a decision to move the Physiological Laboratory from Clement's Inn to the Royal Air Force airfield at Hendon (with just a wooden hut containing a workshop and an office, the services of a flight sergeant and access to one pilot and an aircraft), nothing appears to have been done.

Then, in May of the following year, Livingston, while conducting an eye test on a Member of Parliament, a Captain Lampugh, happened to bemoan Britain's backwardness in aviation medicine and the RAF's failure to appreciate its importance. Shortly afterwards, Lampugh reported Livingston's views to a friend on the Air Council, the immediate upshot of which was a carpeting for Livingston for having bypassed normal channels! This was passed down to him through the Chief of the Air Staff to the new DMS, Air Vice-Marshal Victor Richardson (later Sir Victor, but known to his subordinates as 'King Dick'). However, Livingston's indiscretion may have stimulated matters, for that November a meeting of the Medical Advisory Committee of the Air Ministry was held, specifically to discuss the provision of adequate medical research facilities for the Royal Air Force. The meeting was chaired by the DMS and was attended by Sir Joseph Barcroft, Professor F.C. Bartlett, Dr J.J. Conybeare, Professor W.W. Jameson, Professor Sir Edward Mellanby, Sir John Parsons and Dr C.P. Symonds – all eminent men in the medical world. Their deliberations and recommendations were to be of momentous importance for the future of aviation medicine in the United Kingdom.[2]

Richardson told the Committee about Livingston's visit to Germany and how it had become apparent that Britain lagged far behind Germany in aviation medicine research. He pointed out that, although the Physiological Laboratory had been moved to Hendon in order to give better access to aircraft, shortages of staff, accommodation and equipment meant that no work was yet being done. Equally seriously, there was little co-operation with other medical departments at the CME, and in the scientific field there appeared to be no clear idea of what work needed to be done. Clearly, with war against Germany now seemingly inevitable, this dismal state of affairs could not be allowed to continue. It was proposed, therefore, that an independent committee under Air Ministry authority should be set up, composed of outside specialists representing psychology, physiology, neurology, general medicine, vision and hearing, and that its Secretary and Chairman should be the Commanding Officer of the CME and the DMS respectively – i.e. serving officers in the RAF so that the full military benefit of the committee's work could be extracted. Because the suggested responsibilities of the proposed committee extended beyond purely medical matters to the problems of the applied physiology and psychology of flight, it was also recommended that the new committee should be called 'The Flying Personnel Research Committee'. Just one week later these proposals were given official blessing by the Under-Secretary of State for Air, Captain H.H. Balfour MC, MP.

The next few months saw the DMS busily engaged in gathering together the necessary medical specialists, but by March 1939 all the necessary arrangements had been made. On the 10th of that month, Air Ministry Communiqué No. 6213 proclaimed: 'As announced in the House of Commons yesterday, the Secretary of State for Air, Sir Kingsley Wood, on the recommendation of the D.M.S., R.A.F., has appointed a standing committee to investigate and advise him on the medical aspects of all matters concerning personnel which might affect safety and efficiency in flying.'

This direct access to the Secretary of State for Air was of crucial importance and was to provide the Flying Personnel Research Committee (FPRC) with a powerful weapon which it could use in its dealings with other bodies. It was made possible by a change to the originally proposed post of Chairman. The Chairmanship was offered not to the DMS but to Professor Sir Edward Mellanby, the Secretary of the Medical Research Council. During the war Mellanby's contacts (he was, amongst other things, a member of the Scientific Advisory Committee of the Cabinet) gave the new committee access to the highest echelons of government – access that would certainly not have been countenanced had the DMS been the Chairman, since he would have been expected to report up the normal service chain through the Air Member for Personnel. The Communiqué went on to say:

> The Committee will be constituted as follows:
> Professor F.C. Bartlett, M.A., F.R.S.
> E.A. Carmichael, F.R.C.P.
> C.S. Hallpike, M.R.C.P., F.R.C.S.
> B.H.C. Matthews, Sc.D.
> Sir John Parsons, C.B.E., F.R.S., F.R.C.S.
> Professor L.J. Witts, M.D., F.R.C.P.
> The representatives of the Air Ministry on the Committee will be:
> Air Vice Marshal A.V.J. Richardson, C.B., O.B.E., K.H.S. Director of Medical Services, and
> Air Commodore H.E. Whittingham, C.B.E., F.R.C.P. (E), K.H.P.

The Committee consisted, respectively, of a Professor of Psychology from Cambridge University, the Director of the Neurological Research Unit at the National Hospital for Nervous Diseases, an ear specialist from the MRC, a physiologist from Cambridge University, an Emeritus Professor of Ophthalmology from the University of London and the Nuffield Professor of Clinical Medicine at the University of Oxford. Air Commodore Whittingham is also worthy of further note. A founder member of the RAF Medical Branch, he was Consultant in Pathology to the RAF and the founder of the RAF

Institute of Pathology and Tropical Medicine. In 1938 he filled the posts of both Consultant in Pathology and Director of Hygiene at the Air Ministry; he had also previously been Commanding Officer of the CME. He had carried out much valuable research for the RAF, including a study of sandfly fever in Malta in 1923; this work had won him many awards and an international reputation. A glutton for hard work, he did not (and at the time of writing still did not!) suffer fools gladly. Indeed, while still a squadron leader, he had made it his practice to visit the flights on any station that he happened to be passing; at the end of his visit, he would go to see the station commander to tell him what was wrong with his station! For some time, Whittingham had seen the inevitability of war and had persuaded a number of able, young, medical research workers to join the RAF Volunteer Reserve, with the idea of forming a uniformed cadre of first-class scientists. One man with whom he had made contact, and whom he had convinced of the importance of applied physiology in the RAF but had been unable to dragoon into uniform, was Dr B.H.C. Matthews. Bryan Matthews was already a physiologist of international repute – a reputation gained by work on hypoxia in the Andes and on neurophysiology with Dr (later Lord) Adrian. In addition, he was a first-class electronics engineer who made most of his own equipment; indeed, he had made himself one of the earliest, battery-powered, portable electrocardiograph machines for recording the electrical activity of the heart during experiments. In the late 1930s Matthews was working for Sir Joseph Barcroft at Cambridge. Barcroft, who was on the Medical Advisory Committee of the Air Ministry, had himself been invited to serve on the new committee (the FPRC). However, pleading old age and knowing of Matthews' interest, he had suggested that the younger man should take his place.

Such was the gravity of the situation in those hectic months before the outbreak of war that the first two meetings of the FPRC had been held before the announcement in the House of Commons of the Committee's appointment. These had been concerned with considerations of the terms of reference for the FPRC* and with reviewing the outstanding medical problems facing the RAF.[3] Struan

* 'To advise the Secretary of State on investigation into the medical aspects of all matters affecting personnel which might conduce to safety and efficiency in flying, including research into problems associated with the scientific selection of flying personnel, and into measures designed to maintain their physiological efficiency.'

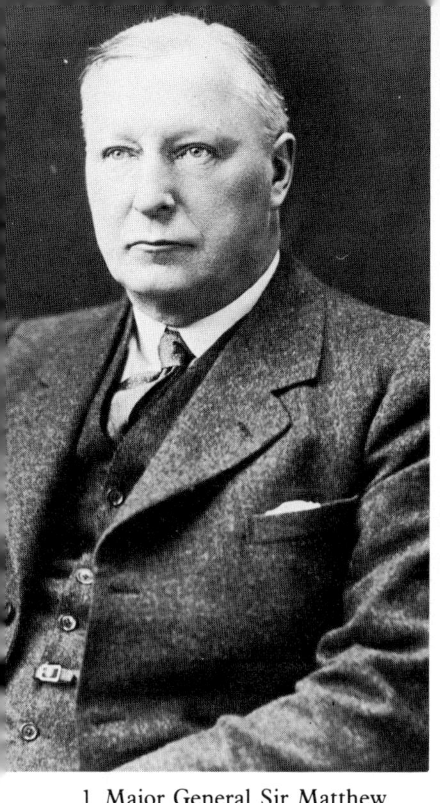

1 Major General Sir Matthew Fell KCB CMG

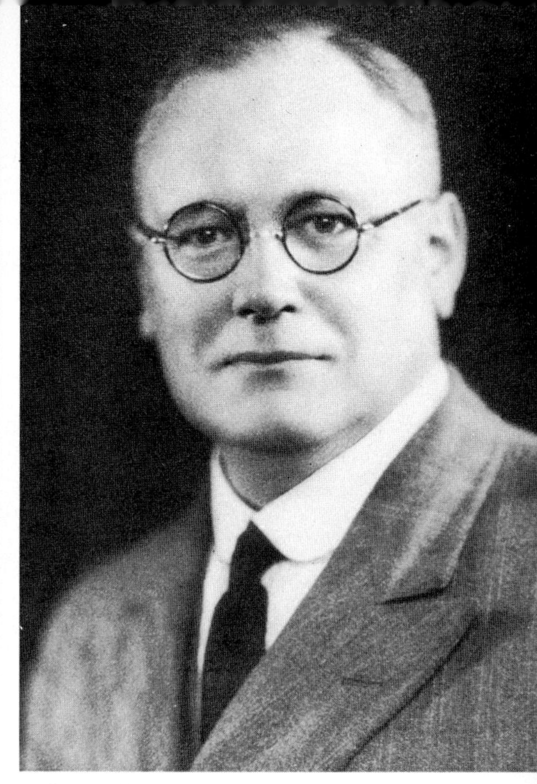

2 Group Captain Martin Flack CBE

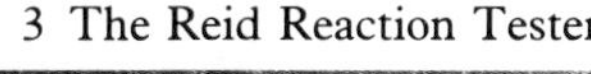

3 The Reid Reaction Tester

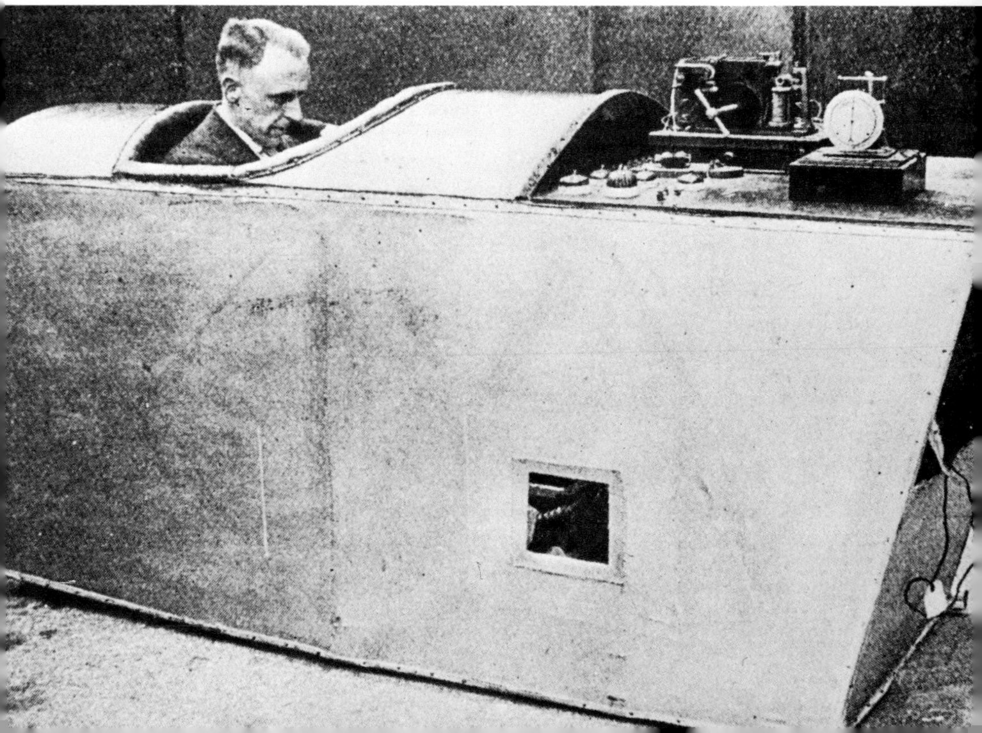

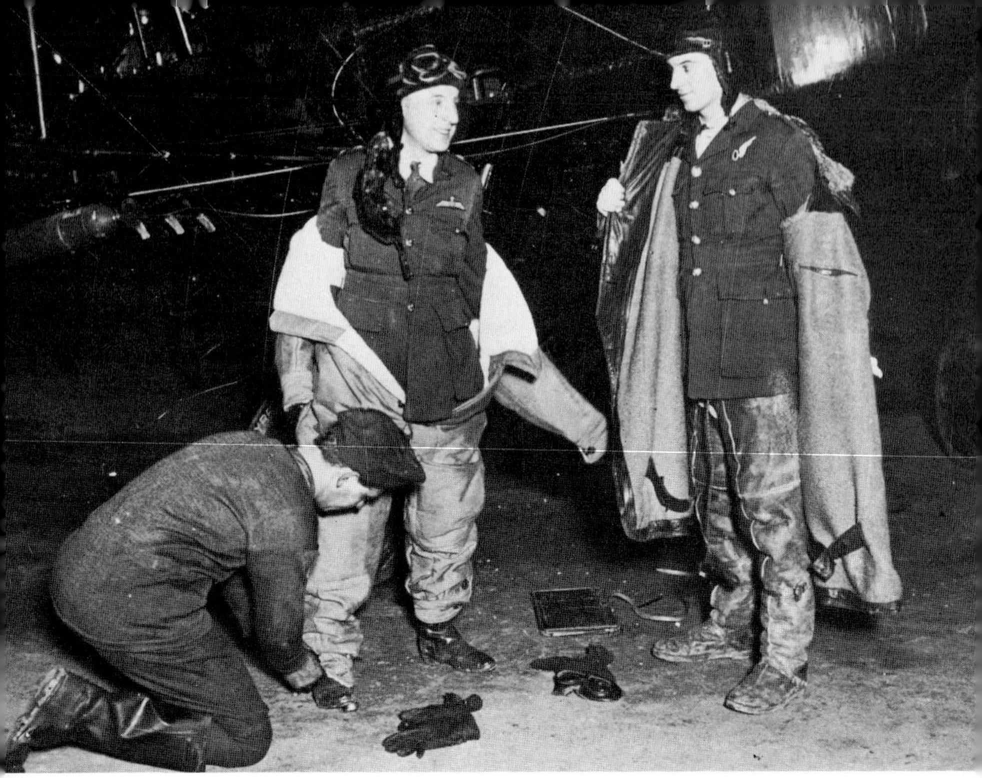

4 Flying clothing. On the right, the official issue leather flying coat and thigh-length 'fug-boots'; on the left, the Sidcot Suit

5 Left to right: Squadron Leader F.D.R. Swain, the inflated but unoccupied pressure suit and Flight Lieutenant M.J. Adam, 1937

6 Air Marshal Sir Harold Whittingham KCB KBE

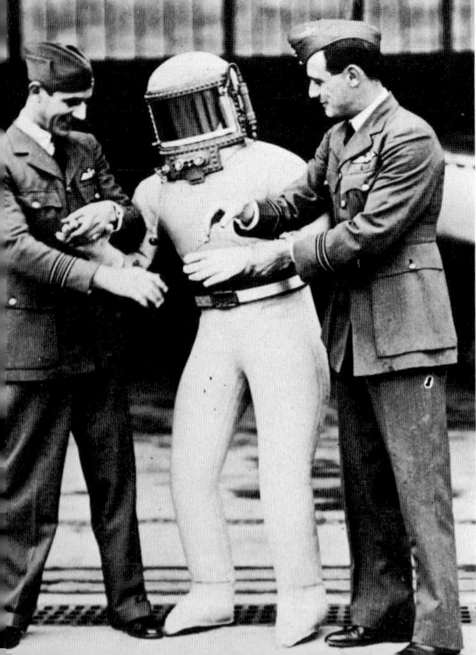

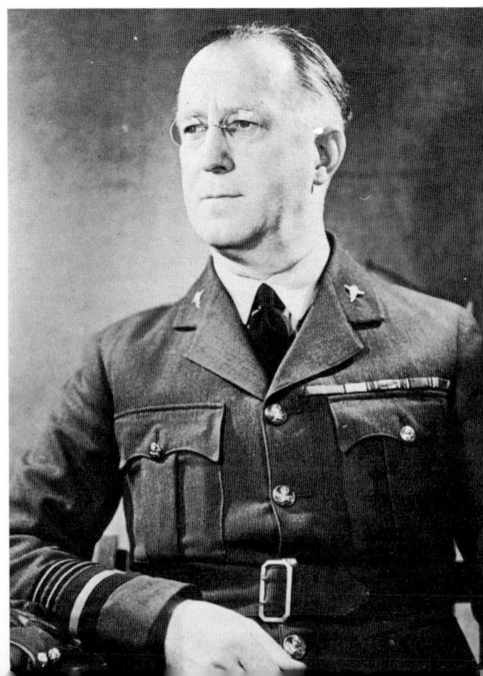

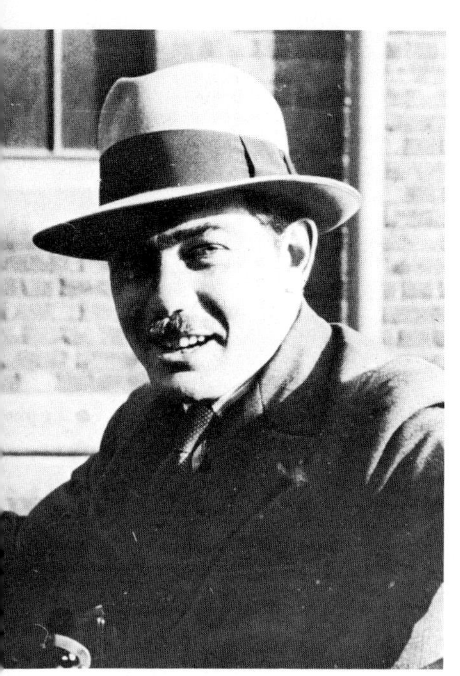

7 Dr B.H.C. Matthews, 1938

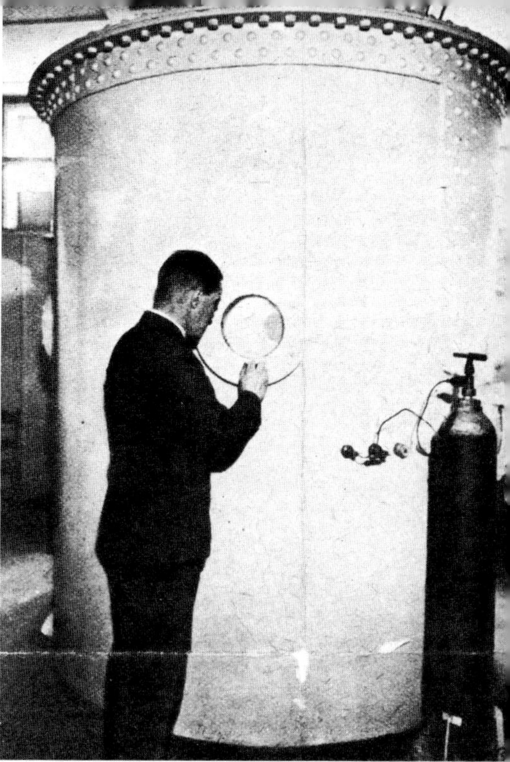

8 The RAE Instrument Department's vertical decompression chamber

9 Left, the Beta Shed, RAE, and right No. 3 Building. The RAF Physiological Laboratory occupied the lean-to behind the bicycle shed on No. 3 Building from August 1939 to January 1940

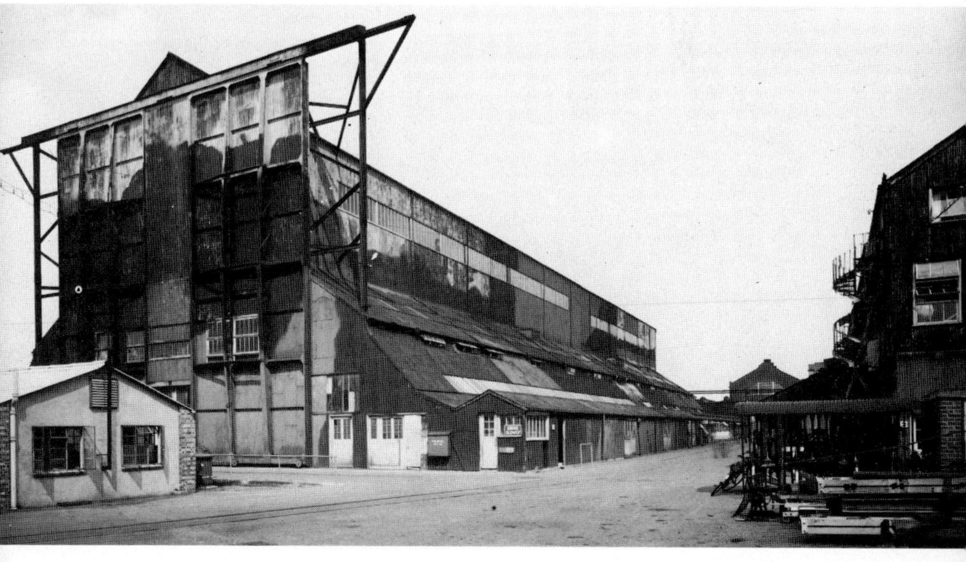

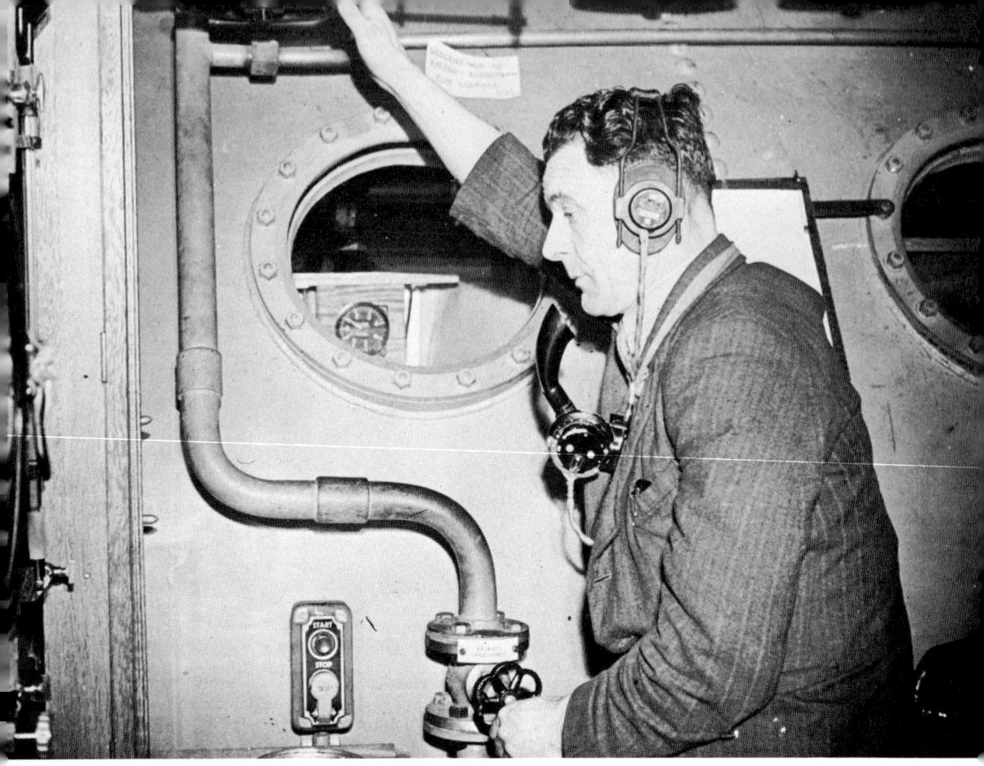

10 'Happy' Day, operating the Physiological Laboratory's new chamber

11 Whittingham's team at the Lab early in 1942. Left to right: Dr B.H.C. Matthews, Flying Officer H.L. Roxburgh, Dr E.A.G. Goldie, Flight Lieutenant J.C. Gilson, Wing Commander R.H. Winfield, Flying Officer E.A. Pask, Squadron Leader W.K. Stewart, Air Marshal Sir Harold Whittingham

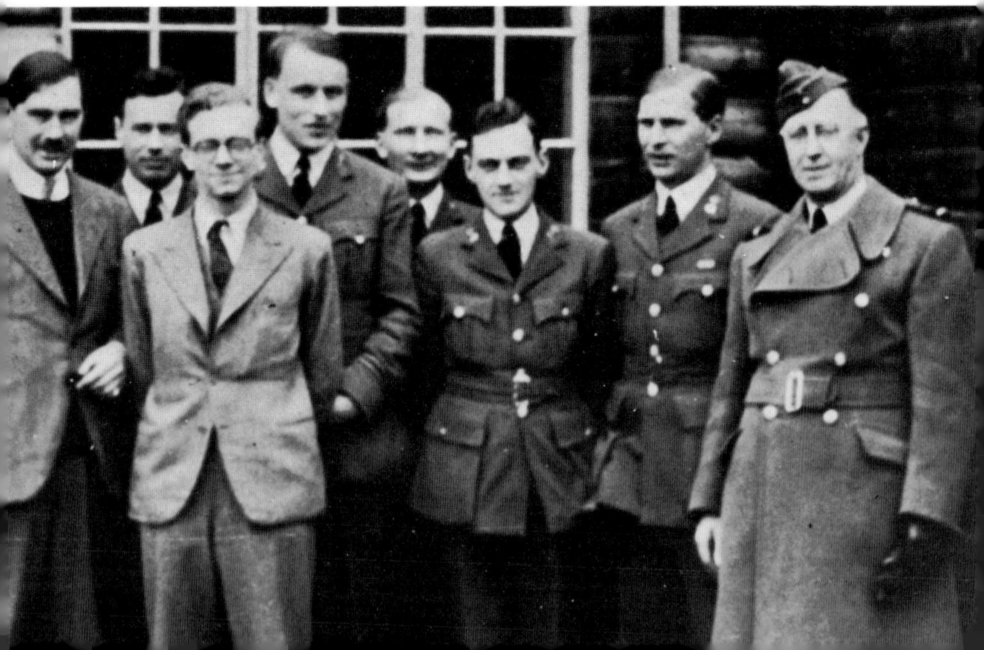

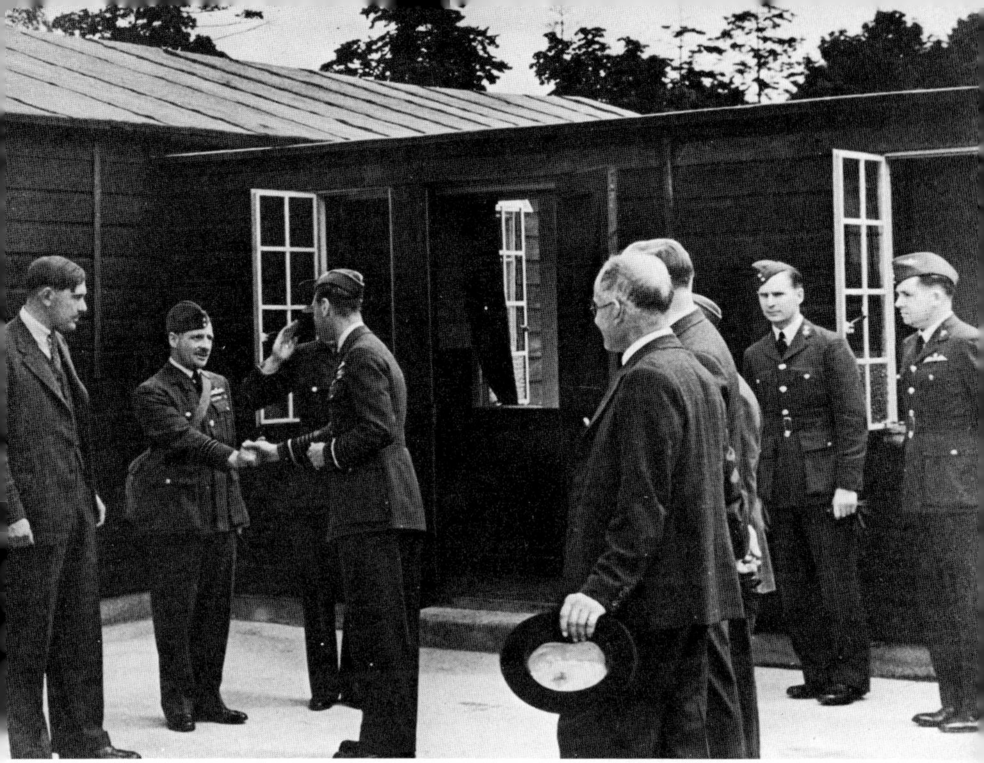

12 Visit of HM King George VI to the Lab, 1940. Left to right: Dr Matthews, Wing Commander B. McEntegart (Experimental Flying Department, RAE), unknown (obscured), the King, Mr Swan, Mr W.G.A. Perring (obscured), Air Marshal Sir Victor Richardson (obscured), Flying Officer W.K. Stewart, Squadron Leader T.C. Macdonald

13 The Lab, 1942. Left to right: cold chamber, decompression chamber, store, library, dark-rooms

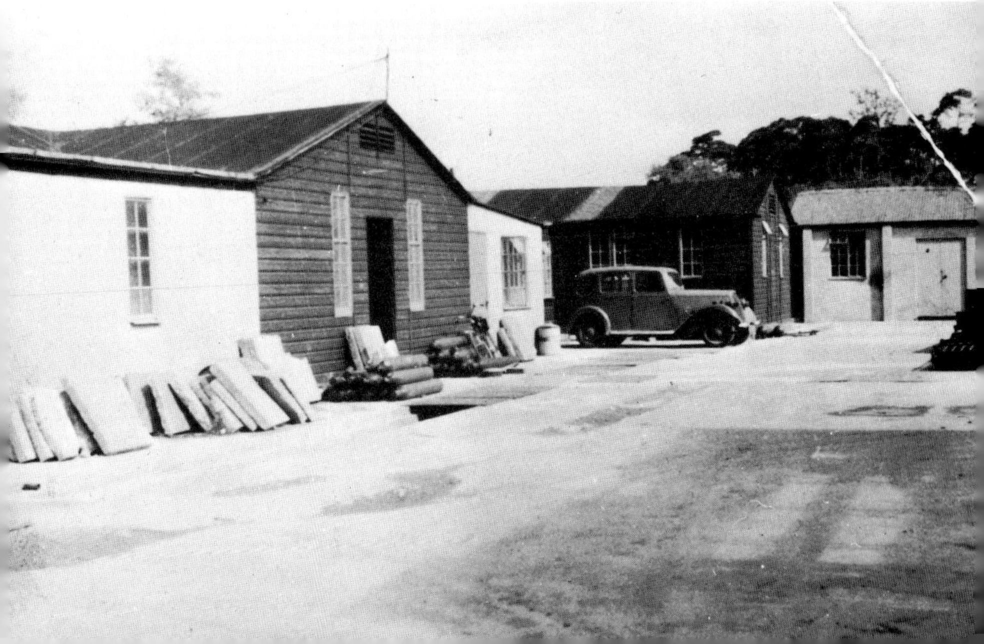

14 Wing Commander R.H. Winfield before the first snatch, and stages in a human snatch

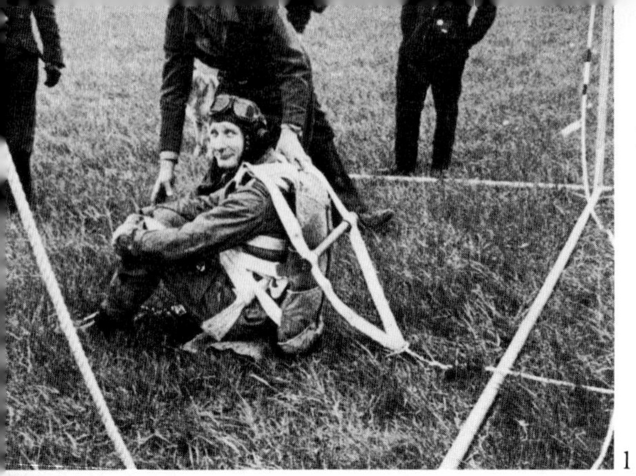

1

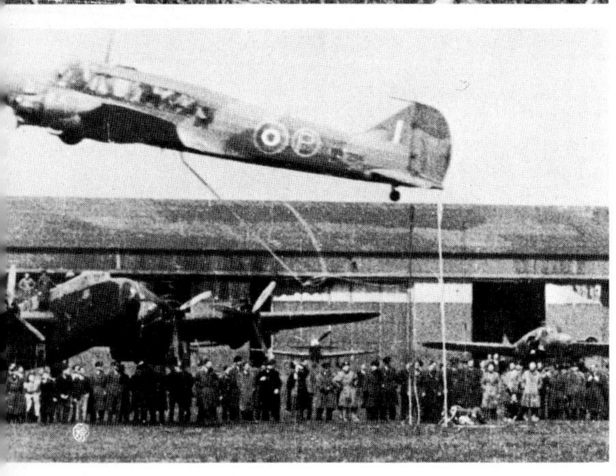

2

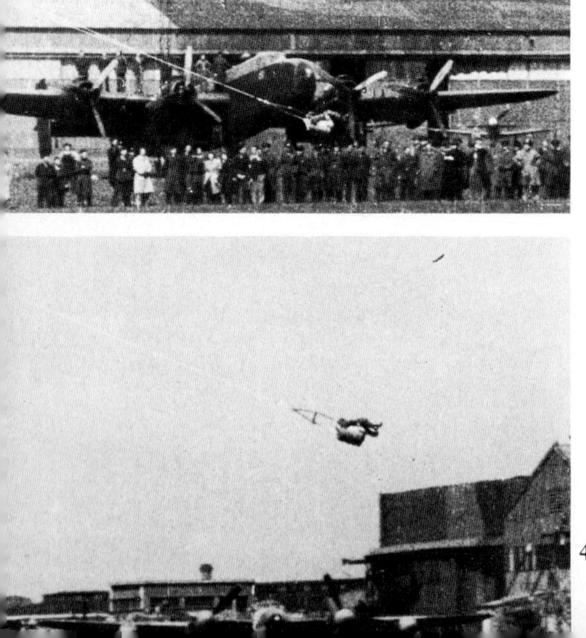

4

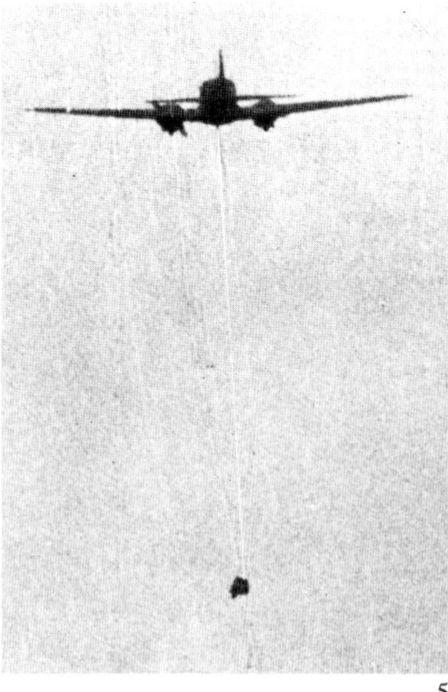

5

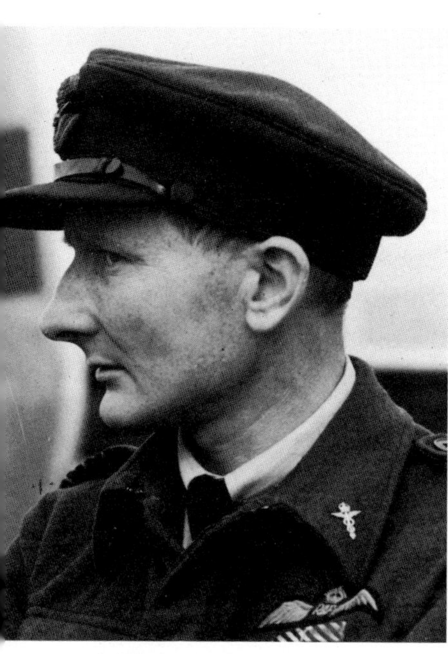

15 Wing Commander R.H. Winfield DFC, AFC

16 Air Vice-Marshal W.K. Stewart CB, CBE, AFC. Head of the Institute 1946-67

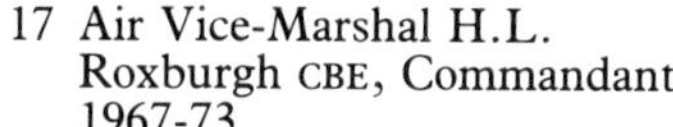

17 Air Vice-Marshal H.L. Roxburgh CBE, Commandant 1967-73

18 Air Commodore P. Howard OBE, Commandant 1975 to date

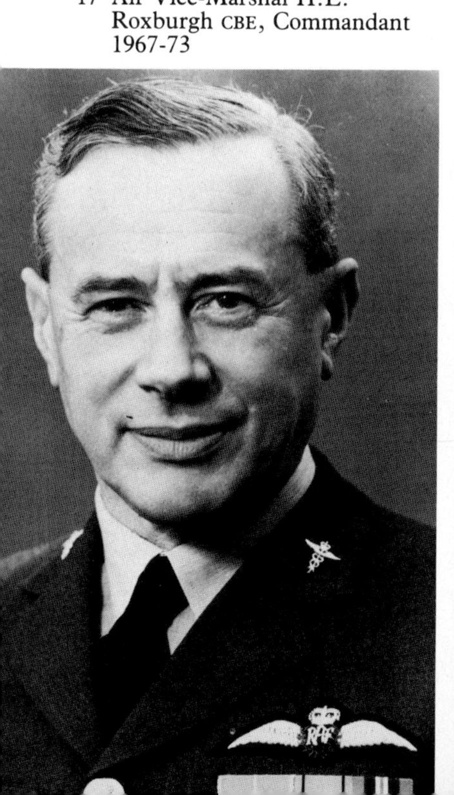

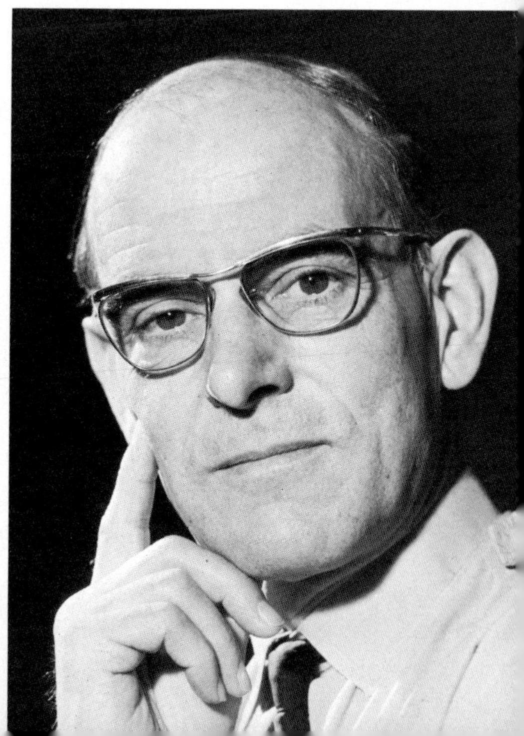

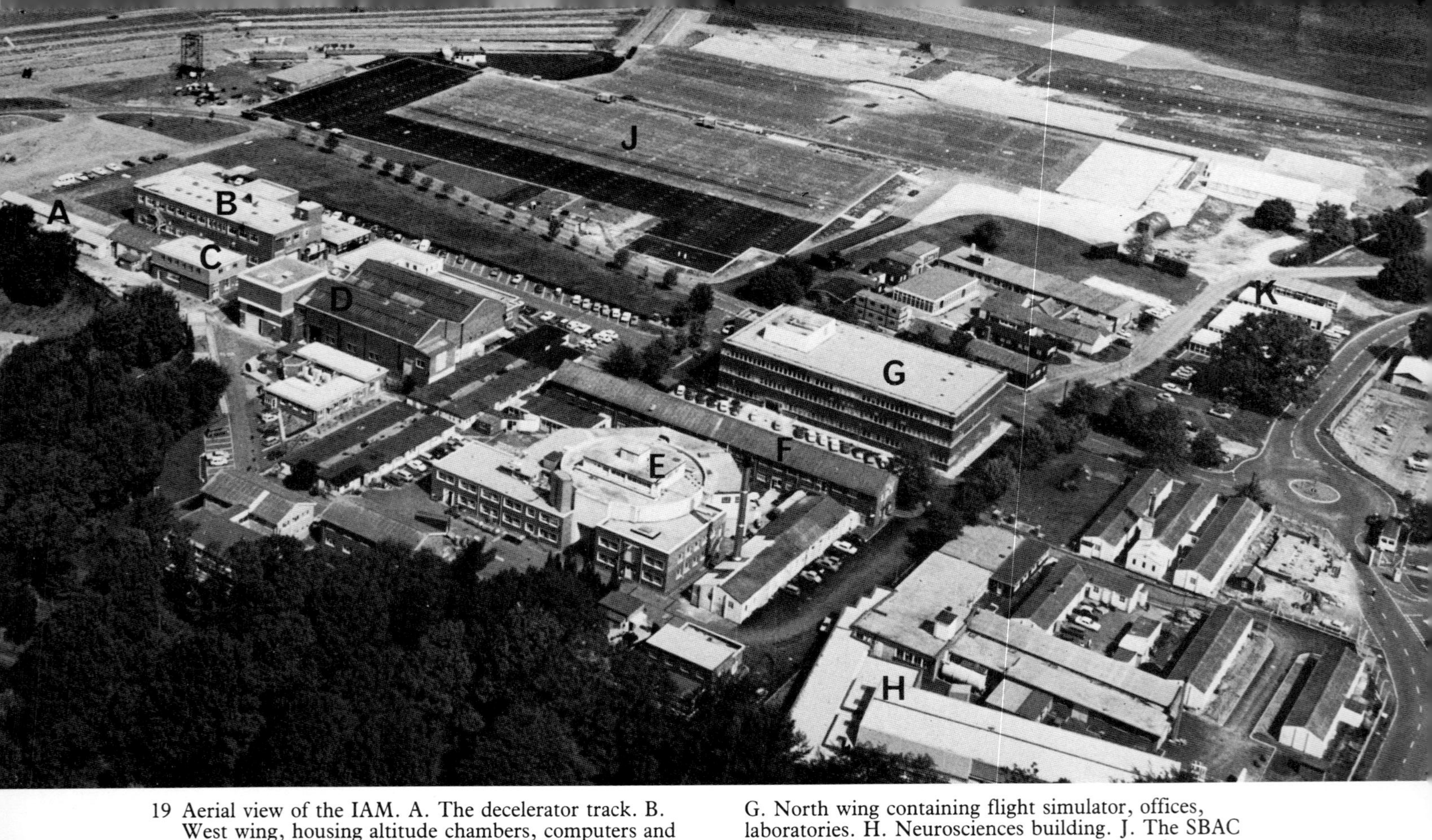

19 Aerial view of the IAM. A. The decelerator track. B. West wing, housing altitude chambers, computers and teaching section. C. Vibrator and offices. D. Climatic G. North wing containing flight simulator, offices, laboratories. H. Neurosciences building. J. The SBAC display area. K. The Army Personnel Research

Marshall had been asked for his views, and the advice of Charles Heald sought. However, the Committee failed to make any specific recommendations, much to the disquiet of the Secretary of State for Air.[4] So, at its fourth meeting, on 7 June 1939, the Committee was obliged to do something constructive. It did, defining exactly what work was needed.[5] The most urgent problem was considered to be the prevention of hypoxia – the inadequacies of the in-service oxygen equipment were well recognized. But only slightly less urgent in the Committee's view was the need to protect against increased g. Other important areas for research were selection procedures for aircrew, reducing cockpit noise, improving visual standards and identifying the causes and consequences of fatigue. The latter had important implications for accident prevention, and the Committee felt that a far greater medical impact was needed into accident investigation. As will be seen, all of these problems are still very much with us today.

Next the Committee had to decide who should carry out the necessary research and where. Because of the urgency of the work to be done, it was decided that a research team should be formed at once. The Committee proposed that the work on oxygen problems, together with 'any other physiological problems arising in that connection', should be carried out under the supervision of Dr Matthews, whose services should be obtained from the University of Cambridge for six months. The Committee also proposed that Group Captain Struan Marshall should concentrate his attention on the problem of blacking out, as arrangements had already been made for a special aircraft to be fitted out for the researches that he had suggested at an earlier meeting. In addition, Flight Lieutenant T.C. Macdonald, a medical officer with wings (who was in the process of completing an MD thesis on the subject of carbon monoxide poisoning in aircraft), was to be attached to the team. But where should this work be carried out? Although the Physiological Laboratory at Hendon was the obvious choice, this was still not operating satisfactorily at its new location. In addition, it appeared that Hendon was not a busy enough airfield for the Laboratory to obtain either the flying it needed or sufficient direct contact with aircrew. The DMS therefore told the Committee that he intended to ask for authority to move the Laboratory from Hendon to the Royal Aircraft Establishment at South Farnborough. In fact, there is evidence of some anticipation here, for the Committee's Chief Executive Officer, Air Commodore Whittingham, had already set the necessary wheels in motion. Sir Bryan Matthews' later appreciation of the situation was that, whilst the DMS was a stickler for doing things the right way, Whittingham could see that there was a war coming and was prepared to act accordingly. Whittingham and Matthews had therefore already been down to Farnborough to meet the Superintendent of the Royal Aircraft Establishment (RAE) and to discuss the possible use of RAE facilities, before the June meeting of the FPRC. It had been agreed then that a corrugated iron lean-to shed, opposite the Balloon Shed, could be used by the research team and that they could have access to the Instrument Department's vertical decompression chamber nearby. The lean-to shed had a glass partition to divide it into a workshop and an office; apart from the partition, the shed was totally empty. Arrangements were made for the research team to become an administrative part of the RAE – an arrangement which would prove to have advantages and disadvantages. The CME Physiological Laboratory became, in due course, 60 (later 17) Department, RAE, although the RAF Medical Branch were careful to retain executive command of the Laboratory. A new wooden hut was ordered, and arrangements were made for a larger, low-pressure chamber, already on order for the Laboratory but destined for Hendon, to be erected on the new site. And all this took place *before* the DMS advised the FPRC that he was to seek authority to move the Physiological Laboratory to Farnborough. Presented with a *fait accompli* by Whittingham, the Committee solemnly endorsed his actions. It was decided, however, that researches into flying aptitude would continue at the CME under Squadron Leader Williams and that follow-up work would be carried out at the Central Flying School, Upavon, by Wing Commander Hugh Corner and Flight Lieutenant D.J. Dawson, both of whom were physicians and pilots. Nevertheless, aviation medicine in the UK had at last found a permanent home – at the birthplace of British aviation.

At the last meeting of the FPRC before the outbreak of war, the appointment of Bryan Matthews as Head of the RAF Physiological Laboratory was confirmed. Within a matter of weeks he was down at Farnborough, carrying out with Marshall and Macdonald the first experiments, or 'runs' as they were called, in the Instrument Department's decompression chamber. The accommodation in the lean-to shed was spartan. Marshall, presumably exercising his right as senior (but not commanding!) officer, had commandeered the office, leaving the other two to make themselves as comfortable as they could in the workshop.[6] The decompression chamber too was hardly ideal – it was noisy and cramped and the Instrument Department had priority in its use. However, a start had been made on the new wooden hut, and the new decompression chamber was expected at any time. In the event, the vagaries of the English weather so delayed building and installation that it was to be March the following year before the new facilities were ready.

In the meantime, the Laboratory started to gain a few recruits. The first was Miss Margaret Worthington, who had been one of Matthews' students at Cambridge before obtaining a job at the RAE. When she discovered that her old tutor was also working at Farnborough, she successfully applied to be transferred from the Instrument Department to the Physiological Laboratory. Her duties were to act as observer for experiments in the decompression chamber and to carry out chemical analyses. She was (and is) a colourful personality and an accomplished artist; two things that most early colleagues remember of her are that she usually wore trousers and that she drove a Frazer Nash sports car which she maintained herself. Shortly afterwards she was joined by Mr J.L. Parkinson, who had previously been personal technician to the eminent physiologist Professor A.V. Hill. Marshall's seventeen-year-old Boy Scout son also came down to Farnborough to give a hand, but he lasted only two days. Matthews remembers that John Marshall kept testing the oxygen bottles to see if they were empty by turning the taps fully on; very soon they were empty! Marshall senior also supplied a treadle lathe which stayed for the entire war; apart from that, the workshop contained just a six- inch lathe, a drilling stand and a brazing hearth.

Then came a young man named Alan Hodgkin, who was a fellow of Trinity College, Cambridge. Hodgkin had been awaiting instructions to join a top-secret establishment, but while he was kicking his heels, Matthews invited him to Farnborough. In later life this young man would become Sir Alan Hodgkin OM, share the Nobel Prize for Medicine in 1963 and, from 1970 to 1975, be the president of the Royal Society. So for about six months the Lab, as it came to be called, had the future President and Vice-President (Matthews) of the Royal Society working together within its corrugated iron walls. In those few months they both spent many hours in the decompression chamber assessing different oxygen systems and suffering, regularly and acutely, from the effects of decompression sickness. This condition is caused by nitrogen, dissolved in body fat, coming out of solution as bubbles of gas. If the bubbles become trapped around joints, severe pain results. Bubbles in the blood-stream can block the small blood-vessels in the lungs, causing difficulty in breathing, coughing and a choking sensation; hence the name 'the chokes'. More alarming still is the partial paralysis which can be caused by obstruction of blood-vessels supplying the brain. Matthews was particularly susceptible to decompression sickness – or 'the bends' as it was known in those days – and was to suffer permanent damage to his vision. Carmichael, the neurologist on the FPRC was appalled at the risks the Farnborough team were taking.[7] Unfortunately, there was simply no other way of evaluating different oxygen systems nor of trying to discover what factors made some individuals so much more prone to the bends than others.

The next arrival was to stay at the Lab rather longer; Bill Stewart arrived at the beginning of 1940 and was to remain until his death in 1967. From 1946, after the departure of Matthews, he was to be the Head of the RAF Institute of Aviation Medicine. In 1938, as a research student, Stewart had come up to Cambridge from the National Hospital for Nervous Diseases at Queen Square to work for a few months with Matthews in Professor Adrian's laboratory. He and Matthews took to each other immediately. Both were easy-going, extrovert types, individually brilliant and sharing a common love of the sea. Matthews recollects sailing across to Dunkirk with Stewart in the summer of that last year of peace and seeing the large formations of Nazi bombers familiarizing themselves with the coastline. A platoon of utterly slovenly French conscripts were being drilled on the quayside by an equally slovenly sergeant-major. Stewart expressed grave reservations about their ability to stop any German invasion. His misgivings proved entirely justified!

Shortly afterwards Stewart returned to Queen Square, whilst at the same time joining the RAF Volunteer Reserve. He and Matthews then lost contact for a while. By late 1939 Stewart had been called up and, as Flying Officer Stewart, was serving as medical officer with a balloon unit based in Northumberland, where his contribution to the war had amounted to treating a broken ankle and one case of VD! Entirely by accident Matthews learned of his whereabouts from Professor Carmichael, who had known Stewart at Queen Square. With Whittingham's connivance, a delighted Stewart was soon heading south to take up his new appointment as head of the acceleration research programme at the RAF Physiological

Laboratory, a position which had fallen vacant with the somewhat mysterious departure, shortly before, of Marshall to Coastal Command Headquarters as Deputy Principal Medical Officer, a position he was to hold until his retirement in 1944. The mystery concerns precisely why he was posted. After all, he was the RAF specialist in applied physiology, an Honorary Physician to the King and, as a Group Captain, a very senior officer. However, it seems likely that he did not find the new arrangements at the Physiological Laboratory entirely to his liking.

When, in July 1939, the FPRC decided that acceleration research was to be carried out using aircraft, Marshall had been put in charge of the programme. From Marshall's point of view this must have been, to say the least, unsatisfactory. Apart from the brief foray in the early thirties, already described, it had not been problems of acceleration which had been earlier his main interest or concern but problems of oxygen supply. Even more galling was that all the oxygen work, and command of the Laboratory, had been given to Matthews – an outsider nearly twenty years his junior – and a civilian to boot! He did, therefore, have some cause to feel aggrieved – for he *had* been pushed aside, despite his senior RAF rank.

Despite the fact that there appears to have been little personal animosity between the two men, something obviously had to give, and inevitably it was Marshall. Even though by late 1939 an aircraft had been made available for g research, little had been accomplished. To be fair to Marshall, this was not entirely his fault. To begin with, he had been allotted a Harvard training aircraft which, according to Squadron Leader Stainforth, was '... most unsuitable for experiments in acceleration'.[8] Then, after it had been fitted out with the necessary instrumentation by the RAE, the Air Ministry said that the aircraft was required for other, more urgent work. Although shortly afterwards a Fairey Battle was delivered, it too was almost immediately temporarily withdrawn. However, some attempts were made to determine whether the degree of acceleration required (4g) could be sustained long enough for meaningful measurements to be obtained – attempts which were regularly thwarted by poor weather. Nevertheless, it was this lack of progress with the acceleration programme[9] coupled with his apparent abhorrence of the decompression chamber (perhaps because of ill health) which were almost certainly responsible for his early departure from the new Laboratory.

Early in 1940 Matthews' personal assistant at Cambridge, Mr

'Ossie' Blunt, joined his former boss at Farnborough, and a general 'labourer' was provided by the RAE. 'Ossie', with Parkinson, was to be in charge of all mechanical construction. The labourer was Mr 'Happy' Day, an ex-Navy cook and adept scrounger, a talent which proved of inestimable value to the Lab. He also learnt to operate the decompression chamber, eventually taking over this job from Macdonald. Since RAE bureaucracy could not permit a mere labourer to undertake such a responsible task, he was officially promoted to the important grade of Engine Driver, Stationary! And bureaucracy presented Matthews with his fair share of problems too. When he arrived to begin work, he found that none of the equipment ordered in July had been delivered. In frustration, he told Whittingham that, if this sort of thing was to be commonplace, he was not going to achieve much during his six-month secondment from Cambridge. Matthews' attitude annoyed Sir Edward Mellanby, the Chairman of the FPRC, who complained about it to Whittingham. However, Whittingham was on Matthews' side, which annoyed Mellanby even more. So Mellanby wrote a stern letter to the DMS complaining about Whittingham's attitude too! (Nevertheless, Matthews' tenure of office was first extended by six months and then, in September 1940, the FPRC unanimously recommended 'in the strongest possible terms' that Matthews' services be retained for the entire war.)[10] To enable some work to be carried out, Matthews received permission from Sir Joseph Barcroft to borrow equipment from the University of Cambridge, and he ran six car-loads of apparatus from Cambridge to Farnborough during August. Another problem was that the question of Matthews' salary was not settled for some time; to start with, he was still receiving his fellowship stipend from King's College but, eventually, he was awarded the sum of £6 a week for being the Head of the RAF Physiological Laboratory.

Later in the war, when he could take a far more relaxed view of things, Matthews would 'play the system', for example by having the decompression chamber classified as a chapel so that it qualified for the thick blue, sound-deadening carpet normally laid only in chancels! On another occasion he requested, and eventually received, authority to buy mousetraps, which were not available through RAE stores, on the pretext that mice were nibbling away the insulation round the pipes in the decompression chamber. This led, of course, to the opportunity of further annoying the system a week or so later by requesting permission to buy a weekly supply of cheese to bait the traps! Matthews' sniping eventually paid dividends, for he was finally given the funds to buy equipment for the Lab on his own authority.

In November 1940 a certain Flight Lieutenant Winfield arrived at the Lab, and things were never quite the same again. Roland Winfield had joined the RAF early in 1939, having previously been a ship's surgeon and then a civilian general practitioner. He was with the Air Component of the Allied Expeditionary Force in France at the time of the German breakthrough and was one of the many who had to be hurriedly evacuated back to England. He never forgave the Germans for the undignified manner of his departure from France; from that point on, Winfield harboured a deep hatred of everything German, a hatred that goes a long way to explaining his subsequent exploits.[11]

On his return to England, Winfield gained his 'wings', and it was shortly afterwards that serendipity saw him sitting next to the DMS, Air Marshal Sir Victor Richardson, at a Mess luncheon. Richardson asked Winfield if he had come across any problems in the physiology of flying and, in Winfield's own words, 'That of course unloosed the floodgates.' The next day he was posted to Farnborough, initially as an ordinary member of the team; however, shortly afterwards Macdonald was posted to Fighter Command, and so Winfield became the Deputy Head of the RAF Physiological Laboratory.

Winfield's first problem was that Richardson had posted him to Farnborough without telling Air Commodore Whittingham, who regarded the Lab as his own property. But Winfield soon got the chance to win his spurs with an investigation into the problem of airsickness amongst crews of Coastal Command. This, Winfield's first major assessment in the field, established his reputation both as a valuable member of the Farnborough team and as a hog for flying hours – he flew in Lerwicks and Sunderlands from Mountbatten, Stranraer and Oban. More importantly, the report Winfield gave found him favour in the eyes of Whittingham. Soon he was flying other sorties as second pilot, navigator or air gunner, not only in Coastal Command but also in Bomber Command, where he flew in most operational types of aircraft and on many sorties including an attack on the German cruiser *Prinz Eugen*. In all, Winfield flew ninety-eight sorties against the enemy with the crews of Bomber Command, studying problems of night vision, dazzle, fatigue, airsickness, hypoxia and cold. Often he flew with crews of suspected 'low moral fibre', partly to assess their capabilities and also to bolster their morale. He flew also with the American 7th Bomber Group to assess their oxygen equipment and body armour, and in

Beaufighters and Vengeances in India, where he had been sent by Whittingham to see how the efficiency of the air and ground crews of South-East Asia Command could be improved.

One of Winfield's more memorable airsickness studies involved gliders. Because piloting a glider under tow was very difficult, requiring considerable training, the RAE were doing experiments with a Hotspur glider to see if an automatic pilot would make matters easier. Winfield was interested in seeing whether the use of the automatic pilot would increase the likelihood of airsickness, and his chance came one hot day in June 1942. As it happened, on that particular day, two factors made it very likely that Winfield's pet remedy for airsickness, a cocktail of hyoscine and other drugs, would be severely tested. First, cumulus clouds were forming in the sky, a portent of turbulent conditions. And second, Winfield had a monumental hangover as a result of a party the previous night to celebrate his award of the Air Force Cross. (The hangover was caused by drinking masochistic cocktails called 'Doctor's Blood' – double rum and a bottle of Guinness topped up to one pint with draught bitter!)

Winfield was unique at Farnborough in being allowed to keep his own parachute in his room. This, combined with the fact that the glider captain had forgotten to tell the Ops desk that Winfield was to be second pilot on this flight, led to the authorities assuming that there were only four people on board the glider instead of five. Because of the heat, Winfield stowed his hat and jacket under the seat, putting on his parachute harness over his shirt. The stage was set for a course of accident and misunderstanding. To begin with, the hawser from the Whitley towing aircraft to the Hotspur glider snapped at 6,000 feet in severe turbulence; whipping back, it sliced off the nose of the glider and wrapped itself around the tail plane. The crew baled out one by one; fortuitously one of the men, in baling out, fouled the broken hawser, dragging it free of the tail before managing to free himself and deploy his parachute. By the time that Winfield and three others had gone, the glider was responding to control again, so the captain began a leisurely descent to the RAE and made a perfect landing – much to the amazement of watchers on the ground who, having seen the expected four parachutes deploy, had assumed the glider to be devoid of any crew! Winfield's troubles were merely gathering momentum, however. He forgot he was not attached to a static line, only remembering to deploy his parachute at low altitude after a dangerous freefall. Then, on landing, he was roughly accosted by two workers who had seen the Whitley and the glider land but had missed seeing anyone bale out and therefore assumed he was a spy. Winfield, it will be remembered, had no jacket or cap to identify himself as an RAF officer. The two workers were being exceedingly threatening, so, to save himself from being pitchforked to death, he suggested that they should all retire to the nearest pub while the police and the RAE were informed. The police were duly summoned, and Winfield was allowed to make a telephone call to the Chief Test Pilot at the RAE. Not having heard what was going on, he naturally assumed that Winfield was still on the binge from the night before and was now coolly requesting transport back to base! Eventually everything was straightened out. The only good thing about the morning's activity was that Winfield was not sick!

Winfield had a great interest in parachuting, making many jumps at Ringway Aerodrome, near Manchester, in the furtherance of research into the causes of parachuting injuries. Eventually he persuaded the authorities that the problem required a full-time medical officer – and even arranged for his younger brother, Flight Lieutenant B.J.O. Winfield, to carry out the duties. Out of the elder Winfield's parachute work at Ringway arose his association with the Whitley flight at Newmarket, with whom he flew many sorties dropping agents into enemy territory. It was as a result of this involvement that Winfield was approached, later in the war, to see if he could provide human cargo for the final checks of a system being considered for plucking a man from the ground by aeroplane. The system had originally been developed in the USA to retrieve mail and then later on to pick up gliders that had been used in war operations. However, it also had obvious implications for the recovery of agents from occupied territory. The towing aircraft flew slowly past, trailing a hook at the end of a pole. The object to be towed was attached to a cable, a loop of which was held off the ground on a pair of poles. The pilot engaged the hook on the loop, applied full power and climbed away, while the shock of the connection was reduced by allowing the cable to be paid out from a winch in the aircraft. Finally the subject was winched into the aircraft. Unlike a glider, a man could not be trundled across the ground before he became airborne, so the 'snatch' had to be clean. This required an acceleration of about $5\frac{1}{2}$g; some forty successful pick-ups had already been carried out on dummies, and the time was now ripe to use live subjects. Snatches were carried out at Booker Airfield in Buckinghamshire, using Winfield, Stewart and the originator of the project, a Lieutenant Lee Warner, as the human cargo. Squadron Leader Davidson, a medical officer pilot who joined the Lab in 1943 and who did much of the testing of the early anti-g suits, gave this vivid description of the first two snatches, those of Winfield and Stewart.

> Winfield sat calmly with bowed head waiting for the aircraft. When the jerk came his body was whipped into the aircraft and the immediate impression made on the observer was that the shock was more brutal and severe than he had anticipated by his muscular tone. It was as though he had been tackled very hard, terribly swiftly, when comparatively unprepared. In a second, I thought he had been blacked out and perhaps become unconscious from the sudden g. It was an impression of catastrophe rather than control. When he landed I was not surprised to see that he was pale and, though cheerful and eager to repeat the experience, clearly physically shaken.
>
> Stewart prepared himself by sitting in the same attitude as Winfield but with a deliberate and purposeful tenseness of posture. At the moment of pick-up he seemed rather to sail away at incredible speed but with absolutely no whip or flailing of the limbs. His whole body was swept instantaneously into the air without apparent lag or jerk. The contrast between his ascent and Winfield's alarming and merciless evulsion from the ground was most striking. Stewart's appearance and demeanour on landing confirmed his comparatively smooth passage, which was almost certainly due to the greater degree of muscular preparedness at the moment of ascent.[12]

A further demonstration was subsequently arranged at Farnborough for some important visitors. Much to Davidson's annoyance (for he wanted to have a go too), Winfield again was to be the subject. This time, however, disaster very nearly struck. The event is described in the words of Mr K.G. Wilkinson, who was responsible for the RAE input to the project:

> For the demonstration at Farnborough (the 53rd snatch) I was operating the winch in the aircraft. After pick-up I was winding Winfield back into the aircraft. As the rope came in I could see that the rope had not been caught cleanly in the hook – it had actually caught round the head of the bolt that shackled the hook to the rope, and if it had slipped off, Winfield would certainly have

> been killed. I managed, using the boathook-like tool that we kept for handling the rope harness during wind-up, to coax the loop off the bolt head and into the hook.[13]

This incident was extremely bad luck, for it took three hundred more tests by Wilkinson to reproduce; the hook was then redesigned, and the system was passed for use.

One of Winfield's major tasks was gathering information. It was essential for the RAF Physiological Laboratory to know what was going on 'at the sharp end', in order that Matthews could appropriately direct the research effort. Unfortunately Winfield was extraordinarily secretive about his flying exploits, and almost all of his information went straight to Whittingham. Often, on arriving at the Lab on a Monday morning, tired out after a weekend on operations, Winfield deliberately cultivated the impression that he had been enjoying a dirty weekend in town. However, Matthews did have access to other sources.

In the early days much information was gleaned in the informal atmosphere of the Civilian Staff Mess at the RAE, where eminent scientists and future Nobel Prize Winners rubbed shoulders with engineers and test pilots. These pilots, who lived in the Mess, were the same pilots who carried out the experimental flying for the Physiological Laboratory, and since Matthews, Macdonald and, as they arrived, the rest of the Lab team also lived in the Mess for a while, it was easy to pick their brains and discuss the research programme. Much information also came to the Lab through the FPRC, many of whose members visited the Physiological Laboratory, gave advice and took part in experiments. Information on operational matters came from two men in particular, Wing Commander J.P. Huins, the Flying Personnel Medical Officer (FPMO) of Bomber Command, and Group Captain H.W. Corner AFC, his counterpart at Fighter Command.

Huins had been a pilot in the First World War, gaining his medical degree afterwards, in 1925. In 1939 he rejoined the RAF and was posted to Bomber Command, where he was to remain for the entire war, eventually leaving as a wing commander with an Air Force Cross and OBE. Huins' reports to the FPRC were models of thoroughness, making many recommendations to improve the lot of Wellington, Whitley, Blenheim, Hampden and many other aircrew, particularly in the fields of cold and mobility. He flew on many operational sorties in 'a quiet, modest way without official knowledge'.[14] Late in 1940 Huins was sent to the Gold Coast in HMS *Furious* and thence flew to Egypt to carry out investigations and give lectures on aviation medicine to aircrew in the Mediterranean and Middle East. Surprisingly he was sent to the same area at the same time as Squadron Leader Macdonald from the Lab, to do exactly the same job. However, their reports told a similar story of poor equipment and lack of familiarity with the basic principles of aviation medicine.

In 1939 Hugh Corner already had many years' flying experience with the RAF behind him. He had also served at the RAF Hospital at Halton during the 1920s and whilst there had become acquainted with Harold Whittingham. However, what he did not have was experience of flying fighter aircraft. This he quickly rectified by undertaking a course of operational flying training, so that by 1940 he was able to fly his own, unarmed Spitfire on missions with the fighter squadrons.

Corner's philosophy was spelt out in an early report to the FPRC: 'By keeping closely in touch with the "operational requirements" of fighters, it is hoped that such first-hand knowledge will be of some use to the Farnborough medical research staff, – or elsewhere. It is hoped, too, to get the correct background for such information. This implies, I think, not experimental flying, and not the occasional single flight under experimental conditions, but the more strenuous conditions of Squadron flying.'[15] In the same report he drew attention to the dismissal by the senior staffs of g as an important factor in combat. 'In spite of the "last word" on the subject by the C. in C. Fighter Command, pilots themselves consider that blacking-out is a feature of certain tactics ...' We shall be hearing more of this particular controversy later.

Despite his age, advanced for a fighter pilot (he was in his early forties), Corner flew on many operations. He was in one of the Spitfires that spotted the *Scharnhorst* and *Gneisenau* on their famous Channel dash. Shortly afterwards, however, he was tragically killed on a dawn sweep over the Channel; he was shot down and, although he was seen to bale out, he was never found. Ironically, he was killed on the day that the Royal College of Physicians elected him a Fellow – the first RAF flying doctor to be so honoured. Whittingham in particular felt his loss keenly, for he had singled out Corner for future high office. The man who replaced Corner was Squadron Leader Macdonald, from the RAF Physiological Laboratory. Macdonald's success in the post can be gauged by his being mentioned in despatches, by his award of the Air Force Cross and by his subsequent high rank.

Corner, Huins and Macdonald were just three of a larger, very distinguished, group of medical officers with wings – a group that included men such as Wing Commander MacGown DFC, who earned his Pathfinder badge while studying night vision over Berlin, and Wing Commander H.P. Ruffell-Smith, the only medical officer to win two bars to his AFC. Some, like Corner and Squadron Leader D.A.G. Robson, lost their lives while carrying out medical investigations. Robson was a Scot who had come to the notice of the Farnborough team early in the war with his helpful and constructive reports on oxygen masks. Serious problems were being encountered with the freezing of the oxygen masks used in the B17 Flying Fortress. After modifications to the mask had been made at Farnborough, Bill Stewart arranged with Robson for a flight test in a Fortress from RAF Polebrook. Using his prerogative of senior rank, he managed to claim a place on the flights instead of the squadron medical officer, a Flying Officer A.J. Barwood. At 30,000 feet, over Catterick, the aircraft flew into severe turbulence and was thrown out of control into a spiral dive. Stewart, knowing that the aircraft was likely to break up, struggled up to the tail of the aircraft against the g-forces. On his way he came across Robson, nearly unconscious. Stewart helped him out of the aircraft and then made his own escape as the Fortress broke up. Unfortunately Robson must have been too far gone to pull his rip-cord, for his parachute never opened. Stewart was the sole survivor of the eight-man crew.[16] Barwood, later to have a long and distinguished career at the RAF Institute of Aviation Medicine, thinks that Stewart probably saved his life, since he would have been too inexperienced to know what to do. Shortly afterwards Stewart was awarded the Air Force Cross.

When Winfield arrived at Farnborough, the Physiological Laboratory was already set firm on the course that would make it, by the end of the war, the leading centre for aeromedical research in the world. Research was being directed, in accordance with the wishes of the FPRC, towards improving oxygen-supply systems and identifying the causes of acceleration-induced black-out. However, other commitments were already making deep inroads into the time available for research, and more staff were desperately needed. Winfield, as the senior RAF officer, was obliged to help Matthews with the ever-increasing demands of routine administration. Then there were teaching-duties and the seemingly endless flow of visitors.

The Lab's involvement in teaching and training began innocuously enough with simple demonstration ascents in the decompression chamber to show aircrew the effects of hypoxia, but blossomed into one of its greatest chores. Many of the very senior officers in the Air Ministry had learnt their flying in the previous war, when oxygen had been regarded as more of a luxury than a necessity. Their attitude frequently was that avoiding hypoxia was simply a matter of keeping fit, and this tended to filter down through the ranks, so much so that some aircrew were still implacably opposed to the use of oxygen.[17] Macdonald convinced Whittingham that it was a problem of education, and Whittingham, in turn, persuaded the Air Ministry that Commands should send him a list of all aircrew who claimed to be able to operate at high altitude without oxygen so that they could be tested at Farnborough. A similar arrangement was made for those aircrew who claimed to be unduly susceptible to oxygen lack. Oxygen 'courses' were started at the Physiological Laboratory in March 1940; by December that year, 67 courses had been given to instruct 315 personnel. The highlight of the course was the decompression chamber test, when the course members were taken up to a simulated altitude of 25,000 feet and then one member was disconnected from his oxygen supply. Often he was given a writing or arithmetic task to do, so that he could have a permanent record of his performance, but occasionally pranks were played on him. Hypoxia course members mysteriously lost their wallets, cuff links, RAF identity cards or even their trousers (mysteriously, because they were not aware of what was happening whilst they were hypoxic).

The more remote stations were unable to spare crews for the time that it took to visit Farnborough, and so Whittingham arranged that squadron medical officers should give the courses at their stations, with the aid of mobile decompression chambers which would move from one station to another in turn. Initially twenty mobile chambers were ordered. The Physiological Laboratory had a large say in the design of the chambers but, despite the specifications being decided promptly and the contract being placed quickly, they were delivered from the manufacturer only after a lengthy delay. When Matthews investigated the cause of this delay, he discovered that the blame lay in the very poor relations between the contractors and the Ministry of Aircraft Production quality inspectors. The company (Vickers) had refused to allow the inspectors access during working hours to the chambers under construction; because of blackout regulations, the inspectors were, understandably, having difficulty doing the necessary inspections by candlelight![18]

One of the station medical officers involved in running mobile chambers was Flying Officer Edgar ('Gar') Pask, who proved so useful and enthusiastic that he was posted to the Lab late in 1941. He was to be an invaluable acquisition. Although his medical speciality was anaesthesia, it was in the development of flying clothing and, in particular, survival clothing that Pask would make his greatest contribution.

With the introduction of mobile chambers into service, the load on the Lab decreased, as only aircrew and the squadron medical officers needed to be trained at Farnborough. To assist the Lab during the time that it took to get the mobile chambers into use in the RAF, Whittingham arranged for extra staff to be posted to Farnborough. Unfortunately the Air Ministry decided that, since training was involved, education officers would be ideal for the posts. Accordingly two education officers, knowing no physiology at all, were posted to the Physiological Laboratory. However, they soon settled down and were able to remove a large proportion of the teaching-load from the overworked staff. But there were still the visitors.

The constant flow of high-ranking visitors often proved to be an embarrassment to the RAE, for Matthews and Winfield tended to be somewhat tardy in letting the appropriate authorities know that a VIP was expected. The Chief Superintendent of the RAE, Mr W.S. Farren, wrote to Air Marshal Whittingham, complaining of the lack of notice he was given when the Prime Minister visited the Lab in 1942. Then, only six weeks later, Viscount Trenchard, the 'Father' of the RAF, arrived unannounced in Farren's office to ask his way to the Lab. As if this were not bad enough, Farren and his personal assistant were both out of the office and Trenchard had to wait for half an hour to see them.[19]

That the Lab had already established its reputation after just ten months of war was underlined by a visit in July 1940 from King George VI, who was sufficiently interested in what he saw there to ask for the annual report of the activities of the FPRC to the Secretary of State to be sent to him. On the morning of the visit, Matthews suddenly remembered that there was no visitors' book for His Majesty to sign, so Mr Parkinson was hurriedly dispatched to buy one. The King was the first of many distinguished visitors to the Lab to leave his autograph.

In March 1941 the eminent scientist J.B.S. Haldane, accompanied by his assistant and future wife, Dr Helen Spurway, went up in the decompression chamber. In addition to the letter he wrote shortly afterwards suggesting several possible lines of research (which were not taken up), he enclosed a bill from a Harley Street specialist covering treatment they had both received for decompression sickness! Needless to say, the Air Ministry declined to pay.

Other visitors included Beaverbrook (who complained bitterly to Winfield about being kept waiting for about thirty seconds), the Under-Secretary of State for Air, and Queen Wilhelmina of the Netherlands with Prince Bernhard, as well as most of the high-ranking military commanders of the day. On one occasion a French admiral returning to London after his visit was directed to the bus-stop on the Farnborough Road and given instructions on how to reach Farnborough main-line station. On another a French general, hitherto fairly aloof, was much impressed when Mr Parkinson came up to Dr Matthews and said, 'Excuse me, sir. The Duke of Cambridge is on the telephone for you.' What Parkinson neglected to explain was that Dr Matthews was at the time living in a hostelry called the Duke of Cambridge. Most of the visiting commanders signed the book and added their appointment, for example 'C in C Free French Air Force' or 'C in C Polish Forces in Russia', but General de Gaulle wrote only 'France'.

However, at least as 1941 drew to a close, staff numbers at the Lab were increasing. In addition to Pask there had by then been three notable new arrivals. The first of these was Flying Officer Harry L. Roxburgh, a medical graduate from Edinburgh, who had come straight to the Lab from an orthopaedic post in a hospital. His work was to be concerned with oxygen equipment and decompression sickness. Like Stewart, he was to stay on after the war, eventually becoming Air Vice-Marshal Roxburgh, Commandant of the RAF Institute of Aviation Medicine. Next came Flight Lieutenant John Gilson. He, almost single-handedly, was responsible for the series of oxygen masks developed at Farnborough between 1941 and 1945, for which he received the OBE in 1944. A great friend of Pask, whom he regarded as the 'brains' of the Lab during the second half of the war, he is remembered by Roxburgh as an extrovert enthusiast for whom no experiment was too much trouble. Gilson also became a great friend of Margaret Worthington; they married shortly after the war!

The final member of the trio was Dr E.A.G. Goldie. Goldie was a contemporary of Matthews at Cambridge, and Ossie Blunt worked for him briefly before moving down to Farnborough to rejoin his former boss. When Matthews, with Stewart and Macdonald, started studying the effects of hypoxia induced by exposure to various altitudes and, more importantly, comparing the ability of different oxygen-supply systems to ameliorate these effects, they needed to know how hypoxic the subjects actually became. In theory this information is easily obtained by measuring how much oxygen is carried in arterial blood. In practice the necessary measurements are difficult and tedious to make, and getting the blood out of the artery is a painful, and often nauseating, business. Goldie, whilst at Cambridge, had hit upon the solution. An estimate of the oxygen content of blood can be obtained by measuring the 'redness' of the blood, something fairly easily achieved by passing a light through a sample of blood and seeing how the wavelength changes. And convenient samples of oxygenated blood pass close to the skin surface in the lobes of the ears. So why not pass light through an ear lobe? Contact between Matthews and Goldie was quickly re-established, and Goldie soon found himself spending far more time at Farnborough than at Cambridge. By 1942 a device known as the Goldie Anoxiameter, the predecessor of the ear oximeter of later years, was being used routinely in hypoxia experiments.

Unusually for equipment developed in wartime, the details of the anoxiameter were published in the open literature in 1942,[20] and this led to many requests for advice, and for the equipment itself, being made to the Lab during and after the war. The device was so elegant, and Whittingham so jealous of credit being directed to bodies other than the RAF Medical Branch, that Goldie was dragooned into uniform. Thereafter his interests broadened to include night vision, a field to which he made several important contributions. He ended the war as a squadron leader, with the relatively unusual (for ground personnel) and well-deserved award of the Air Force Cross.

By 1942 the Lab was virtually at full strength, with the value and importance of its work being appreciated not just by the various Commands but also by the allies. There was a constant stream of eminent scientists from abroad, particularly from the United States. The Lab had an excellent liaison with medical officers on RAF stations not just in this country but all over the world, who regularly came up with problems and questions for Matthews and his team to resolve. Stewart had become the recognized authority on all matters relating to acceleration; Pask looked after clothing and survival; Roxburgh and Gilson between them dealt with oxygen systems. Bryan Matthews himself increasingly became just what he had abhorred so much when he first took the job as Head of the Laboratory – an 'organisation man'. But he proved a very good 'organization man', with Whittingham's help keeping red tape and bureaucracy at bay and making sure that deadlines were met and high standards maintained. By 1943 the tide of war had started turning slowly but inexorably against Germany, and thoughts, or at least Air Marshal Whittingham's thoughts, were being directed towards the post-war future of aviation medicine research in the United Kingdom. He was determined that there should be no return to the scientific backwaters from which he and Matthews had so successfully rescued the RAF's Physiological Laboratory, and plans for the future Institute of Aviation Medicine were well in hand by February of that year.[21] Also, as the end of the war approached, so some of the urgency inevitably went out of the Lab's research programme. But there was to be one final fling before the team broke up and its members went on their own separate ways; that was to find out just what the Germans had been up to.

Winfield was the vanguard of the Lab's brief foray into intelligence gathering. He had, in fact, had some experience of this type of work when he had accompanied Churchill on the latter's flight to Moscow in August 1942. The day before that flight the great man had been down at Farnborough for indoctrination in the use of, and need for, oxygen. Churchill was clearly unimpressed with the oxygen systems he was shown, calling the mask he had to wear in the decompression chamber 'this damnable muzzle'. Winfield, who fitted the mask, was understandably nervous, because Churchill became irritable at having to put down his cigar. When Air Marshal Whittingham telephoned late that afternoon to order Winfield to accompany Churchill to Moscow the next day as a member of the crew, solely to look after his oxygen system, Winfield realized that something would have to be done.

Winfield, Parkinson, Blunt, Pask and Gilson worked late into the night to produce an oxygen system for the flight that would be acceptable to Churchill. They prepared a mask so that the cigars could be smoked normally while the oxygen was delivered to the nose. Winfield later described Churchill wearing the mask, with its green nose, green tubes circling the mouth to the green rebreathing bag and a big cigar sticking out of the middle as 'looking exactly like some Christmas party disguise". The only risk of this procedure was of incurring Churchillian wrath when the cigars burned more rapidly because of the oxygen-enriched air! Even so, it was difficult to persuade the Prime Minister to use the equipment; Churchill's great friend Field Marshal Jan Smuts had flown round Mount Kilimanjaro at 24,000 feet without oxygen, and Churchill told Winfield that he could do anything that Smuts could do! Winfield and the rest of the crew managed diplomatically to get Churchill to wear his mask by assiduously wearing their own masks from ground-level upwards.

Winfield also liked to tell the story of Churchill flying the Liberator:

> The pilot asked him if he would care to have a go and he was obviously delighted. He clambered forward along the cat-walk to the second pilot's seat and then, holding the control column in his hands, he beamed like a cherub. Looking around towards us he asked, 'How am I doing, boys?' 'You're doing swell, sir', the American navigator, Ruggles, replied. He didn't have the heart to add that George, our automatic pilot was doing pretty well too!

In that same telephone call Whittingham had told Winfield, 'And when you get to Moscow I'm not going to have you just sitting about on your bottom doing nothing, or possibly worse. You are to get busy at once and find out what the Russians are doing in Aviation Medicine.' The Air Attaché in Moscow could not have been more helpful, and arranged contacts, meetings and the full-time services of an interpreter for Winfield. But it proved very difficult to extract any information from the Russians – indeed they were deviously obstructive, just showing him a series of hospitals and pathology laboratories and saying that the only officer of sufficient rank to do justice to Winfield's high rank of wing commander was presently out of Moscow. It was only on the last day of his visit that he had an interview with the Director of Hygiene of the Russian Army, only to be told that there was nothing he could be told because the Russian Air Force was used merely for low-level flying.

However, it was to be in Germany that Winfield carried out his most important intelligence-gathering work. His brief was to seek out all German centres of aviation medicine and physiology research, interrogate the workers there and acquire any items that seemed to be of great operational significance.

Winfield started the job enthusiastically but soon discovered that the Germans had little knowledge in applied physiology that was not known at Farnborough. Eventually he came to hate the job as it deteriorated into a series of manhunts. It soon became apparent that several eminent German scientists had been involved in unnecessary, grisly experiments on inmates of concentration camps. One man in particular surrendered personally to Winfield; he had conducted experiments into the effects of windblast to simulate baling out at high speed, exposing prisoners to higher and higher speed jets of air in a wind tunnel until their faces were torn off. Winfield turned him over to the American authorities in that sector but was, and remained, outraged at the fact that the Americans did not put him on trial but instead shipped him back to America and offered him a job!

Other Nazi scientists, however, did not fare so well. One professor in Hamburg committed suicide shortly after being interrogated by Winfield. The man's laboratory contained some recording equipment that Winfield thought might be useful back at the Lab. On his return to Farnborough, Winfield arranged for Stewart and Pask to visit the centre in Hamburg to organize the transfer to Farnborough of any equipment they thought suitable. The equipment taken needed four Lancaster flights to bring back; on examination, Winfield was puzzled to see that everything, down to light bulbs, light switches and door knobs had been taken. When Stewart and Pask arrived back from their tour of other centres, with only one further crate of carefully selected material, Winfield asked them what they had been up to in Hamburg. They replied that it was obvious that the professor had been involved in Himmler's experiments. The only way they could think of demonstrating their contempt for the professor and his work was by stripping the place bare and telling the laboratory staff why. Winfield was appalled at the thought that two of his officers could be 'done' for looting, although sympathizing with their gesture. There was nothing he could do save tell the DGMS and face his wrath; and wrath there was! Then, after the savage carpeting, Whittingham suggested, unofficially, that Winfield should add each item to the official inventory of the Lab, to be held in reserve for the possible setting-up of an ancillary Institute of Aviation Medicine. As Winfield left the DGMS's office, he received another broadside of Whittingham's ire, but this time Whittingham was polishing his pince-nez and the blue eyes were twinkling! Some of the German apparatus is still in use at the RAF Institute of Aviation Medicine.

Roxburgh and Macdonald too became involved in interrogating German prisoners. Roxburgh's job was to find out as much as he could about German oxygen equipment, and it soon became clear that in the design of oxygen regulators the Germans were far ahead of the British. However, this was an isolated case, and during the six years of war the Germans had, by and large, been left well behind. For example, they never developed an anti-g suit, relying on a crouching posture to increase g-tolerance. And, as Tom Macdonald discovered whilst in Norway, their sea-survival clothing was grossly inferior. He brought to the Lab at Farnborough for evaluation two examples of the German 'foam suit'. This garment consisted of a separate jacket and trousers, closed at the neck, wrists and ankles by a drawstring. Front closure was by a zip. Three layers of fabric were used in its construction, the intermediate layer being a form of coarse-pile towelling into which a large quantity of power (sodium bicarbonate) had been rubbed. On becoming wet, which inevitably happened with the drawstring arrangement (the British immersion suit and flying overall had tight rubber seals), the powder produced a foam of bubbles which became entangled in the interstices of the fabric – hence the name. The idea was that this layer of bubbles served as heat insulation. However, when tested, the suit was no better at protecting against immersion than some of the ordinary British flying suits which were not intended for immersion protection. What is more, the foam quickly escaped and the suit lost its buoyancy.

In 1945 and 1946 Winfield became involved in several 'firsts', including the Aries project, when a Lancaster flew to the magnetic and geographic North Poles, to Alaska and then back to the UK, to pioneer the transatlantic polar route for post-war civil flights. Another record set on this project was by the wireless operator, who announced over the aircraft intercom, with his mouth full, 'First man to eat a banana over the North Pole!' However, with the war now over, the staff of the Physiological Laboratory had to start making some decisions – whether to go or stay, remain in the service or return to civilian life. It will be remembered that the Head of the RAF Physiological Laboratory, Dr Matthews, had been appointed for the duration of the war; six years of what in 1939 had promised to be a most distinguished academic career, had been lost. Was it likely that he could be induced to stay at Farnborough? Matthews was offered an appointment as head of the IAM at a rank of Deputy Chief Scientific Officer with a salary of £1,500 a year – a considerable advance on the £10 a week he was getting at the end of the war. However, he stayed on at the Lab only a short while before deciding to return to Cambridge as Reader in Physiology. Despite his departure, however, Matthews was to retain close links with the IAM through the FPRC, of which he was still a member and which he later chaired for some years.

On the service side, not one of the RAF officers at the Lab was on a permanent commission; thus not a single one of them was under obligation to stay when demobilization came around. In the event Winfield accepted a position at St John's College, Cambridge, and Gilson went to the MRC Pneumoconiosis Research Unit near Cardiff. Goldie chose to return to research with the MRC but tragically died of cancer soon after. Pask, after some hesitation, elected to resume his career in anaesthetics. Squadron Leader Davidson, the medical officer pilot at the Lab during the later war years, went to Birmingham to become a consultant in obstetrics and gynaecology. This left Stewart and Roxburgh. Unlike the others, they had not completed their post-graduate training before the war. However, they were well established in the field of aviation medicine, where their post-graduate qualification was wide experience. In addition, Roxburgh wanted to complete his flying training. It is fortunate indeed that these two decided to stay, for without them the corporate experience so painfully and slowly gained would have been lost altogether.

5 Growing in Stature

When, in 1943, Air Marshal Sir Harold Whittingham was laying his plans for the future of aviation medicine research in the United Kingdom, he was aware that the then current arrangement, with the Lab being an administrative part of the RAE whilst remaining under the operational control of the DGMS, was not a very convenient one. Not only did Matthews quite often find it difficult to obtain administrative support from the RAE, but also the Lab was on a site which was too small for further development and which also belonged to the Ministry of Aircraft Production (MAP). Air Marshal Whittingham therefore proposed to the FPRC that a new 'RAF Institute of Aviation Medicine' should be built. By the beginning of 1944 he had obtained the necessary approval of the Air Council, and he was able to tell the FPRC that the plans were already going out to contract.[1] Land on the south side of the airfield, the opposite side from the RAE, had been chosen and released by the MAP, and £32,000 had been made available for construction work. The new building comprised offices and laboratories, the decompression and cold chambers which had been removed from the old Physiological Laboratory, a small pool for immersion experiments, and a library.

The new Institute was opened on 30 April 1945 by the Princess Royal. There were separate sections for acceleration, altitude, biochemistry, biophysics, personal equipment and teaching. The research itself was to be in both pure and applied physiology and included psychology, development of equipment, investigation and testing of personnel and teaching, although it was specially stipulated that the last 'must not be allowed to choke the growth of research'.[2] Dr Matthews, in particular, had strong feelings about the balance of research to be carried out; his idea was for part of the workers' time to be spent on pure research, not necessarily closely connected with aviation. This was a fine concept which led to one of the most cherished privileges of the Institute and which certainly attracted many members of staff of very high calibre, but which naturally became a focus of attack whenever the workings of the RAF establishments came under financial scrutiny.

With Matthews' departure for the academic cloisters of Cambridge in 1946, Stewart was appointed Head of the RAF Institute of Aviation Medicine. By the end of the year, of all the 'old originals', only he and Roxburgh remained, and there was a real concern that the RAF would be left, as it had been less than ten years before, with no one of the right background, experience or interest to carry on the traditions established by the Physiological Laboratory. However, the fears proved unfounded. To the fledgling Institute flocked talented research workers and medical officers doing their National Service, all keen to enter the new and exciting world of aviation medicine. Several of them were to remain at the Institute for many years thereafter, either as permanent serving officers or as civilian medical or scientific officers. From some dozen professional staff in 1946, the establishment increased constantly during the fifties and sixties and then gradually declined with the economic cutbacks of the seventies.

The decompression chamber from the Physiological Laboratory had been removed from the RAE in 1945 and installed in the main building of the new Institute. Although another chamber was obtained in 1963, the old war-time chamber is still used today. In 1952 the much-needed Climatic Laboratory was built alongside the main building, and in 1955 the human centrifuge was completed. The final additions to the Institute's capital facilities were made in 1968, with the commissioning of a second climatic chamber, and in 1972, with the construction of a decelerator track.

The immediate post-war problems were related specifically tò the greater speeds and heights attainable by aircraft. In association with the Martin-Baker Aircraft Company, the Institute conducted pioneering research into tolerable accelerations for election. Research continued into methods of increasing protection against the effects of acceleration, with the emphasis being placed on anti-g suits and on altering the flying-position of the pilot. Also, throughout the fifties and into the sixties, attention was focused on methods of preventing hypoxia. Extensive research was conducted, particularly by John Ernsting, into the physiological and psychological effects of hypoxia and into the consequences of rapid decompression.

During the war years the problem of providing protection against the severe cold encountered during high-altitude bombing and reconnaissance missions had, as we shall see, received much attention from the staff of the RAF Physiological Laboratory. Although research in this area continued at the IAM, heat stress was to become an equally serious problem.

The twenty years after the war can now be seen as a period of unparalleled expansion of aviation medicine research in the United Kingdom. As the Institute grew, so did its reputation, reaching the point when 'aviation medicine' and 'the IAM' became almost synonymous throughout the world. The high calibre of the scientists the Institute attracted was one reason, and the inspired leadership provided by Bill Stewart was another. All who have ever worked at the Institute recall Stewart with admiration, affection and respect. His premature death in 1967, at the age of fifty-three, represented a tragic loss not just to the IAM but to the RAF and to aviation medicine. In addition to his acknowledged ability as a scientist of the first rank, he was also an excellent administrator and planner, whose papers on future requirements for aviation medicine research were models of clarity and common sense. He got the better of most people with whom he argued because of his tenacity of purpose, but this was done in the most pleasant way possible, and his counsels were valued by all. It is a measure of the man that, when in the final stages of his illness he developed incurable hiccups, he proposed an experiment on himself to elucidate the cause.

Stewart's death marked the end not just of an era but of the 'Golden Age' of British aviation medicine. His successor was a fellow Scot, Air Vice-Marshal Harry Roxburgh, who for so many years had been in Stewart's shadow. His researches were, perhaps, less exciting and spectacular than Stewart's had been, but they were of no less benefit to the RAF. From 1941 until his retirement in 1973, Roxburgh maintained a special interest in all matters relating to oxygen equipment and was largely responsible for insisting on the safe engineering standards in the design and manufacture of oxygen systems that are taken for granted today but which were revolutionary in the 1950s. Roxburgh had performed a difficult task under Stewart, even acting as the Head of the IAM for a year while Stewart was on study leave at McGill University in Canada. Being a perpetual number two makes considerable demands on tact, diplomacy and loyalty; it says much for the characters of both men that they worked for so long in such harmony and that there was little discernible change in either emphasis or policy when Roxburgh took over.

When Air Vice-Marshal Roxburgh retired, the obvious heir

apparent, Group Captain Peter Howard, was too junior to be appointed Commandant. Instead, Air Commodore C.J. Soutar, later to become PMO of Strike Command and then DGMS, was appointed for two years. It would have been totally unfair for a non-scientist to direct the scientific work, so Group Captain Howard was appointed Director of Research, the two jobs being combined once again when he became Commandant in 1975.

The period under Roxburgh and Soutar saw both extensive internal reorganization of the Institute and a change of emphasis away from basic research and towards applied research directly in support of operational requirements of the services. Although this trend has continued, the distinction between basic and applied work is often a fine one. Some years ago Group Captain Glaister was carrying out some experiments to determine the benefit to pilots of using reclined seats to protect against increased g forces. A senior RAF officer, who was visiting the Lab, asked which aircraft the seat was intended for. Glaister's reply was, 'If I could tell you that, it would be several years too late.' While the work was obviously applied, it was also of long-term value to the RAF.

In 1974 the research staff of the Institute was cut by twenty per cent. This was the second establishment cut in two years, for in 1972 there had been a five per cent staff reduction. As a further economy the Institute's Canberra aircraft was relinquished, leaving only a single Hunter T7 aircraft – all a far cry from the halcyon days just after the war; in 1953 alone, the Institute used twelve aircraft types regularly.

A major development in the Institute's organization came in January 1970, with the establishment of the Aircrew Equipment Group (AEG). From the very beginning a significant proportion of the Institute's work has involved ensuring that the many varieties of equipment used by aircrew are well designed and meet the necessary physiological, physical, psychological and anthropometric requirements. The AEG serves to co-ordinate all research activities involving aircrew clothing and equipment and to ensure that appropriate advice is offered by the Institute to the Ministry of Defence. Its most significant and important task during the 1970s has been the organization of research into, and the submission of recommendations for, the development of the UK aircrew chemical defence clothing assemblies. This period also saw a change of emphasis in the Institute's basic and applied research programmes. For example, the development of effective anti-g suits during the fifties and sixties meant that there was less need for research into protection against prolonged accelerations. The emphasis instead has been placed on more abrupt accelerations. An expanding research area has been the study of the effects of the flight environment on the central nervous system and, in particular, the problems of irregular rest and activity in sustained air operations. New laboratories were built in 1974 and 1975 for studies into the physiological and psychological consequences of sleep disturbance and deprivation and of the effects of certain drugs.

The Institute's status as a teaching organization was enhanced in 1967 when it was authorized by a conjoint board of the Royal College of Physicians of England and the Royal College of Surgeons of England to hold courses in preparation for a Diploma in Aviation Medicine. These courses are of six months' duration, with one course per year. Other courses, of two or three weeks' duration, are run on a regular basis. The specialist staff of the Institute also carry out teaching commitments on graduate and post-graduate courses for several universities, some as either honorary professors or lecturers.

Despite the staff cuts of 1972 and 1974, the Institute's research programme in the early and mid seventies was, quantitatively at least, little different from that of the mid and late sixties. From 1975 onwards, and coinciding with the appointment of Peter Howard as Commandant, repeated demands for yet more economies have had inevitably adverse effects not just on the total research effort but on morale too – and morale is crucially important to an establishment which has to use its own staff as subjects in its research programmes. As virtually all the Institute's research is concerned with human performance, the demand for subjects is insatiable. The trouble is that the primary interest is in human performance under stress, and if subjects are to suffer considerable discomfort and even pain, often for no reward whatsoever, then they have to be pretty highly motivated – and, perhaps, not a little crazy!

Of course, some experiments are far worse than others. Fairly innocuous, even if the stress is hypoxia, noise or vibration, are those concerned with monitoring charges in performance at some specific task over a period of time; boredom is frequently the subject's greatest problem. Equally innocuous is the extension of this type of work to look at effects of drugs or of disturbed sleep, except that then the subjects find that their personal lives are disrupted. Problems start to arise when an experimental procedure, however brief, causes discomfort, nausea or pain. For example, whilst some people love to ride the centrifuge, it makes others sick. Decompression to 30,000 feet is virtually without discomfort. Yet the return to 'ground-level' can be a painful business if air cannot ventilate the sinuses or the middle ears. And few who have experienced the agonies of rewarming severely chilled hands and feet would willingly undergo the experience day after day. Next come the experiments which are classed as 'invasive'. If there was a popularity poll for experiments, these would come at the bottom. To many the very thought of needles in veins, let alone tubes being pushed up veins, is anathema. Then to lose perhaps a pint of blood during the course of a series of centrifuge runs, or during a long run on a treadmill in the heat, is understandably considered by some to be asking just a little too much. A somewhat milder version of the 'invasive' procedure is the 'intrusive' procedure, when electrodes are attached to various parts of the body, or devices for measuring body temperature inserted into the ear, down the throat or up the rectum. However, even intrusive techniques are not without discomfort. Sticking needle electrodes into the scalp, or touching the ear-drum with a temperature sensor, can be excruciatingly painful.

Finally, there are the experiments which are downright dangerous. We have already described one of these – the 'bends' runs conducted by Matthews, Macdonald and Hodgkin in the vertical decompression chamber – and we shall be describing more. There were Bill Stewart's g studies in the Battle aircraft (Chapter 7) and John Rawlins' underwater ejection experiments (Chapter 8). In some of the centrifuge experiments conducted by Peter Howard and David Glaister, to tubes in veins were added tubes in arteries which were pushed up towards the heart and lungs. Needless to say, apart from themselves there were few volunteers, and since the late 1960s procedures of this sort have, thankfully, been actively discouraged. The most dangerous experiments of all were carried out by Edgar Pask, on himself, at the Physiological Laboratory during the war (Chapter 10). His philosophy neatly captures the spirit which has driven the Institute's scientists to explore the limits of human endurance with almost complete disregard for their own safety and welfare. Pask believed that no sacrifice was too great to enable the aircrews of the RAF to fly in greater safety, and, fostered by the example of men like Howard, Ernsting and Glaister, this belief has echoed down the years. It should also be remembered that not all of these brave and dedicated scientists are RAF officers. Many are civilians, whose working life is far removed from the popular image of the civil servant. Ironically, although they do everything that their uniformed colleagues do, they are paid less – and they are even paid less than their counterparts in the executive and administrative branches of the civil service. So it is hardly surprising that, with the stringent cuts and other 'economies' now being imposed, morale is suffering, the camaraderie for which the Institute was renowned is vanishing, and Pask's admirable philosophy is being forgotten.

However, if the Institute is no longer exactly thriving, it is still surviving, which is more than can be said of the FPRC; in 1979 it suffered the same fate as so many other 'quangos'. Not everyone mourned the Committee's passing. It had seemed to some that in more recent years the FPRC had become detached from the realities and practicalities of aviation medicine (an accusation from which the Institute itself is not immune!). Nevertheless, since 1939 its regular meetings had provided an expert and critical advisory service at all stages of research projects, and opened avenues to contacts outside the IAM which could also be used for advice and guidance. In addition, the FPRC acted as an important outlet for research reports, especially those with some security restriction. Without the FPRC there would probably have been no IAM, and certainly Britain would not have acquired its outstanding reputation for aeromedical research. But, most important of all, for forty years the Committee acted as guardian and protector of its creation against the predations of others.

Various bodies and agencies have occasionally cast covetous eyes on the Institute, notably the MRC and the RAE. However, the most sustained and serious challenge to the Institute's autonomy came from the Ministry of Supply (MOS). It started in 1950, shortly after Professor Sir Edward Mellanby had resigned as chairman of the FPRC.[3] His place was taken by Air Marshal Sir Harold Whittingham, who was then the Director of Medical Services of the BOAC. Also remaining on the Committee, and succeeding Whittingham as chairman in 1967, was Professor Sir Bryan Matthews. Neither man was likely to take kindly to a take-over bid for the Institute by a bunch of civil servants from London, and the MOS's first attempt was resolutely and successfully rebuffed. Relationships between the Ministry and the IAM became increasingly difficult over the next four years, however, and eventually Tom Macdonald by then an Air Commodore and Director of Hygiene and Research (DHR), was obliged to express his deep concern to the FPRC about the delays in developing and introducing new personal flying equipment into service.[4] The main problem was the absence of any direct feedback to the MOS regarding faults and problems with equipment already in use. For some years after the war the IAM had continued, with the RAE, its war-time job of testing and evaluating personal and survival equipment for the RAF and Fleet Air Arm. Most development work, however, even of items of physiological significance, was left mainly to industry working under contract to the MOS. When, in the 1950s, the RAE became solely a research organization, an important channel by which the IAM had access to equipment for appraisal was severed. Consequently the expert opinion of the IAM was rarely sought either by Industry or by the MOS, and so personal equipment could, and did, enter service without medical scrutiny. The Air Staff were frequently compelled to accept inferior or untried equipment in order to allow aircraft to fly without too great a delay.[5]

Despite attempts to improve co-operation between the IAM and the MOS by holding regular, joint meetings, in 1957 the FPRC was still 'gravely concerned that present and future aircraft could not be operated at the full ceiling and range without unwarrantable disregard for the efficiency and safety of their crews owing to delayed development and faulty production of aircrew flying equipment, especially oxygen regulators'.[6] A year later the DGMS, Air Marshal Sir Patrick Lee Potter, was forced to complain to the Chief of the Air Staff about the poor quality of the personal equipment.

By this time it was evident that the only solution was for the MOS to set up its own organization, and this it, or rather its successor, the Ministry of Aviation, proceeded to do. A fifty-two-strong Human Engineering Division was formed within the Mechanical Engineering Department of the RAE with specific responsibility for development and testing of aircrew personal equipment. The notice promulgating the establishment of the new Division proclaimed:

> The staff of the Division will include a number of doctors whose task it will be to give medical advice within the Division itself and to other parts of the Department as well as to the Royal Aircraft Establishment in general. Although these doctors will be Serving Officers, they will also be expected to contribute advice in the field of civil aviation. We hope to see the new Division become a centre for the application of aviation medicine to all the various problems of aircraft design for which it has relevance.[7]

This was strong stuff for the IAM to have to swallow. First, because of the shortage of suitable medical officers, those required by the new Division would have to come from the IAM, which could ill afford to lose staff of the required calibre. Second, there was the implied intention of the Ministry of Aviation to develop its own rival Aviation Medicine Department somewhat on the lines of the IAM. And, as if this were not unpleasant enough, the Ministry of Aviation appointed a mathematician to head the new Division, instead of a biologist or doctor. However, hurt pride was eventually assuaged when the Secretary of State confirmed that biological research and development would still take place at the IAM, that the Ministry of Aviation would be responsible for production contracts and that the IAM would be authorized to inspect systems and to make recommendations.[8] After a few teething problems, the new arrangements started to work well and, especially over the last few years, there has been very close co-operation between the RAE's Human Engineering Division and the IAM, notably in the development of chemical defence clothing for aircrew.

Since 1971 communication and co-operation between the IAM and other government defence departments has been greatly assisted by the formation of the Ministry of Defence, with its own purchasing organization, covering all three service arms, the Procurement Executive. Procurement in this context means not only the purchase of all military equipment but also the processes of research, design and development which were excluded from the terms of reference of the MOS and of its 1959 successor, the Ministry of Aviation. In other words, there are now avenues of direct contact between all agencies involved in the production and testing of aircrew clothing and equipment for the RAF.

It is not just in the personal equipment field that the Institute has sought to exert an influence. As we have seen, during the war one of the most demanding of the Lab's tasks had been the indoctrination of aircrew, and this had led to the inauguration of training at unit level using mobile decompression chambers. However, with the introduction of pressure clothing and the need for specialized training, instruction became concentrated at a few centres. With the shift to advanced oxygen systems and other complex items of personal equipment, the trend to centralized training continued. In 1960 the Aeromedical Training Centre was established at RAF Upwood and moved to RAF North Luffenham in 1964. Now named the RAF Aviation Medicine Training Centre (AMTC), it is a unit of the RAF's Strike Command. The recent transfer of the IAM from Support to Strike Command has facilitated exchange of equipment and the direction of aviation medicine training of aircrew by the IAM, and co-operation between the two units is close and effective.

Despite the occasional admonishment that the Institute is far removed from the world of flying, aircraft have always been one of the Lab's main capital facilities, and airborne research forms an important part of the overall research programme. At present the Institute's aircraft is a Hunter T7, although since 1945 the IAM has used no fewer than twenty-four aircraft types in the prosecution of airborne research.[9] Many of the aircraft used were actually on the Lab's inventory instead of merely being borrowed for the occasion. The 1950s were the golden years of flying at the Institute, with many different types of aircraft, including the most modern, and with many medically qualified pilots to fly them. Pre-eminent amongst these were Wing Commander Pat Ruffell-Smith, Wing Commander Howitt and Squadron Leaders Wambeek and Bazarnik.

Ruffell-Smith initially came to the Institute for a two-week attachment and ended up staying for thirteen years! From 1946 to 1958 he and Dr Geoffrey Morant were involved in the cockpit ergonomics of every military aircraft produced in this country. When jet aircraft were first introduced into the RAF, many aircrew complained of feeling 'woozy' in the air, and the term 'ultrasonic sickness' was coined to describe the symptoms. On hearing of the disquiet, Ruffell-Smith flew a Meteor 4 at high speed 'solidly for one week' without experiencing any symptoms at all, and the scare died down.[10] Shortly before this, he had been involved in the Berlin airlift with Squadron Leader Bob Maycock, another Medical Officer Pilot (MOP) at the Institute. The airlift crews worked seven days on and two days off, with poor food and disturbed rest conditions; often they had time only to grab a bun and a cup of tea between sorties. Not surprisingly, they became tired and mistakes were made. As a result of their investigations, Ruffell-Smith and Maycock recommended changes, especially a reduction in flying time by ten per cent, and better food and accommodation. Maycock, in attempting to convince a senior officer of the urgent need for radical improvements for the aircrew, coined a phrase for which he earned a certain notoriety in the RAF. 'Sir,' he said, 'you can't fly, fight or f*** on buns!'[11]

Another large research programme conducted in the 1950s was on high-speed, low-level flight, initially in a Meteor 7 but later in Javelin and Hunter aircraft. The Hunter proved to be relatively unsuitable for the work since it kept losing rivets out of its tail! The early flights proved to be unacceptably noisy for local residents so the trials were moved to Libya, where Tony Barwood's air-ventilated suit, described later (Chapter 10), proved invaluable. The inhabitants of the United Kingdom have since become more tolerant of aircraft noise!

With such a large amount of flying going on, it was inevitable that there would be crashes. Ruffell-Smith broke two aeroplanes in one week; according to Group Captain Barwood, that week happened to be the one when Ruffell-Smith was attempting to wean himself away from his beloved pipe! Somewhat shaken, he resumed smoking. Howitt bent a Spitfire, and Konrad Bazarnik, with Tony Goorney as a passenger, had a nasty accident in a Meteor. Bazarnik, whilst battling his way around the circuit after losing an engine and part of the canopy, had looked round and seen Goorney slumped in his seat, bleeding and apparently unconscious. After crash landing, the Meteor caught fire but, to Bazarnik's consternation, there was no sign of Goorney anywhere; it later transpired that Goorney's exit from the crashed aircraft had been even faster than his own, and he had continued running until he was out of sight! The first casualty was a German pilot flying the IAM Meteor on a low-level sortie in Germany, he was diverted to help another aircraft, which meant that he had to climb. He plugged his oxygen hose into a connector he expected to be the oxygen supply but which was, in fact, a suit-pressurization air supply; he became hypoxic at altitude and crashed. More recently, in 1974, Squadron Leader Gordon Lamont Smith was killed while doing continuation training in a Meteor at the RAE. His death underlined the desperate shortage of MOPs in the RAF, the Institute eventually being helped by the attachment of first an MOP from the USAF and then a US Navy equivalent.

Throughout the 1960s the flight research load was carried mainly by Javelin, Canberra and Hunter aircraft, the latter two remaining longest. The Canberra was removed from the fleet in September 1974 and was not replaced. Since the Hunter was too small for the equipment being used in some of the flight programmes, space was found in several of the RAE's aircraft to allow the research to continue. However, advances in technology in the last few years have allowed far greater miniaturization of electronic components in experimental apparatus, so, by and large, the Hunter has coped. The problem now is the aircraft's age; at twenty-five, it is nearing the end of its useful life. A Hawk would be the ideal replacement, although in these days of financial stringency the struggle to obtain one may be long and hard.

Much to the disappointment of many of its staff, the Institute has not been much involved in space medicine; the Germans provide the European lead in this field. However, there have been some areas of space research where the IAM has been able to help both the National Aeronautics and Space Administration (NASA) and the European Space Agency (ESA). In the early days of the American manned spaced programme, when the Project Mercury missions were being flown, the Institute carried out research in cardiovascular, respiratory and vestibular physiology specifically for NASA, and in 1972 Squadron Leader Mike Whittle was seconded from the IAM to NASA's Manned Spacecraft Center at Houston, Texas, where he was to be actively involved in the Skylab project for two years. He was replaced out there by Group Captain Peter Whittingham who, on his return, helped ESA to define the methods and criteria for selecting European payload specialists for the Spacelab project. Throughout Western Europe, many candidates had applied for the distinction of possibly being the first West European in space; in the United Kingdom alone, more than five hundred candidates put themselves forward. Each participating country eventually supplied five names to ESA, and the resulting sixty names were reduced to eleven after further stringent medical and psychiatric tests by ESA. The remaining candidates were then subjected to a battery of special tests – a physical fitness test, a test of resistance to fainting, vestibular tests, centrifuge runs and 'roller coaster' flights to simulate weightlessness. Five candidates were tested at the IAM and six at a sister establishment in Germany. Despite the huge number of visitors from the Press and from ESA, the programme ran so smoothly that the entire schedule of tests was completed in under four days instead of the fourteen allowed.

Over the last few years, Dr Alan Benson from the Institute has been closely involved in the development of the 'vestibular sled', a device whereby precisely controlled stimuli can be applied to the vestibular systems of weightless astronauts. Unfortunately, after much work the sled was dropped from the programme for the first of the Spacelab flights allocated to ESA, in order to accommodate other apparatus which the designers had failed to make sufficiently light. At very short notice, the Institute produced a provisional design and model of a simpler and lighter alternative sled, which would at least allow some of the experiments to be carried out. The new system has been greeted with enthusiasm, and the Americans have adopted it for their own programme.

Despite its peripheral involvement, the Institute is often approached for advice on matters pertaining to problems of man in space, and in the late 1960s Squadron Leaders Sharp and Nicholson appeared frequently on the rival TV channels answering questions about the Apollo space flights. Various scientific programmes for TV have been filmed at the Institute, and assistance and advice are regularly given to the Open University. Just as in the days of the Physiological Laboratory, requests for visits still far exceed the capacity of the Institute to oblige. Sometimes these are from scientists in allied fields who want to find out what goes on at the Institute, and sometimes from people with a specific problem they think the Institute can help them solve. Often they are from representatives of the Royal Navy, the Army or the Civil Aviation Authority (CAA), with each of which the Institute co-operates closely on a variety of aeromedical problems of mutual interest and concern. For example, several staff at the Institute are, or have been, wholly or partly funded by the CAA to work on general problems related to flight safety in civil aircraft. Other staff have received both financial and material support from the CAA to study in-flight pilot workloads and to make recommendations on the most effective way of scheduling aircraft so as to minimize problems of jet-lag. The Institute exists not just to serve the RAF.

6 Too Little Oxygen …

At the outbreak of the Second World War, aircraft were flying at ever higher altitudes, even though the in-service oxygen-supply system was dangerously inadequate and wasteful of oxygen. The reason why the endeavours of Struan Marshall, the RAE and the Siebe Gorman Company had come to nought during the mid 1930s was that the concepts being incorporated into the designs of new equipment were too advanced for the technology then available. Consequently, virtually no new oxygen equipment had entered service with the RAF since the end of World War I. Yet all the indications were that the Germans had made considerable advances and that in any combat at altitude, and for high-altitude bombing, they would have a significant advantage over their British adversaries. Little wonder, therefore, that the FPRC decreed that a research programme into the development of a new oxygen-supply system should have the highest priority and that in August 1939 Bryan Matthews moved post-haste down to Farnborough to get the research underway.

Throughout the war attention was to be concentrated upon four specific problems: first, how to produce and carry the oxygen; second, how to ensure the reliable, controlled delivery of oxygen to the aircrew; third, to design a mask to ensure that the oxygen went where it was supposed to – into the lungs; and finally, how to minimize the effects not just of hypoxia but also of the decompression sickness which can accompany flight at high altitude. From March 1940 much of this research was carried out in the Physiological Laboratory's new decompression chamber.

Decompression chambers provide a very convenient means of exposing people to simulated altitude under carefully controlled conditions, whilst at the same time allowing physiological measurements to be fairly easily made. The Lab's new chamber was twenty-seven feet long and eight feet wide, with a door two-thirds of the way along which divided it into two compartments. There were doors at either end, and portholes along each side, so that observers could see clearly what was going on inside. Evacuation of air was by means of an electrically driven vacuum pump, and the two compartments could be used either separately or together. When used together, the chamber could reach a simulated altitude of 42,000 feet in 4 minutes and 90,000 feet in 30 minutes; the small end used alone could reach 10,000 feet in 20 seconds and return to ground-level in 18 seconds. Because the machinery had been placed in a separate room, the chamber was very quiet, especially compared with the Instrument Department's chamber used by Matthews and his team for the first six months of the war.

The only way of testing the effectiveness of any oxygen system is to measure the amount of oxygen in arterial blood but, as we have already noted, taking blood samples from arteries is not a procedure to be encouraged – it is difficult, painful and not without risk. A more convenient, although indirect way is to determine the amount of oxygen in the last part of each expired breath, which reflects the oxygen content of the blood in the lungs. However, measuring the amount of oxygen in small samples of expired air is a tedious, time-consuming and finicky process – or at least it was with the techniques available in 1939. Gas analysis was performed with the 'Haldane' apparatus, a complex arrangement of taps and glass tubes containing mercury, alkali (to absorb carbon dioxide) and reducing solution (to absorb oxygen). Not only does the apparatus require skill and persistence to obtain accurate results, but also it is all too easy to make a mistake and end up with a useless mercury-alkali mixture. From 1939 to 1945 Margaret Worthington had the dubious pleasure of carrying out the gas analyses for the Lab. Considering that an average chamber run would yield about twenty samples for analysis and that each sample was measured until three consecutive estimations agreed very closely, it can be seen that she must have carried out thousands of analyses.

Between 29 August and 31 December 1939, Matthews spent over 8 hours above 30,000 feet on 26 separate occasions, experiencing 'bends' 16 times. Some runs sought to define the extent of Dr Matthews' alarming symptoms while suffering from bends (including partial blindness and paralysis of one arm) and attempted to alleviate them by making him breathe pure oxygen for some time before ascent. A routine chamber log was maintained by Margaret Worthington, and, in addition to technical data, it contained enlightening memos to herself such as 'Bucket required next time. Routine equipment!' and 'Storm pot required'; it also contained messages which were obviously held up to the chamber window for the occupants to read, such as 'We are changing the battery', 'Only 11 samples?' and, optimistically, 'Everything is under control' and on one occasion, the note that mosquitos were still flying happily at 30,000 feet.

Some of the early decompression chamber tests were interrupted by air-raid alerts. The drill was to bring the chamber back to 'ground-level' as smartly as possible and then to file out of the building into a trench outside. Later on, the team decided that the chamber was probably a safer place to be in than the trench, and further tests were uninterrupted. Other dangers arose not so much because of enemy action but rather from friendly action; on one occasion Macdonald was making a film record of a hypoxia run for training purposes, and to get adequate illumination inside the chamber, he placed a very powerful lamp bulb next to the chamber window. Needless to say, the window cracked with the heat, pieces of broken glass flying across the chamber, and the chamber itself making an unscheduled and hurried return to ground-level.

At altitudes above 10,000 feet the aviator needs to be supplied with oxygen if his performance is not to be impaired. If a pilot becomes hypoxic, the consequences can be highly dangerous – albeit amusing too, as the navigator of a Halifax aircraft returning from a bombing mission discovered.

> The captain became very talkative and resented any suggestions that he was behaving abnormally. On seeing the marker flares over the target, he found he could not take his eyes off them and forced the aircraft into a steep dive. Afterwards, he said that he could only read the large figures on the instrument panel and these appeared far away. When we realised that the aircraft was out of control, the engineer trimmed the aircraft. The pilot resented this and assaulted the engineer. He then gave the order to bale out, which we cancelled. He opened the window to look out, and was only prevented from falling out by the engineer who hauled him in. He said that he felt very happy, and had no feeling of fear, even when he tried to force land on a cloud thinking he was near the ground. On one occasion, he informed us we were below ground. After being forced to take oxygen from the spare

helmet and mask, he gradually recovered his senses and was able to fly the required course to base, although he suffered from headache which persisted after landing.[1]

Although in this instance the cause of the hypoxia was a malfunction in the oxygen equipment, there were occasions when the oxygen equipment could be inadequate for quite different reasons. For example, when the pilot has to abandon his aircraft, he also abandons his oxygen supply. Some aircrew, who were known to have baled out at relatively high altitudes, had not opened their parachutes, and there was a suspicion that this was because they had lost consciousness through hypoxia.

At that time there were two schools of thought about the best way of surviving a high-altitude bale-out without oxygen. The first was that, as soon as possible after leaving the aeroplane, the rip-cord should be pulled; then, even if consciousness was lost during the relatively slow descent to altitudes where oxygen was not needed, the parachute would be safely deployed. The detractors of this scheme argued that death from hypoxia could occur during the slow descent and that injury from frostbite was very likely. They proposed a free-fall to a safe altitude before deploying the parachute. But then it was argued that consciousness would be lost during the free-fall and perhaps never regained. Flight Lieutenant Pask devised an experiment to simulate descent from high altitude in an attempt to settle the argument.

The experiment involved subjects breathing oxygen/nitrogen mixtures, with the oxygen concentration being gradually increased to simulate the change during descent from high altitude. At the start, therefore, the oxygen concentration was very low, and the subjects inevitably became hypoxic and lost consciousness. The end point of the test was taken to be when the hypoxic subject showed signs of recovery and therefore might be expected to think about opening a parachute. Because the experiments were so hazardous, they were carried out at the Nuffield Department of Anaesthetics in Oxford with the assistance of the RAF Consultant in Anaesthetics, who also happened to be Head of the Department, and Pask's former boss, Air Commodore R.R. Macintosh. The subjects were Winfield, Stewart, Gilson, Roxburgh and Pask himself. At first, tests were carried out with subjects lying down, but they soon escalated to subjects sitting, and final runs were carried out with the subjects hanging in a parachute harness to simulate the slow descents after parachute deployment. Descents were made from 'altitudes' as high as 40,000 feet, with Pask reserving the most dangerous exposures for himself, also eliminating from the higher runs those subjects who had shown adverse reactions to descents from the lower altitudes. Even so, the margin of safety was very slight. Pask discovered that suspended subjects became so limp when they lost consciousness that their heads flopped forwards to produce respiratory obstruction. Neither was descending free-fall safe, since some subjects, had they been doing it 'for real', would have hit the ground before they had recovered consciousness sufficiently to pull the rip-cord.[2] Not surprisingly Pask received a letter of congratulation from Whittingham for this courageous piece of research, for he had confirmed the absolute necessity for a bale-out oxygen set and had defined the total volume and flow of oxygen required. Within a very short time a design had been agreed and the RAE was working on engineering details. The production version of this 'emergency oxygen set' is still in use in only slightly modified form.

The oxygen equipment in large aircraft, such as bombers, was also inadequate on occasions when crew members had to move around the aircraft whilst it was flying at oxygen-requiring altitudes. Since it would clearly have been folly for the airman to disconnect himself from his oxygen supply, long tubes were provided which connected the supply and the mask. The trouble with these tubes was that, being so long, they were difficult to stow and easily damaged, and they hampered movement around the aeroplane. Also, although it was not appreciated at the time, the oxygen flow was inadequate for the type of physical activity the crew engaged in. There was, therefore, a requirement for a portable oxygen set that would not inconvenience the crewman and would have a realistic endurance.

In September 1939 such a device, giving ten minutes' endurance at 20,000 feet, had been tested for the Ministry of Aircraft Production at Boscombe Down; the set, designated the Portable Oxygen Set Mark 1A, was accepted for service. However, it was far from satisfactory, being bulky, heavy and awkward and having inadequate endurance. Experiments in a Stirling bomber at 18,000 feet demonstrated that the flow was insufficient to maintain adequate oxygenation of the body. The Ministry of Aircraft Production decided in 1943 that design of a new set was therefore to be 'Priority A'.

Because the Physiological Laboratory was, at that stage, overstretched, the design work for the new set was carried out in

Canada after extensive discussions with Farnborough. What eventually emerged, although, despite the high priority, only in August 1945, was a lightweight portable oxygen set which was compatible with the current RAF oxygen masks. By that time, of course, for the bomber crews for whom it was primarily intended, the war was over.

Neither was it just the aircrew who were at risk from the effects of hypoxia. So too, at least early on in the war, were the poor passengers on the long transatlantic flights. The aircraft most commonly used was the Liberator, an American aircraft with American oxygen equipment. The aeroplane had to fly high to obtain maximum range, and this exposed the passengers to the twin perils of cold and hypoxia. Add to that the unaccustomed discomforts of cramped condition, noise and vibration, and it can be easily be imagined that the unfortunate passengers often arrived in a fairly poor physical state. But when the passengers were delivered 'practically unconscious', with one passenger 'having to have both hands amputated because of frostbite', clearly something had to be done, and urgently.[3]

In October 1941, just two weeks after the ordeals of the passengers referred to above had been related to the FPRC, Flying Officer Pask visited RAF Prestwick, the terminus for transatlantic flights, and the home of Scottish Aviation Ltd, who were involved in fitting out aircraft for Ferry Command. Pask found that the problems stemmed from an appalling mixture of incompetence and neglect. The passengers were given American masks to use which required the wearer to breathe through the nose; unfortunately no instructions about this were given to passengers. Pask even found one crew who did not know how to use their own system, so advice from that quarter could have been misleading to say the least. Moreover, the masks were very susceptible to freezing in cold conditions, the oxygen inlet easily becoming blocked; yet it was well known that the heating system for the Liberator passenger compartment was barely effective above an altitude of 17,000 feet.

On examining Scottish Aviation's plans for fitting an oxygen system to Liberators used on other routes, Pask found that the supply that they intended to install would satisfy only one quarter of the requirement. But worse, in the transatlantic Liberators the oxygen bottles for the passengers were not joined together in parallel, so cylinders had to be changed in flight. This was highly dangerous for several reasons. First, all the passengers' masks were fed from a single oxygen delivery point; thus, while the cylinder was being changed, the passengers would be totally without oxygen. Second, no instructions were issued on how to change the bottles. Third, in some of the aircraft examined, there were no spanners supplied for changing the bottles, and in others the spanners did not give sufficient leverage to move the tightly applied nuts. And if this were not enough, Pask found that some of the oxygen delivery points were partly or completely blocked by debris and that the flowmeters supplied to monitor the flow of oxygen were intended for ground use only, being unreliable and inaccurate at altitude! In one new Liberator, which had just been delivered for service, there were no regulating jets at the oxygen delivery points (to limit the flow of oxygen to that which was manually set) in the crew compartment, giving the aircraft an 'oxygen endurance' of between twenty and forty minutes.

In his report, Pask commented, 'Scottish Aviation officials seemed not to know much about oxygen systems'! Pask's recommendations included the necessary redesign of the passengers' oxygen system, the provision of a greater flow of oxygen from larger supplies, the supply of written instructions to the passengers on the use of the oxygen system and the rigorous checking of the oxygen apparatus in all newly delivered aircraft.[4] This advice was apparently all that was required, for there is no record of similar problems arising in Ferry Command during the rest of the war.

Whatever the oxygen equipment is to be used for, it has three basic components: the oxygen source in the aircraft, the regulator controlling the supply the oxygen from the source to the man, and the face mask to which the oxygen is delivered. The source can be either a gaseous or liquid store or a device which manufactures oxygen during flight. Most modern aircraft oxygen systems depend on liquid oxygen (LOX). Indeed, the RAF was using a form of LOX storage for a while after the First World War. Unfortunately the technology of that time was unable to devise a storage container that prevented loss of oxygen by evaporation. This inefficiency forced the discontinuation of the LOX system in the late 1920s, ironically, just when more aircraft than ever before were required to have oxygen supplies because of their ever-improving altitude ceiling. From then on, oxygen was supplied in gaseous form from steel bottles where it was stored under pressure. Each bottle weighed just over 14 lbs and was vulnerable to enemy fire, exploding when hit. During the war Mr Eric Taylor, of the Instrument Department, RAE, developed a system of winding wire around the bottles to prevent them from fragmenting when punctured, but this resulted in a further increase in weight, to 19 lbs. When one considers that a Wellington carried up to 9 oxygen cylinders, a Whitley up to 13, a Stirling or Halifax up to 22 and a Manchester up to 24 the weight penalties of gaseous oxygen systems become apparent. Later in the war the York, an unpressurized passenger aircraft, needed up to 45 cylinders of oxygen.[5] Larger charging bottles had to be transported from the nearest British Oxygen Company plant to the airfield – a considerable administrative and logistic chore.

It is hardly surprising, therefore, that the FPRC considered that alternative methods of oxygen supply should be closely studied. Dr Matthews initially favoured development of a LOX system and, to this end, the FPRC resolved, in June 1939, to seek the aid of the Royal Society Mond Laboratory at Cambridge. Professor (later Sir John) Cockcroft suggested that a young physicist, Dr J.F. Allen, should assist the Farnborough team with their researches. Dr Allen had, in fact, a device which he thought might be suitable for development; its principle of operation was as follows. If you compressed a large quantity of air, it heated up; the heat was then dissipated in a heat exchanger. The compressed but cooler air was then passed through a valve which allowed it to expand. Rapid expansion causes cooling, and with Allen's apparatus this cooling was enough to liquefy the gas. The liquid air was then distilled into its constituent gases by warming it with the incoming air, which was thus itself cooled. The nitrogen and inert gases went to waste, the carbon dioxide was removed by passing the gas through soda lime, the remaining oxygen being produced at low pressure.

By mid-March 1940 Allen's first separator had been installed at the Lab, and a second was under construction. However, the Mond Laboratory had received neither money nor any details of the financial arrangements for the work over the previous eight months, and Matthews complained to the FPRC, 'It would be easier to execute the work and get the staff concerned to do their best if the financial side of the Air Ministry part in it were not a stock laboratory joke.'[6] Two months later, the Mond Laboratory had still not received payment for work or materials, and Allen, who had been employed by the Air Ministry since January, had not yet been given any salary.[7] Yet the first separator was to prove an extremely valuable acquisition. From mid 1940 to the end of the war it was uniquely reliable and trouble-free, providing a daily supply of oxygen for the decompression chamber.

The second, slightly smaller separator, intended for use in an aircraft, was delivered at the end of 1940; it was 34 inches high with a diameter of 10 inches, weighing 32 lbs. Unfortunately the motor and compressor, at 18 cwt. were too heavy even to contemplate installing in an aircraft, and the team were unable to obtain permission to run the compressor off the aircraft engines. A new, much lighter motor and compressor therefore had to be obtained. Matthews approached Mr H.R. (later Sir Harry) Ricardo, who ran a small engineering developing company at Shoreham.

Despite Ricardo's company being moved shortly afterwards, lock, stock and barrel to Oxford, the machine was delivered just ten months later. It was petrol-driven and, with the water and carbon dioxide separators, weighed 524 lbs (4.7 cwt). Bench tests with the equipment proved sufficiently encouraging to start installation in an aeroplane. Modifications were undertaken to decrease the weight of some of the components, a total weight of 450 lbs (4 cwt) being achieved. The aircraft allocated for the tests was a prototype Wellington based at the RAE, and flight testing took place between October and December 1941. It was found that the system satisfactorily produced oxygen thirty minutes after the system was started; for the Wellington, if the compressor was started at the same time as the aircraft engines, breathable oxygen would be available ten minutes after take-off. Overall, the apparatus worked well up to 25,000 feet, but above this level, performance tailed off because the compressor was unable to maintain the required flow of compressed air to the separator. The team for the flights usually consisted of a pilot from the Experimental Flying Department at the RAE, Flying Officer Harry Roxburgh, Margaret Worthington and a Mr Worley from Messrs Ricardo. Mr Worley was found to be an essential member of the flight team since he was the only one who could reliably crank the compressor into life.

At the end of January 1942 the team reported that further modifications were needed to make the system practicable. First, a method of obtaining a greater output from the compressor at altitudes above 25,000 feet was necessary. Then ways of lightening the system were recommended, the most important of which was that the compressor should be driven from the aircraft engines.[8] Not surprisingly, perhaps, the team neglected to mention in their report the fact that the aircraft had been written off earlier in the month, a story best told in Air Vice-Marshal Roxburgh's words:

On board were Flight Lieutenant A. MacCracken the pilot, Mr Worley of Ricardos, Winfield and myself. About an hour had been spent at 27,000 feet with the experimental equipment working normally. Cloud covered the country and, with a failing radio on which he was relying for navigation, the pilot decided to descend. We came through cloud and after a square search, during which nothing was recognised to define our position, the pilot decided to land in a field of reasonable size. This he did with the undercarriage down and with some skill. It is surprising how quickly in these circumstances that the things at the far end start coming towards one; these included a house. Fortunately, there was a corrugation across the field which lifted the undercarriage evenly and quickly and the aircraft came to rest gently on its belly. The field was at Corburton in Nottinghamshire and, in that area, I reckoned it bad luck that we had not found an airfield.

Now, in 1942 to arrive unheralded in a field in England caused local interest at the very least. When it was done in an aircraft not typical of anything that had been seen before (the Wellington was a prototype without the fore and aft gun turrets which gave it much of its character in side view) and manned by a mixed group of servicemen and a civilian, interest quickly changed to suspicion. Or should I say that initial natural suspicion was confirmed. In any event, we spent the next few hours in a cell of the local police station while the matter was resolved by telephone calls with the R.A.E. Then we moved off to the hospitality of the local military which was most welcome. This proved to be a unit of the R.A.C. stationed at Thoresby Hall, which is one of the stately homes of England. I can still see the expression of pained surprise on the face of the Colonel when our pilot, an extrovert Australian, asked him what R.A.C. stood for. After his answer, the pained surprise increased steeply when my Australian friend said 'Royal Armoured Corps? I thought it meant the Royal Automobile f****** Club!' However, despite this start and our clothing, which was quite unsuitable for an Officers' Mess, we had a pleasant evening and set out for Farnborough by train the next morning.

Although the aircraft was written off, the oxygen-producing apparatus, or 'ice-cream machine' as most people called it, was undamaged; it was returned to Farnborough but was not destined to fly again. The weight penalty was the main reason, although the development of pressurized aircraft which did not have the massive requirement for oxygen that non-pressurized aircraft had was another. Matthews thought that the Ministry of Aircraft Production was mistaken in its steadfast refusal to allow the compressor to be powered by the aircraft engines, but, to be fair, the increasingly sophisticated radio and navigation equipment was by then making very considerable demands on the limited aircraft power. Also, the British Oxygen Company must have been aware of the threat to their monopoly that the Mond separator presented, and some behind-the-scenes lobbying of the Ministry may well have taken place. In the end the system was sent to the USA for evaluation, but all they managed to do was to increase the weight further by insisting on more fire-proofing.[9] However, in the 1970s it was to be the Americans who took the lead in the development of On Board Oxygen Generating systems (known, somewhat indelicately, as OBOGS), and now a British company is developing a version to specifications laid down by a member of the Institute staff, Group Captain John Ernsting.

In 1939 the greatest disadvantage of the continuous-flow oxygen system then in service was the tremendous waste of oxygen. Not only was oxygen delivered when it was not needed – during expiration – but also at rest and at low altitude, when more oxygen was available than was physiologically necessary to meet the body's metabolic demands. On the other hand, at high altitudes and when physical activity greatly increased the metabolic demand for oxygen, the flow could be inadequate. However, it was the fact that aircraft were having to carry far more oxygen than was actually required that made the need for an alternative system so important. There was a pressing requirement for relatively small aircraft to carry bomb loads for very great distances, and these simply did not have any room for carrying several large oxygen bottles. Some slower aircraft could not carry sufficient bottles to enable them to carry out long sorties – and anyway there were not enough oxygen bottles generally in the RAF. Also, as new and more powerful aircraft became available, and altitude ceilings were raised still further, aircrew would have an even greater need for oxygen.

Matthews' team quickly identified four main ways of improving oxygen economy. These were:

1. Admit oxygen only during inspiration.
2. Cut off the oxygen supply during expiration.

3. Divert the oxygen supply to a reservoir, or economizer bag, during expiration.
4. Increase the amount of expired air re-inspired.[10]

How the team went on to develop a new oxygen supply system for the RAF incorporating these suggested improvements, and all in a matter of a few months, is one of the great wartime success stories of the RAF Physiological Laboratory. It is the story of the 'Oxygen Economizer', otherwise known as the 'Puffing Billy'.

The idea of an economizer bag was not original, having been suggested many years before by Professor J.S. Haldane. As already noted, Messrs Siebe Gorman produced a simple version, but this had no valves to control the flow of oxygen out of the bag. In the Physiological Laboratory's Economizer, oxygen flowed from a regulator into a rubberized fabric bag maintained under pressure by a spring-loaded plate (or 'bag crusher'). The bag outlet was controlled by a valve which remained closed either until the bag was so full that bag pressure began to rise or until there was suction in the mask at the beginning of inspiration. Once the bag outlet valve was open, it stayed open until either the bag was empty or the mask pressure rose with the start of expiration. Expired air was vented through an expiratory valve in the mask. If the system was operated with no one breathing from it, it puffed oxygen at you – hence the name 'Puffing Billy'.

Alan Hodgkin was the first to test the new device, being accompanied by Bryan Matthews breathing from a standard RAF oxygen system, in an ascent to 30,000 feet. The event was made all the more memorable by the telephones in the chamber going out of action, which detracted somewhat from scientific observation. Nevertheless, the results of the test were encouraging, and others quickly followed. By 20 March 1940 the team was able to report to the FPRC that the device was satisfactory from a physiological point of view. The PB Economizer ('Puffing Billy' was obviously too flippant a name for formal use, but the initials PB were retained for a short time) was reported to need only half the oxygen flow of the standard RAF oxygen system, even when working at a level considered equivalent to flying a heavy bomber. For example, in the Wellington aircraft, the reduced requirement for oxygen bottles meant a weight saving of 500 lbs.

Next, Blunt and Parkinson set to work to make six more Economizers for endurance, vibration and flight tests. These took place throughout April and resulted in several modifications, mainly to the oxygen mask. Matthews himself carried out the first flight test. He flew as a passenger in a Blenheim to an altitude of 29,000 feet and was able to collect expired air samples from himself to confirm measurements made in the decompression chamber. The Blenheim had a nominal service ceiling of 27,850 feet, and it had been stripped down to enable it to fly higher. Then the pilot, Flight Lieutenant (later Group Captain) Johnny Kent, made a second flight, breathing from the Economizer himself. Matthews was left behind so that an extra 2,000 feet of altitude could be squeezed out of the aircraft. Matthews remembers Kent saying, 'This rotten thing, it's like trying to fly it on the point of a needle up here.'

The first major conference on the Economizer was held at the Physiological Laboratory the following month. The meeting had been called because the time had come for the RAE to decide whether to recommend the use of the Economizer to the service on the basis of the physiological tests carried out at the Lab, and the limited flight experience, or whether to recommend that more formal flight trials should be carried out before a decision was made. The meeting was attended by representatives of the Lab, the Air Ministry and the Instrument and Radio Departments of the RAE. A measure of the importance he attached to the development of the system may be gauged from the fact that Whittingham (now an Air Vice-Marshal) himself attended the meeting.

It was agreed that the Lab would manufacture eighteen Economizers and obtain suitable masks for service trial. Squadron Leader Macdonald was to organize the service trials and supervise installation of the equipment in the aircraft. Since the Lab still felt uneasy about the fact that no low-temperature tests had been carried out at altitude with a man breathing from the system, the Instrument Department was directed to do the necessary experiments on the equipment.

During May and June the Instrument Department carried out flow checks on the Economizer at normal temperatures and down to minus 40°C, and also during vibration. Only minor, easily remediable, defects were found, although the Department did reinforce the Lab's warning of the possibility of the mask icing when worn at low temperatures. By July 1940 a draft specification, entitled 'Specification for Oxygen Economizer Mk I and Economizer Adapter Tube', had been drawn up by the Instrument Department for the Air Ministry. At the same time, further flights were being carried out, by the Photo Reconnaissance Unit (PRU) at Heston, the Economizers being used on 6 sorties totalling 17 hours 26 minutes over 30,000 feet. The Medical Officer at Heston reported that, 'After an initial suspicion of the Puffing Billy, the pilots are now very keen and trust it implicitly. On long trips, they refuse to go without [it] unless a further [oxygen] bottle is carried.' During June and July further flight tests were carried out, and, without exception, all the units and the individual aircrew involved were enthusiastic about the new equipment. As one Commanding Officer wrote, 'It would appear, therefore, that the whole idea is one which should be adopted and fitted to all aircraft.'

So that September a meeting was held at Thames House in London to decide the fate of the Economizer. Despite the success of the laboratory and flight trials, the Air Ministry representative, a Squadron Leader Cooper, thought it premature to rush into production, since the design had not been finalized. This objection was swept aside by Whittingham, who wanted a thousand Economizers to be ordered immediately, stressing the importance placed by the Air Officers Commanding-in-Chief of Fighter and Bomber Commands on early improvements in oxygen equipment. Despite some heated discussion, the meeting agreed to order the thousand Economizers that Whittingham had asked for; to go with these Economizers, which were to be made in the Farnborough area as soon as possible, Messrs Roberts were to supply fifteen hundred Type E masks, at the rate of five hundred a week. As the minutes of the meeting, otherwise laconic and impersonal, observe, 'Squadron Leader Cooper finally agreed with this decision under pressure', a brave man to attempt to withstand such a forceful man as Whittingham, who was also four ranks senior to him.

It was decided that the thousand Economizers should be fitted mainly to Spitfires, and possibly also to long-range bombers; all new Spitfire aircraft were to be fitted with Economizer sets during manufacture. In addition, another version of the Economizer (the Mark II) was expected to be available in another six months. This was essentially a Mark I in which many of the aluminium parts were made of moulded material to facilitate mass production. It was decided that the Mark II Economizer be approved without service trials because it was a production version of the Mark I and that it should be fitted mainly to bomber aircraft.[11]

Despite some frustrating delays, by the end of January 1941 four hundred Economizers were in use; production was described as slow.

By the end of March 1941 nine hundred sets had been made and were in service and a further order had been placed with the RAE for a thousand more. There were some inevitable 'teething' problems, however. For example, in December 1940 the Economizers at Heston had to be grounded because of a failure. The cause appeared to be the very low temperatures being met at altitude (down to minus 50°C). The Economizer had already been tested down to minus 25°C by the Lab and to minus 40°C by the Instrument Department without malfunction. However, on retesting to minus 60°C by the Physiological Laboratory, the bag became very stiff and would not collapse. Dr Goldie, who was by now seconded to the Lab from Cambridge, managed to find a doped material which remained supple at minus 50°C. Freezing of the expiratory valve of the mask was prevented by a modification to the mask; the Lab made the point rather plaintively that, 'as in the case of other equipment, inadequate cabin heating has caused unnecessary difficulty in the design of oxygen equipment'.[12]

However, the failure at Heston may have been nothing to do with the Economizer, for the Lab found eleven times the permitted amount of water in the oxygen used by Heston. Elimination of this impurity and the modification of the equipment quickly cured the PRU's problems, and their Economizers then functioned satisfactorily even at very low temperatures.

The Lab was quick to point out that it needed a cold chamber that could be decompressed, so that oxygen systems could be properly evaluated. Eventually this was provided, but in the meantime Flight Lieutenant Stewart compromised by building a box of sheet steel into which he could just fit; the box had hollow walls into which Stewart put carbon dioxide snow. The device produced very low albeit uncontrollable, temperatures. To withstand the tests, Stewart used electrically heated gloves and boots, but even so one test had to be terminated because of incipient frostbite in one toe.

The Mark II version of the Economizer was supposed to enter service about March 1941. In the event, frequent changes to the specification caused delays, and flight tests were still being carried out later that year. Just who was responsible for the delays is not clear, although the blame was laid squarely at the Lab's door. The seriousness with which the Ministry of Aircraft Production viewed the situation is indicated by a threat to place an official complaint of RAE procrastination with the Secretary of State for Air. It seems that the Ministry thought that the RAE, and therefore the

Physiological Laboratory too, were trying to achieve 'a state of perfection which is probably not essential, and certainly not obtainable at the outset'.[13] Mark II Economizers were made by various companies in the UK including Hoover, for whom their motto, "It beats, as it sweeps, as it cleans," took on a new meaning!

It was to be April 1942 before all aircraft in Britain on the production line were being fitted with Mark II Economizers. By early 1943 the Economizer was well established in service and proving to be very reliable. In the United States, however, there had been very considerable advances in the design of demand oxygen regulators. These are regulators which allow oxygen to pass only in response to the suction of inspiration. The Physiological Laboratory favoured the principle of the demand regulator to the Economizer, provided the former could be made reliable. However, on the principle that the devil you know is better than the devil you don't, the Lab advised, '... the difference is not sufficiently great to recommend an immediate change-over in the face of the difficulties of this and the lack of any experience with demand valves.'[14] Thus the Economizer was to be regarded as a short-term rather than a long-term solution to the problem of oxygen economy, the demand regulator being planned to go into more and more new aircraft.

Although Matthews subsequently applied for financial recognition of the success of the Economizer on behalf of Hodgkin, Worthington, Parkinson, Macdonald and himself, under the scheme whereby inventors of equipment particularly useful to the war effort could be so recompensed, they received nothing.[15] Perhaps Matthews had upset too many people; perhaps it was recognition of the fact that all they had done was to refine an idea that was already there; or perhaps the Economizer was just thought to be of little significance – after all, it was intended to be only a temporary solution to an urgent problem, although that 'temporary solution' is still being used in Shackleton and Jet Provost Mark 3 aircraft. On the other hand, the Economizer enabled airmen to fly higher and further in greater safety.

After the war, the Americans were able to take advantage of the German experience of demand regulators. The American D-1 regulator was a modified version of a German regulator, and it was this version that the RAF bought for use in the Sabre and other aircraft. Air Commodore Howard recalls taking part in one assessment of the acceptability of the resistance to breathing of the new regulator: 'The RAE flew a Valetta, equipped with four D-1 regulators for passengers, to Malta and back. After one hour, it was agreed that we should have a five-minute break from the high breathing resistance; this was later modified to ten minutes of rest in every thirty minutes! On the journey home, we hardly used the regulators at all, but conscientiously kept the masks (with dangling unconnected hoses) on our faces.' Further development of the D-1 and alternative regulators followed, the first series of regulators being panel-mounted in the cockpit; then followed miniature, man-mounted regulators which obviated the need for a separate emergency regulator after ejection from the aircraft. The most recent regulators have been seat-mounted, combining some of the advantages of the man-mounted with some of the advantages of the panel-mounted regulators.

The great contribution British aviation medicine has made to aircraft oxygen systems since the war has been the definition of acceptable characteristics for breathing-equipment. This has involved not only putting steady flows of gas through the system to measure the resistance, as the Americans do, but also changing flows. When a man breathes, he does not instantaneously pull a set flow of gas into his lungs and then out again; instead, the flow builds up to a peak before decaying to zero. The peak flows can be far greater than the flows integrated over a minute; for example, the peak inspiratory flows during speech can be nearly 200 litres a minute (L/min) during normal breathing at a rate of 20 L/min. This can result in an item of breathing apparatus having a subjectively high resistance to breathing even when the resistance to lower, steady flows has been assessed as tolerable. The proper definition of breathing characteristics of aircraft oxygen equipment is an area in which Britain leads the world, thanks to the careful work of Roxburgh and Ernsting of the IAM and Jack London and Geoff Allen of the RAE.

The poor reliability of the early panel-mounted regulators led to the RAF instructing aircrew not to fly with the regulator set to 'airmix'[16] – the setting that allowed oxygen to be added to the inspirate automatically in increasing proportions as the altitude rose until 33,000 feet was reached, at which altitude hundred per cent oxygen was supplied to breathe. From 1945 onwards, reports started coming in from RAF stations of chest pain and bouts of coughing after a sortie. It soon became apparent that the pain was associated with two particular things: first the breathing of hundred per cent oxygen, because when airmix was selected on the regulator, as some aircrew did in defiance of the regulations, symptoms were far less common; and second, high levels of g, because the aerobatic team of 111 Squadron, the Black Arrows, was particularly badly affected. Ernsting suggested possible causes for the symptoms,[17] but it was a newcomer to the Lab, Flight Lieutenant (now Group Captain) David Glaister, who demonstrated conclusively, in a series of elegant experiments, the precise physiological mechanism.[18] Briefly, the application of g, together with pressure from the g-suit, led to closing of airways at the base of the lung. When the lobules beyond the obstruction contained a hundred per cent oxygen, this was absorbed, leading to lobular collapse of the lung. The US Navy still fly using a hundred per cent oxygen from ground-level upwards, and significant numbers of aircrew report symptoms of 'acceleration atelectasis'. In the RAF, by the time that the problem had been solved, oxygen regulators were far more reliable, so that the airmix setting could be safely used.

The first Royal Flying Corps oxygen mask was the Type A, followed in the 1920s and 1930s by the Types B and C. At the start of the Second World War, the standard oxygen mask was the Type D, which was made of fabric and chamois leather. It was attached to the helmet by press-studs which were positioned and fitted after the issue of the mask; no further adjustment to mask fit was then possible. The oxygen supply entered through a tube in the side of the mask. Inspiration of ambient air (to top up the volume of oxygen with the gas required for inspiration) and expiration both took place round the side of the loose-fitting mask and through two nostril holes at the front of the mask. There was a very heavy microphone. Overall, the mask was exceedingly cumbersome and uncomfortable.

When the research team at the RAF Physiological Laboratory developed the oxygen Economizer, they realized that the Type D mask would be unsuitable. Because of its poor fit, inspiration did not always give the reduction in pressure necessary to make the Economizer bag deliver its contents. A new, better-fitting mask was therefore essential. This was duly designed, constructed and named the Type E mask. The early masks were made in the Lab and in other RAE departments, but it soon became apparent that more help was needed. In March 1940, therefore, Matthews approached Alfred Roberts & Sons Ltd, india-rubber manufacturers, and they started to make facepieces for the new mask.

By mid July 1940 the development of the E mask and the oxygen Economizer were looking very promising, and Messrs Roberts were instructed to make fifteen hundred masks to go with the thousand Economizers being made by the RAE. Deliveries of the E mask came promptly, the order for fifteen hundred being completed in January 1941 despite frequent modifications. With new equipment available, the Lab was able to conduct more trials in different aircraft. The E mask was generally liked, but there was too high a resistance to breathing at low altitudes. Also, the suspension system was far from ideal, and the mask was very prone to condensation, which tended to dribble into the oxygen inlet and freeze. Despite these limitations, the E mask was put into mass production and used, not only with the Economizer but also in a modified form with the old continuous-flow system, for the rest of the war.

Since it was evident that the Type E mask was by no means perfect, late in 1940 John Gilson started development of a replacement mask, to be called the Type F mask. This new mask incorporated many changes in an attempt to improve the suspension system and the overall comfort. Modifications were also made to ease the drainage of condensation from the mask – a channel being provided, which was, appropriately, called the 'gob duct'.

The Lab had high hopes for the mask, but these were not to be realized because of a flare-up of the bad feeling that existed between the Lab and the MAP. The Ministry decided, unilaterally, that all work on the F mask should cease and that the E mask would be the definitive mask for the RAF.[19] However, eventually there was compromise and the E mask was modified to incorporate some of the improvements intended for the F. The modified E mask became known as the E* mask.[20]

In trials with the modified E mask, pilots commented adversely, yet again, both on the resistance to breathing in at low altitudes and on excessive condensation occurring inside the mask. To overcome these problems, Gilson had designed yet another new mask, the Type G. The most radical difference between the G mask and its predecessors was the introduction of the oxygen at the top of the mask rather than at the bottom, in order that moisture from the breath would not flow into the oxygen inlet, freeze there and block it. The G mask also had features which enabled the area in contact with the face to remain dry – an advantage, in that comfort when the mask was worn for several hours was greatly improved. In a further attempt to add to the comfort, the mask was lined; many linings had been tried, ranging from velvet (which frayed) to chamois (which became too hard after repeated wetting and drying) to suede (which was finally adopted). In addition, the mask had an improved suspension system that permitted adjustment, gave a snug fit, was stable under g forces and could still be removed rapidly for vomiting – a feature demonstrated on several occasions in the Lab's decompression chamber!

The G mask was first sufficiently advanced in design to be allocated a separate letter of the alphabet in April 1941. Production started in 1942, with the priority for issue going to Bomber Command, following the RAF's shift in emphasis from defensive to offensive operations. By the end of January 1943 two thousand a week were being made by six companies; in April 1943 thirteen thousand Type G masks were made. Ultimately, production was limited by the supplies of natural rubber.[21]

The masks were very well received by the aircrew. Unfortunately, as more and more masks came to be used, a problem came to light that is still with us today – mask dermatitis. In this condition, prolonged wearing of the mask gave rise to a painful and irritating rash in the area of the contact of the mask with the face. Some rubber mixes were more prone to cause the problem than others, so initially some relief could be obtained by waiting until the skin eruption had died down and then changing to a mask made by another manufacturer. Finally the Avon India Rubber Company Ltd produced a special anti-dermatitic mask for those who suffered from the condition.

A big problem with all the oxygen masks up to the Type G was that they had to accommodate a large and heavy microphone. However, by 1943 a new microphone, much smaller and lighter, had been developed, and so there was a requirement for yet another new mask. The Type H was based upon the Type G but, in addition to the modification for the microphone, also incorporated several improvements based on experience with the G mask. By the end of 1944 about six hundred H masks were being produced a week, with the limiting factor again being shortage of rubber.

Gilson, with the rubber manufacturers, investigated many mixes of ingredients in an attempt to reduce the content of crude, natural rubber. By 1944 all the hoses were being made in an approved rubber substitute and the proportion of crude rubber in the masks had been reduced to between thirty-five and forty per cent, compared to the ninety per cent of American masks; by the end of the war, the proportion in British masks had been further reduced to twenty-seven per cent. The net result was a comfortable, well-fitting mask that remained on the face even under conditions of high g. The Type H mask is still in service with the RAF – again in the Shackleton and Jet Provost Mark 3 aircraft; indeed, it has a better performance in the cold than the present RAF P/Q masks!

As the war drew to an end, the MAP and the British Overseas Airways Corporation (BOAC) were already making plans for post-war civil aviation. It was clear that civil aircraft would benefit from the great advances made in the design of military aircraft during the war – for example aircraft could now fly higher (and therefore more economically), further and with a greater payload. Until the development of pressure-cabin aircraft, however, the economical cruising altitude of the proposed airliners dictated that passengers would have to wear oxygen equipment.

In February 1945 it was decided that gaseous oxygen supplies would be used combined with a simple, continuous-flow system, delivering oxygen to a light, comfortable and cheap mask to be worn by the passengers. Unfortunately, neither the G nor the H mask developed by Gilson was suitable. Both had large-bore supply tubing with a big connector and needed a helmet for attachment. The BOAC had already asked Siebe Gorman to produce a lightweight mask, and the MAP proposed that the RAF Physiological Laboratory should also pursue a design for a throw-away mask, provided that it cost less than 5 shillings.[22] Matters proceeded slowly, however, and the RAF, faced with the prospect of trying to transport troops home from the Far East for demobilization, arranged for three thousand masks to be borrowed from the Americans for use by Transport Command. However, while willing to support the RAF's request for help, the US authorities refused to release any masks for civilian use by BOAC and so the stage was set for a purely British mask.

By September 1945 it appeared that the Siebe mask, in three sizes and costing between 6 and 7 shillings each, could well be available for the RAF by the spring of 1946, with the title, 'Oxygen Mask Type K'. The IAM had approved the design in principle, although a sample had not yet been tested. One thousand of the Siebe masks had been promised to BOAC by Christmas 1945, and the MAP optimistically expected that the K mask would be in service before the IAM-designed version.

At the IAM, work on the mask was being done by Squadron Leader Basil Kent and Pilot Officer J.D.B. Wilson, with assistance from John Gilson. Many designs were tried, but Kent eventually settled on a moulded polythene mask with a latex rebreather bag, the ensemble being entitled the 'Oxygen Mask Type L'. The mask, complete with tubing, weighed 2 ounces compared to the 10.5 ounces of the borrowed American mask and the 24 ounces of a comparable Canadian mask. Comparative trials of the IAM and Siebe Gorman masks were carried out during the spring of 1946 in long-distance flights by Transport Command. Generally the results of the trials were difficult to interpret. Passengers tended to favour the Type K mask because it was more comfortable, despite being 1.5 ounces heavier than the Type L. However, Transport Command and the Air Ministry preferred the Type L because 'the plastic facepiece type of mask would be considerably easier to clean and reassemble'. The IAM was quick to point out that the Type L was not meant to be cleaned and re-used but to be thrown away after use; the Institute then drew attention to the advantages of the L mask over the K mask. It cost less than the K and was easier to assemble; the reservoir bag was angled forward so that the pipe connecting it to the mask did not become blocked as could happen with the K mask if the passenger's head rotated forward on falling asleep; unlike the K mask, the L had no metal parts directly in contact with rubber so that it would not deteriorate so rapidly in the Tropics; and finally the L mask packed into a smaller space than the K mask. However, there was one feature of the L mask that was distressing to RAF officers – the reservoir bag was a flesh pink, a 'lingerie colour', which was hurriedly changed to a more manly and military blue! Other factors influencing the decision to adopt the L mask were that it gave better levels of oxygenation at altitude than the K mask and that Siebe Gorman was still making improvements to its mask when the design for the L mask was finalized.[23]

The L mask entered service late in 1946 as a passenger mask at a cost of 2/6d each. Even this small cost was resented, especially as the mask was a throw-away item. In 1948, in an attempt to conserve stocks of polythene, the financial branches of the MAP tried to introduce a scheme to salvage, disinfect and re-use the masks. Not surprisingly, this suggestion was resisted by doctors and operators alike, and eventually the idea was dropped.

Although BOAC had originally sponsored the K mask, they eventually came to adopt its rival, particularly as the advent of pressure-cabin aircraft relegated the use of the passenger oxygen mask to that of an emergency device. If you fly anywhere in the world today and the aircraft suffers a loss of cabin pressure, emergency oxygen masks similar to the L mask will automatically deploy in front of you.

The introduction of jet aircraft in 1945 meant that the RAF had even more opportunity to fly at altitudes greater than 40,000 feet – the altitude limit for non-pressure breathing oxygen-supply systems. Even though most aircraft capable of reaching such high altitudes had pressure cabins, and it was therefore unlikely that the cabin altitude would exceed 40,000 feet, cabin depressurization could occur – accidentally, as a result of enemy action or deliberately when preparing to abandon the aircraft at high altitude. For this reason the RAF decided that pressure breathing was required as a 'get you down' system or, better, as a 'stay up' system after an emergency. However, breathing oxygen under pressure was not possible with the H mask because this was unable to hold pressure; it was designed to offer low resistance to breathing, so an increase of pressure in the mask merely opened the expiratory valve. The easiest way to overcome this was to increase the resistance of the expiratory valve when pressure needed to be supplied to the mask. This Gilson achieved by installing a valve in which the resistance could be adjusted by rotating a knob on the valve housing. The resultant mask, differing from the H mask only in its expiratory valve and control, was called the 'Oxygen Mask Type J'; another derivation of the H mask was the 'Oxygen Mask Type R'. In service the J mask had two major disadvantages – first, the mask would not seal effectively against an increase in pressure, and second, it was very uncomfortable when tensioned against the face when trying to make it seal. These disadvantages were sufficient for Fighter Command to declare the mask operationally unacceptable.[24] Clearly a replacement was needed.

It was at this time, early 1950, that the RAF was buying from the Americans their D-1 demand regulator. The mask that went with the regulator was the A13A, and so the RAF decided to buy that too. A contract was placed for 8,500 masks with Mine Safety Appliances Inc. in America, at a price of $24.85 each. Unfortunately the A13A mask was not liked either. It was heavy and bulky, interfered with downward vision and caused extreme discomfort when the harness was tightened enough to seal against increased pressure. Also, there was a large amount of rubber in contact with the skin of the face, which caused unpleasant irritation. There is no evidence that a formal service trial of the mask was ever carried out before it entered service in RAF aircraft; if such a trial had been carried out, it is likely that the adverse comments would have stimulated development of a replacement even sooner. The A13A mask had a short, unpopular period of service in the RAF, but it did bridge the gap until a better pressure-breathing mask, the Types M and N, could be developed at the IAM by Squadron Leader A.B. Goorney. The M mask was designed to replace the J mask for use with the pressure-breathing waistcoat (see below) worn with a continuous-flow oxygen system, and the N mask was to replace the A13A mask used with a demand regulator.

Unlike the masks made during the war, which were made from a high proportion of reclaimed rubber that tended to cause dermatitis, the new masks were made from natural rubber and so did not need to be lined to protect the face. They also had a reflected edge seal, the idea being that the inner aspect of the seal would be forced hard against the face under positive pressure. That this was an effective way of maintaining positive pressure was confirmed in flight trials by the South African Air Force flying combat in Korea, where the pilots found the N mask better than the A13A.[25] This design feature was therefore retained in later masks.

Unfortunately, despite all Goorney's work, neither the M nor the N mask was to see much service. The successful development of demand regulators made the pressure-breathing waistcoat and, therefore, the M mask obsolete – although it was used with the Canberra B2. And there were so many delays and modifications during production of the N mask that it had changed beyond recognition from the original design. So a new identification letter was needed.

Two of the main difficulties with the M and N types had been attaching the masks to the helmets and adjusting the tension in flight. These problems were tackled by Dr J.E. Gabb, a civilian medical officer attached to the IAM from the Civil Aviation Authority. Gabb produced a harness which consisted of two metal bows, the outer adjustable one being attached to the sides of the helmet and the inner one being attached to a plate or exoskeleton overlying the front of the mask. The two bows were hinged together at the front of the mask by a toggle which could be rotated to increase the pressure of the mask on the face. Thus the mask could be held in three positions: standby, with the mask hanging below the chin; normal pressure, with the mask on the face; and high pressure, with the toggle down and the mask pressed tight on the face. Unfortunately Gabb was most reluctant to commit any account of his very considerable successes and achievements to paper; staff at the

Institute still remember Air Commodore Stewart finally losing his patience, recalling Gabb from leave and incarcerating him in the IAM library until the report on the toggle harness was completed!

The new harness was introduced, with new moulded masks, soon to be called P/Q masks, in the late 1950s. Gabb's harness allowed easy donning and doffing of the mask, easy adjustment of tension during flight, even distribution of pressure on the face, and a rapid tensioning system for pressure breathing after rapid decompression; it was the one advance which, more than anything else, contributed to the ultimate acceptability of the new P and Q masks.

The facepiece of the P mask did not provide a sufficiently good seal for pressure breathing on all faces, particularly smaller ones. Accordingly a new, smaller size was introduced. Because a different manufacturer was given the contract from the one who made the P mask (a policy of the Ministry of Supply to encourage competition to prevent the Ministry from becoming too dependent on one particular company), the new mask was called the Q mask. The P and Q facepieces have provided the basis for all recently introduced RAF oxygen masks, different marks of mask being accorded different suffixes depending on the accessories supplied with the mask, and derivations of the basic design being called S, T and V.

As with earlier types, all the design work for the P and Q masks had been carried out at the IAM and not by industry as required by Ministry policy. Part of the reason for this has been that many of the experts in the rubber industry during the war have retired, and part has been that the equipment is being designed to satisfy physiological criteria that are not fully understood by industry. But probably more important is the fact that the development of oxygen masks requires complex test facilities which, as Roxburgh put it, 'would involve a firm in enormous expense for a product which would only bring a small turnover and little profit'.[26] It is perhaps fortunate that relatively little mask development has been carried out since the introduction of P/Q masks – apart, that is, from the Type W.

Some years ago it became apparent that the methods of making the P and Q masks were very labour-intensive and that this added considerably to the unit costs. The Ministry of Defence Procurement Executive (MOD (PE)), the descendant of the MAP, the Ministry of Supply and the Ministry of Technology) approached an engineering design agency with a request for a study to redesign the oxygen mask. While simplicity and ease of manufacture were obviously highly desirable criteria, for they would result in a cheaper mask, the opportunity was taken to change other features in the mask to take advantage of advances in technology. The result was the Type W mask. Although still in development, the mask is narrower than the Type P or Q masks, thus allowing better head mobility in the cockpit, and it is lighter. It is to be hoped that, when it does enter service, it will last as long as the P/Q series, which is still an excellent family of oxygen masks.

Until 1939 the official view in the RAF was that 'bends' could not occur in aviation because the pressure changes were smaller than those met in diving. Flack had disagreed with Haldane's opinion, expressed in 1920, that bends could occur in flight, and unfortunately Struan Marshall had fostered the myth,[27] unaware of the fact that bends were being both predicted and described at altitude by several workers during the 1930s on the Continent. Thus it came as somewhat of a surprise to Matthews that he, Macdonald and Hodgkin experienced joint pains during their early experiments in the vertical decompression chamber; the pains were similar to the joint pains suffered by divers which had been called 'the bends'. And, as we have already seen, symptoms other than the bends afflicted the Farnborough team, the most alarming of which were the cerebral symptoms, such as partial paralysis of a limb, and the visual disturbances, such as partial or complete blindness. The symptoms usually disappeared on descent, but some, especially the visual ones, persisted for some time after return to ground-level. Because symptoms other than the classical 'bends' were involved, Matthews coined the term 'decompression sickness'.[28]

Since all the early decompression chamber work done at the Physiological Laboratory was aimed at evaluating oxygen systems at medium and high altitude, the team had ample opportunity to study their attacks of decompression sickness. Obviously, if the RAF was going to fly as high as this, aircrew would also be susceptible to the condition. It was therefore a matter of some importance that the condition should be properly studied in terms of its incidence, the predisposing factors and any methods of suppressing the symptoms or protecting the pilot from the condition altogether.

Initial experiments were carried out using the Lab staff themselves as subjects. They confirmed that the condition did not occur below 25,000 feet and that the longer the man stayed above this altitude, the more likely he was to experience the symptoms of decompression sickness. They also noted an individual variation, Macdonald being worst affected, Matthews often suffering from disturbing visual symptoms and Hodgkin being least affected.

The team proposed, and Whittingham concurred, that larger-scale tests on aircrew were required. Accordingly, experiments were carried out on pilots from Fighter and Bomber Commands, as well as on volunteers from the RAE – a helpful and reliable source of victims during these early months of the war. The experiments showed that lightly built, fit young men were less likely to suffer from decompression sickness than older, fatter men.

The Physiological Laboratory concluded that the RAF had experienced relatively few problems with decompression sickness so far largely because of the rarity of flights above 30,000 feet and also possibly because the few cases that there might have been had been misdiagnosed as hypoxia. Once the RAF began to fly higher than 30,000 feet routinely, they could expect a considerable increase in the incidence of decompression sickness. It was pointed out that the only sure way of preventing the onset of decompression sickness would be to have pressurized aircraft. However, since the introduction of such aircraft was still a little way off, they suggested that the problem might be minimized by identifying and excluding from high-altitude duties those aircrew in whom a susceptibility to decompression sickness could be demonstrated in the decompression chamber.[29] A programme of testing for aircrew was therefore introduced (known as 'bends runs'), which also gave the Physiological Laboratory the opportunity to carry out more research into factors affecting susceptibility to decompression sickness. The aircrew most usually tested were pilots from the PRUs, but when the American B17 Flying Fortress aircraft, which flew much higher than other bomber aircraft, entered service in 1941, their aircrew were also tested. The exposures were to 35,000 feet for 4 hours and, in 1942, were associated with a failure rate of 45 per cent. Although the failure rate was so high, the tests fulfilled a useful purpose since only three of those who passed the test for the Fortress aircraft had subsequently to be removed from operational flying because of decompression sickness.[30]

The precise cause of decompression sickness was a mystery, however. Mysteries are always a challenge to scientists, and it is hardly surprising that, despite the demands of war, Matthews and his team should have carried out some rather more basic research. Experiments were conducted using anaesthetized goats, to test an American claim that the symptoms were caused by increased pressure in the brain. Matthews suspected that their results could be attributed to pressure transmitted from the inevitable expansion of the goats' trapped abdominal gases which occurred on decompression, so he induced the abdominal distension artificially by a small air-pump connected directly into the rectum of the unconscious animal. However, the first experiment did not go quite as planned. As Blunt later recalled, the goat literally exploded! Gilson was left to clean up the chamber which, according to Matthews, had to be smelt to be believed! One benefit of the experiments was that goat provided a welcome change to the wartime diet. After each subsequent run, and after the appropriate tissue samples had been obtained, the goat was taken to a local butcher for jointing; each of the Lab staff then had a goat joint for his Sunday lunch.

Other research on decompression sickness was undertaken by medical officers operating mobile decompression chambers in the field. For example, Flight Lieutenant Walder did experiments at Poona on the surface tension of the blood (important in decompression sickness because it affects the formation of gas bubbles). In later life, Professor Walder was to retain a special interest in decompression sickness, becoming, as a result of further research at the University of Newcastle, an internationally recognized authority on the subject.

Later work established the benefit of the American suggestion of pre-breathing oxygen to provide some protection against decompression sickness, and the technique became standard practice in some squadrons. In fact, with the introduction of pressure-cabin aircraft, decompression sickness became less of a problem for the RAF. Before pressurized aircraft, however, came pressure suits.

We have already seen some of the problems of using a full pressure suit, such as the one worn by Swain and Adam in 1936–7. When war broke out just over two years later, the state of the art had not advanced much. The full pressure suits were still hot and very clumsy.

In January 1941 responsibility for the development of pressure suits was transferred from the RAE to the RAF Physiological Laboratory. Because the old pressure suit was totally unsuitable for operational flying, the Lab restarted development on completely new lines, but they found that it was not as easy as it first seemed. When the Lab began making experimental suits, Matthews applied to Whittingham for skilled assistance. Whittingham obtained the services of a Savile Row tailor's cutter, who supplied expert help for the remainder of the war. By March 1942 they had tested one suit but found that it hampered movement unacceptably and was also difficult to put on. A second and then a third suit were therefore constructed. The suits were made for the Lab in the Fabrics Department of the RAE from the light, rubberized fabric used to make the standard Sidcot Suits. The helmet of the first suit was made of canvas with a celluloid window; in the second and third it was a dome of perspex. The third suit was in two parts: trousers with boots and a helmet with tunic which was attached to the lower half by a zip-fastener. Inside the perspex dome was a standard C-type helmet with an E mask. Laryngophones were used for communication. With the suit uninflated, there was no undue restriction of movement; inflated to working pressure, the wearer was able to carry out all manual operations save those involving fine finger movements.

Tests in the chamber showed the concept to be physiologically acceptable, although misting of the dome because of condensed expirate proved to be a problem at first. Further development was then passed to the firm of Baxter, Woodhouse and Taylor Ltd, and the Lab moved on to other things. Once again, these full pressure suits never entered service; that they did not can be ascribed to two main factors – the success of the partial pressure suit, and the introduction of pressure-cabin aircraft.

In 1941 German Ju86 aircraft on reconnaissance missions were crossing the United Kingdom at heights that our aircraft could not reach – between 43,000 and 46,000 feet. The reason they could do this was that the Ju86 had a pressurized cockpit. And the RAF still had neither a pressure suit nor a pressurized aircraft to counter the threat. Although Spitfires stripped down to the bare essentials (Operation Windgap) could just about reach an interception altitude, the pilot was at great risk from hypoxia. Could oxygen therefore be breathed under pressure without a pressure suit? In December 1941 Matthews discussed the problem with Gilson and Pask. They came to the conclusion that applying pressure to the air passages only would result in respiratory fatigue and could cause damage to the lungs; the only possible solution would be to apply pressure not only to respiratory tract but also to the outside of the chest and abdomen. But this might cause problems in the return of the blood to the heart, the extent of which could be determined only by experiment.

The problem was taken up by the Canadians, notably Professor H.C. Bazett, who had been involved in aviation medicine during the First World War. Over the next year he built a prototype

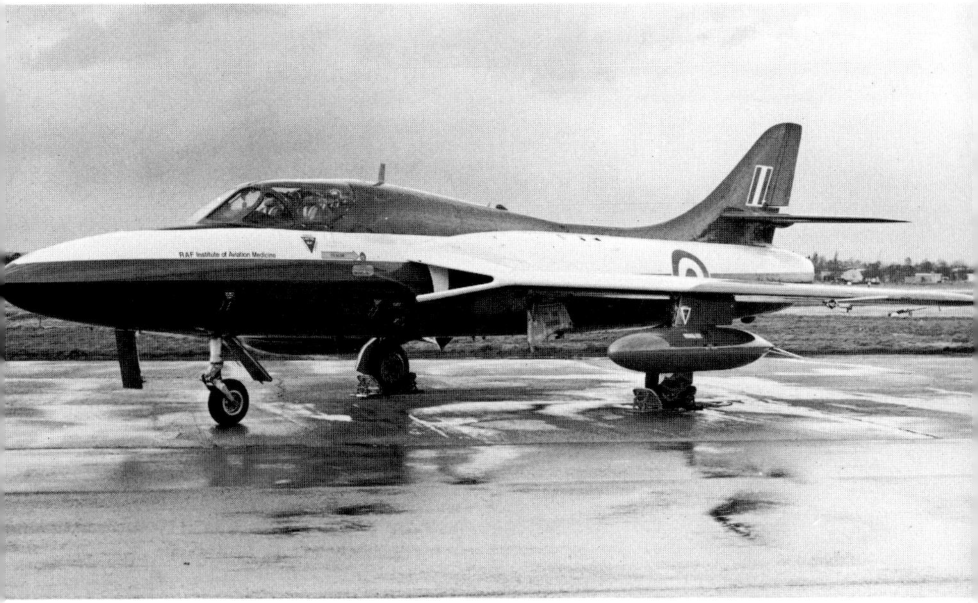

20 The IAM Hunter

21 Special testing of ESA astronaut candidates at the IAM. Left to right: Pilot Officer P. Sowood, Dr Franco Malerba preparing to run on a treadmill, Dr M.H. Harrison, Squadron Leader T.M. Gibson

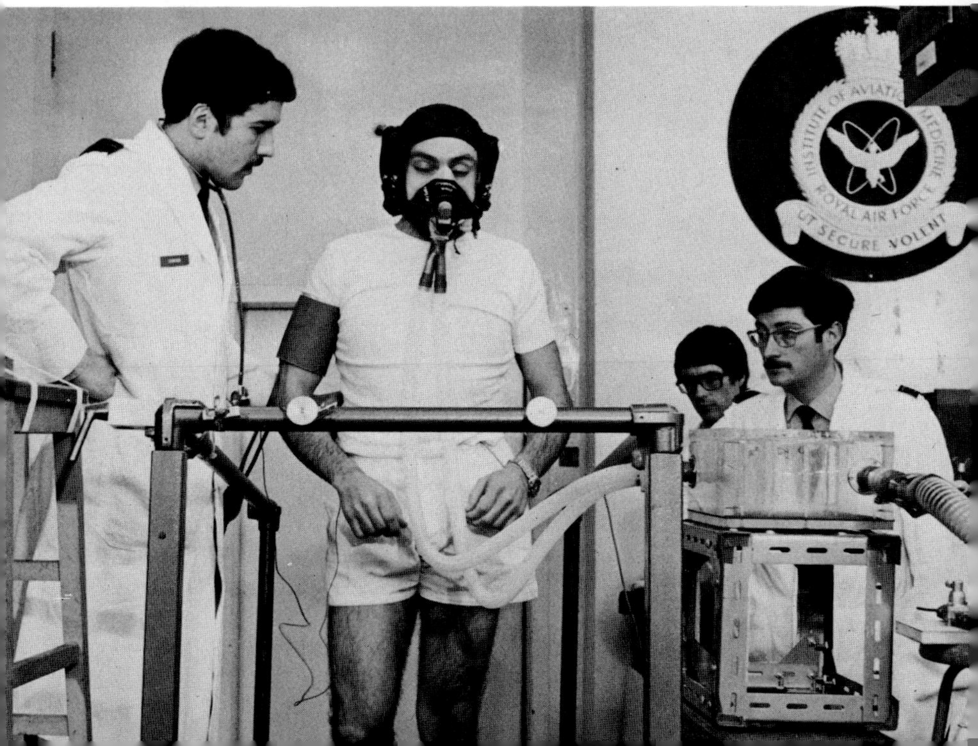

23 *Right:* Oxygen mask Type D with goggles Mark IIIa

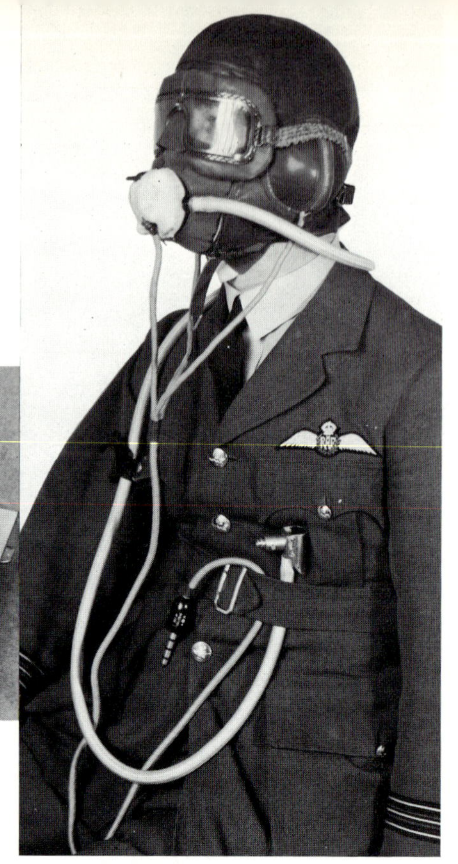

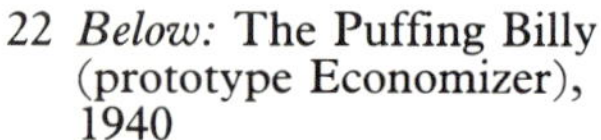

22 *Below:* The Puffing Billy (prototype Economizer), 1940

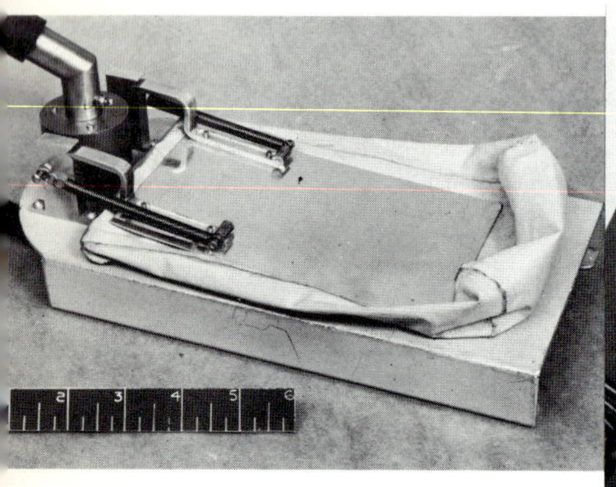

24 *Below:* Oxygen mask Type E with goggles Mark IV which had a flip-down tinted visor

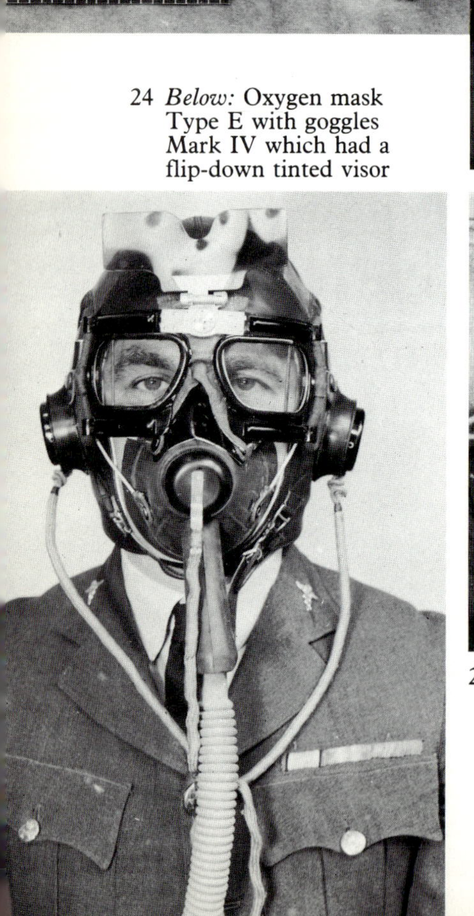

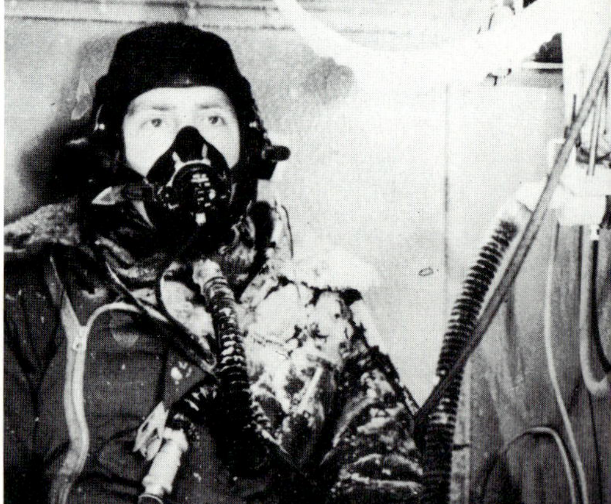

25 *Above:* Stewart in his home-made cold chamber, testing the oxygen mask Type F. Note the Economizer mounted on the right

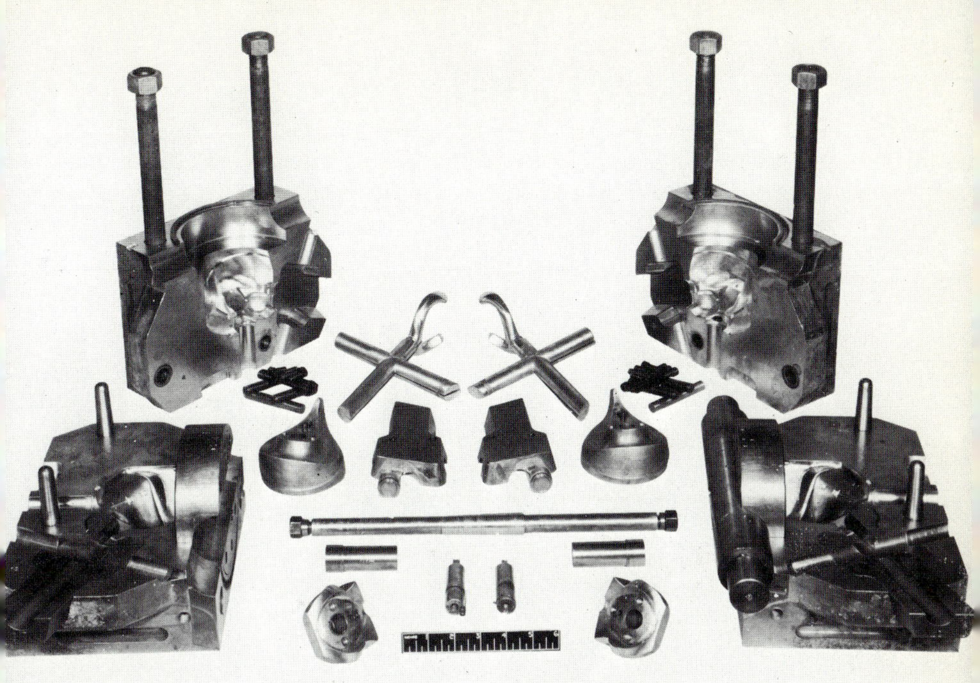

26 The moulds required to make one H mask. The pieces fit together, and liquid rubber is forced into the spaces that have been left

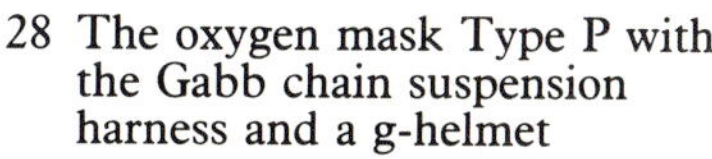

28 The oxygen mask Type P with the Gabb chain suspension harness and a g-helmet

27 The oxygen mask Type L

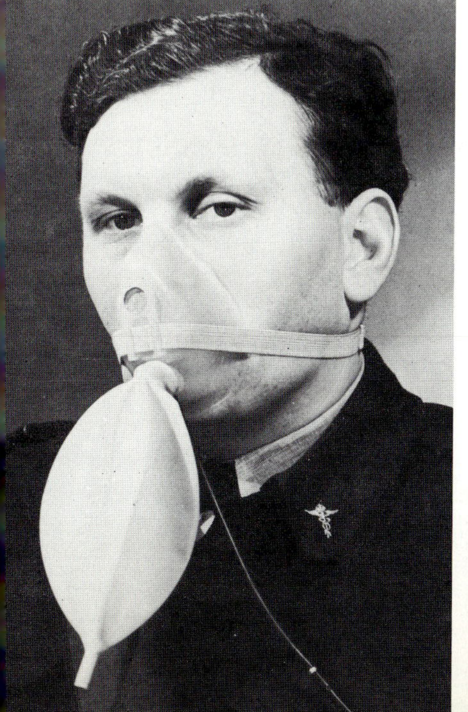

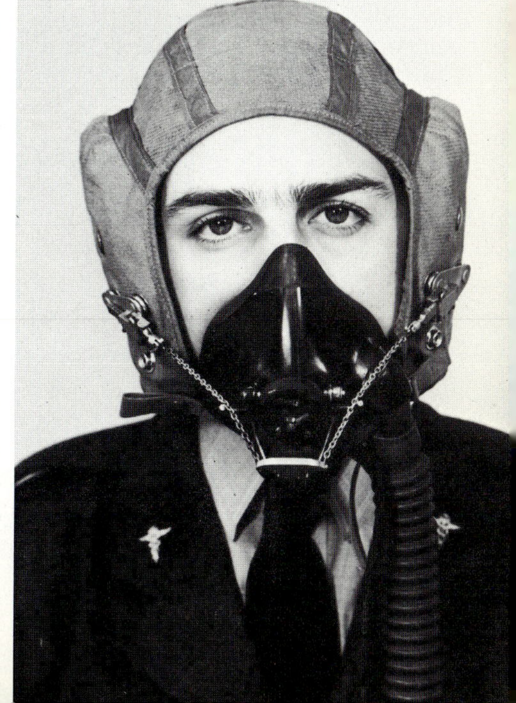

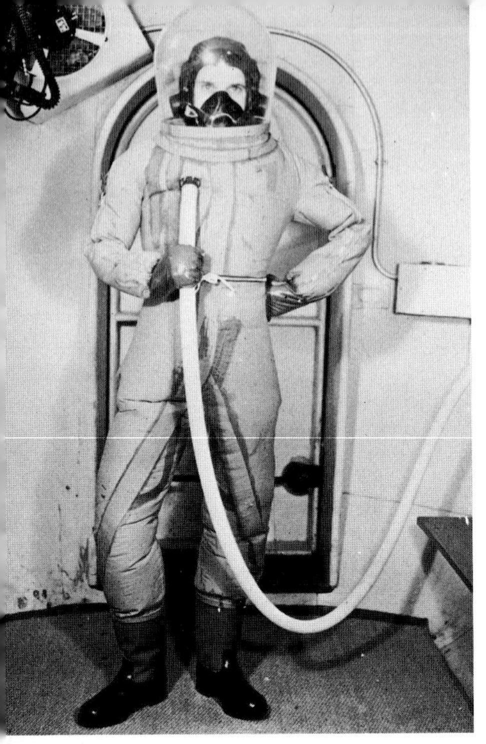

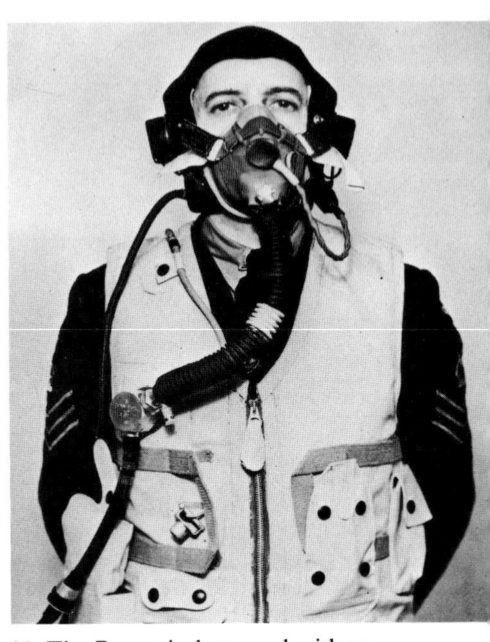

29 Squadron Leader Stewart in a prototype full pressure suit, 1942

30 The Bazett jacket, used with an oxygen mask Type J

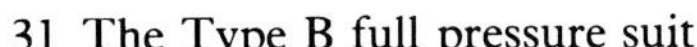

31 The Type B full pressure suit

32 The Type 51 full pressure suit

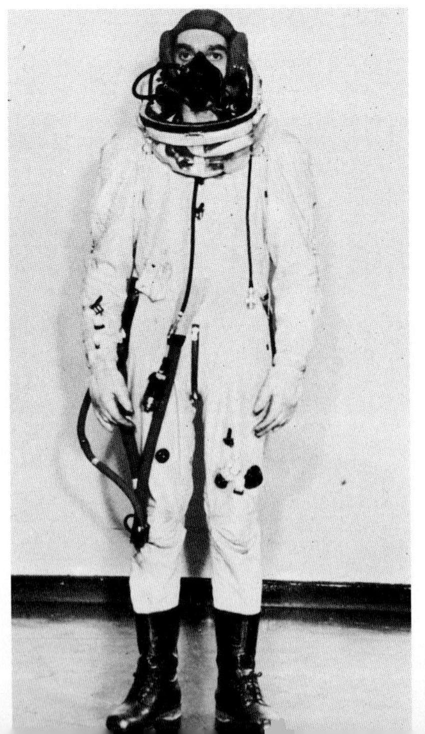

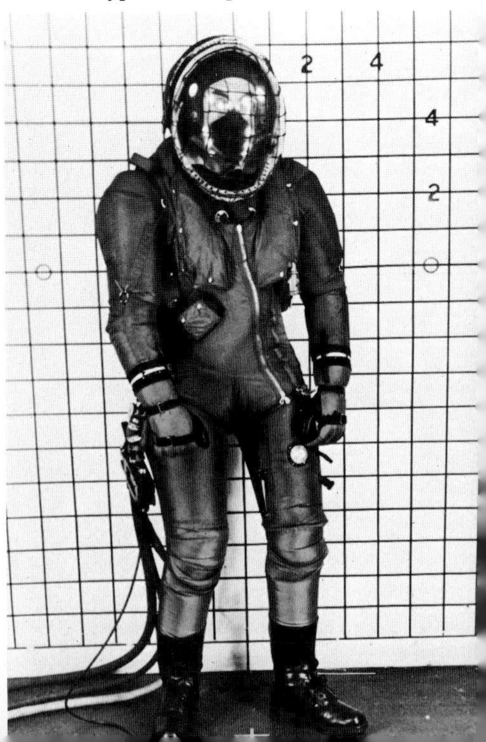

33 *Right:* The partial pressure jerkin with sleeves, Mark 4 anti-g suit, and Type C partial pressure helmet. The subject is pressure breathing at 110 millimetres of mercury

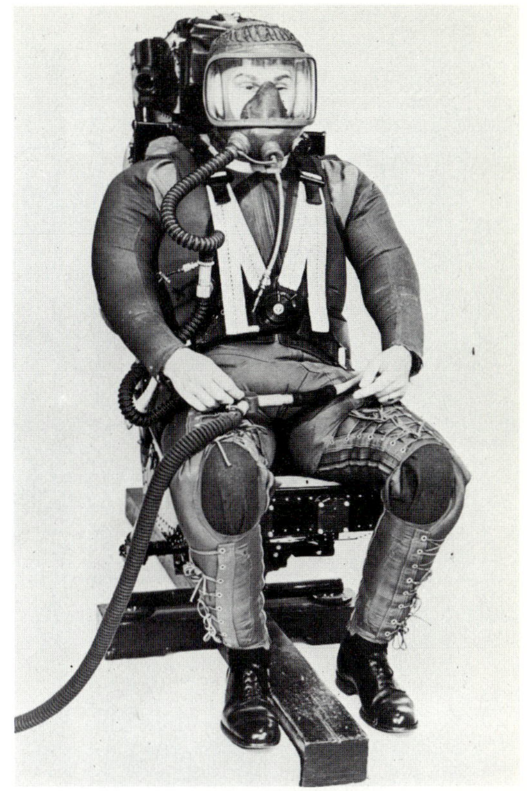

34 *Below right:* The Franks Flying Suit, worn by Squadron Leader W.R. Franks

35 *Below:* The Franks Flying Suit being filled

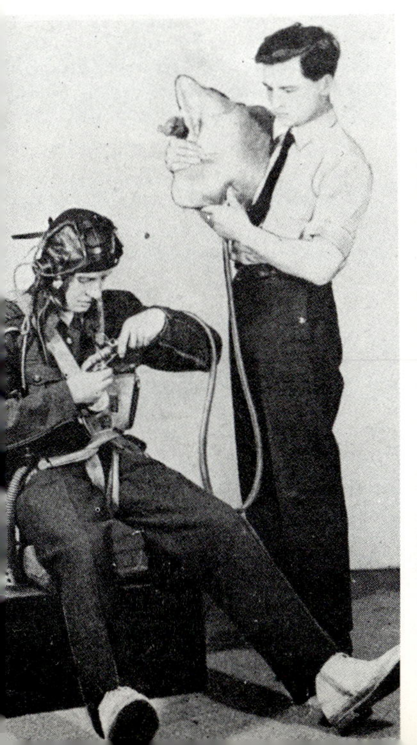

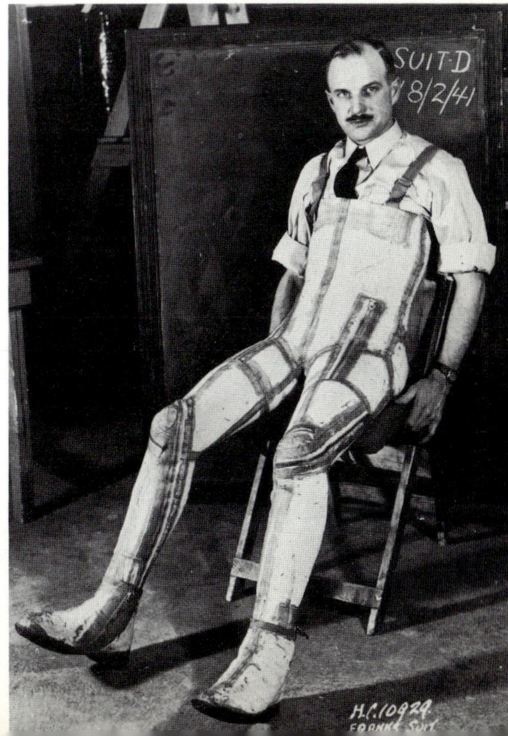

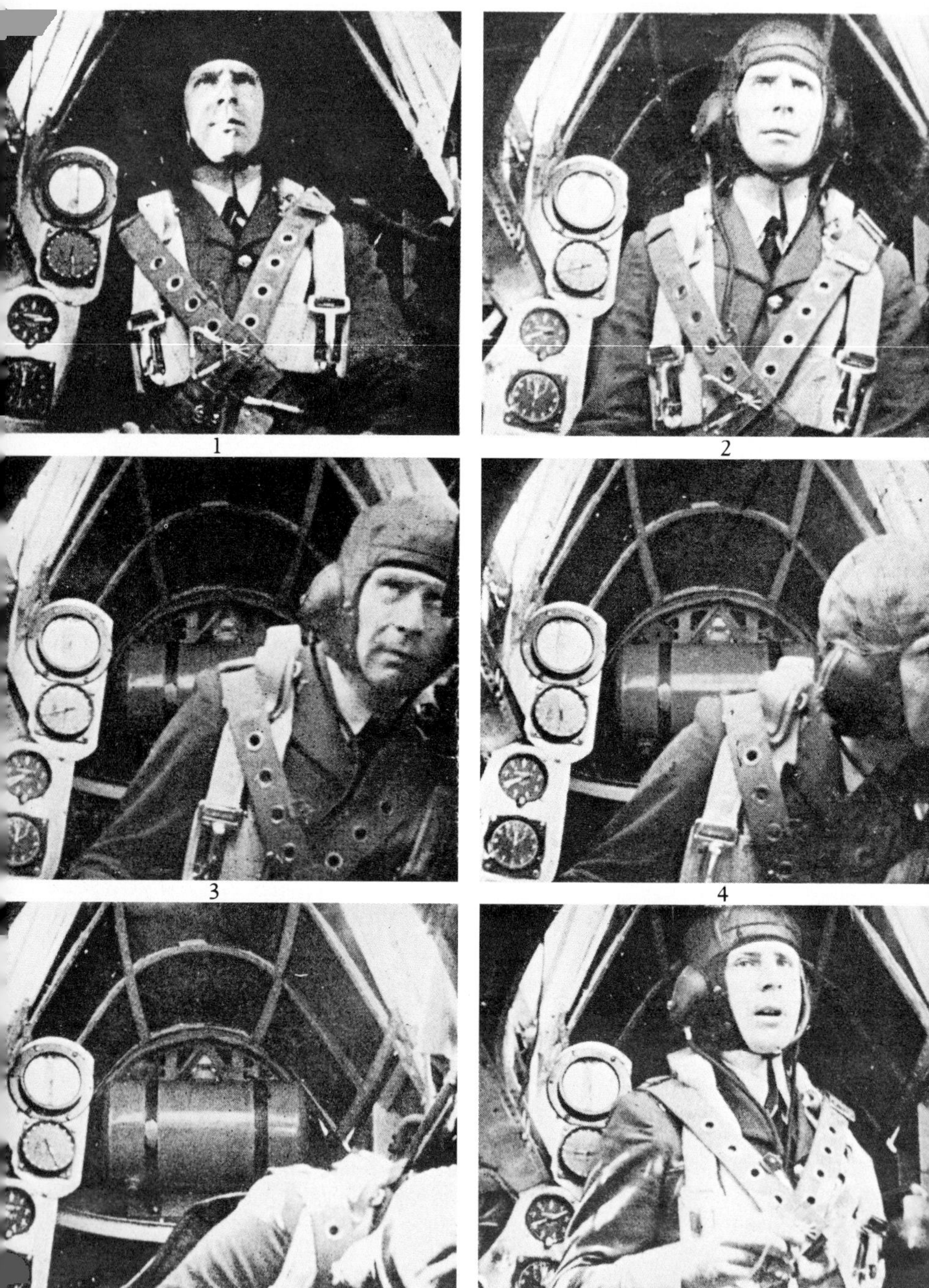

1 2

3 4

5 6

Left: Stages of unconsciousness under the influence of g. The subject is Stewart.
1 g = 2.0. Time = 2 secs
2 g = 6.2. Time = 8 secs
3 g = 6.0. Time = 10 secs. Definite loss of position with marked upward gaze
4 g = 6.0. Time = 11 secs. Marked rotation of head to left
5 g = 5.6. Time = 13.5 secs. Complete loss of posture and memory. Totally unconscious
6 g = 1.0. Time = 21 secs. Recovery

Below: Squadron Leader Konrad Bazarnik from the IAM waiting to be fired up the ejection-seat rig; Mr James Martin is checking his harness

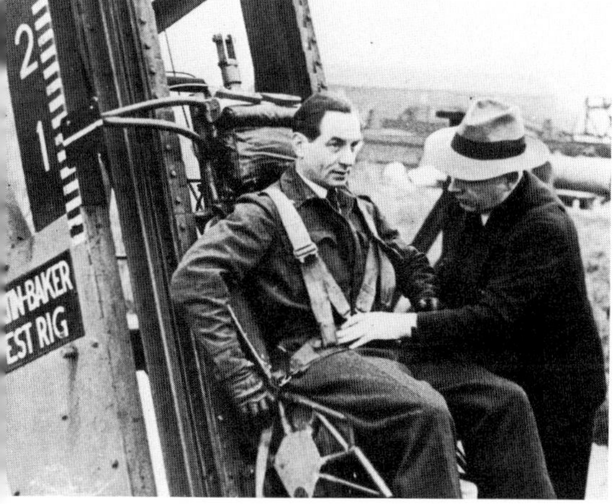

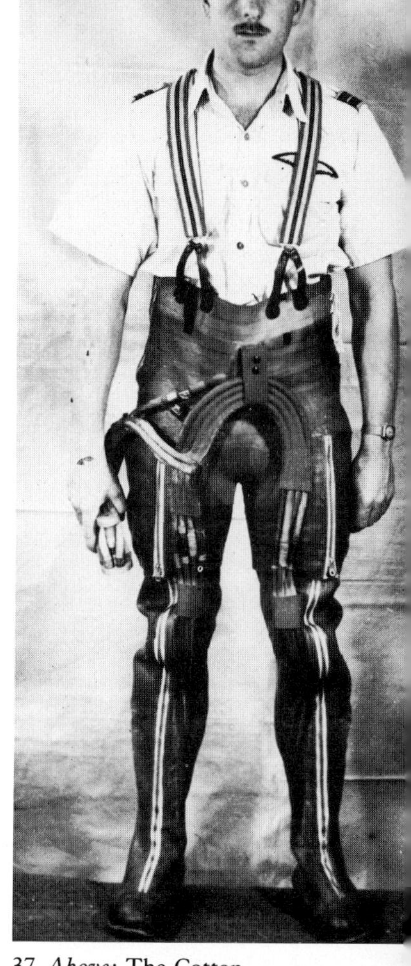

37 *Above:* The Cotton gradient pressure anti-g suit

Below: View of the double-cockpit arrangement of the prone-position Meteor

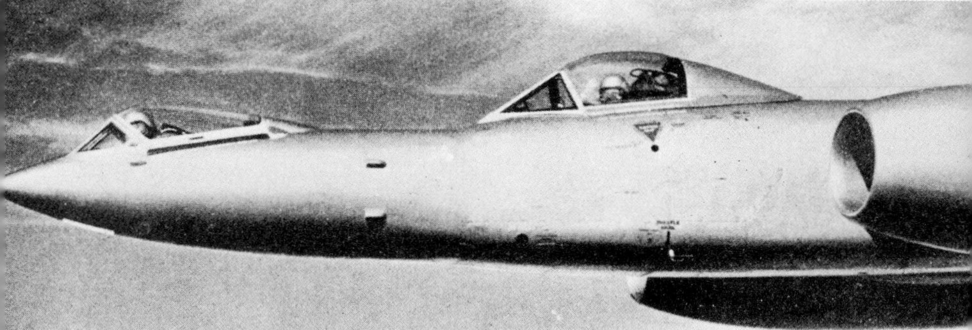

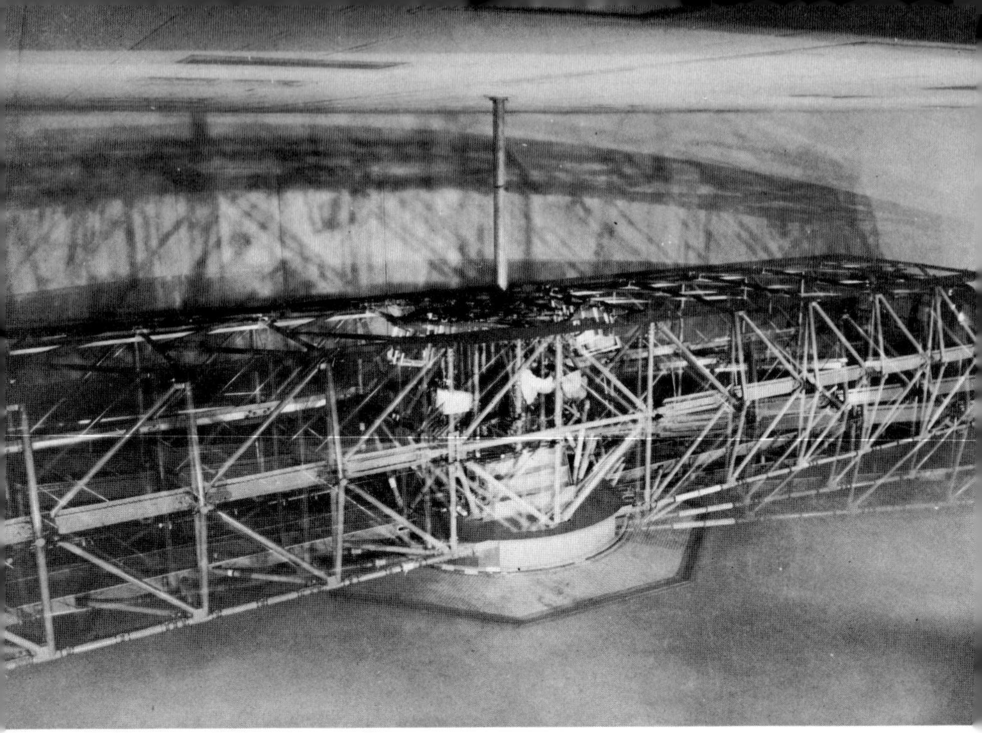

40 The IAM centrifuge

41 Squadron Leader Peter Howard being congratulated by Mr James Martin after the world's first human rocket-seat ejection

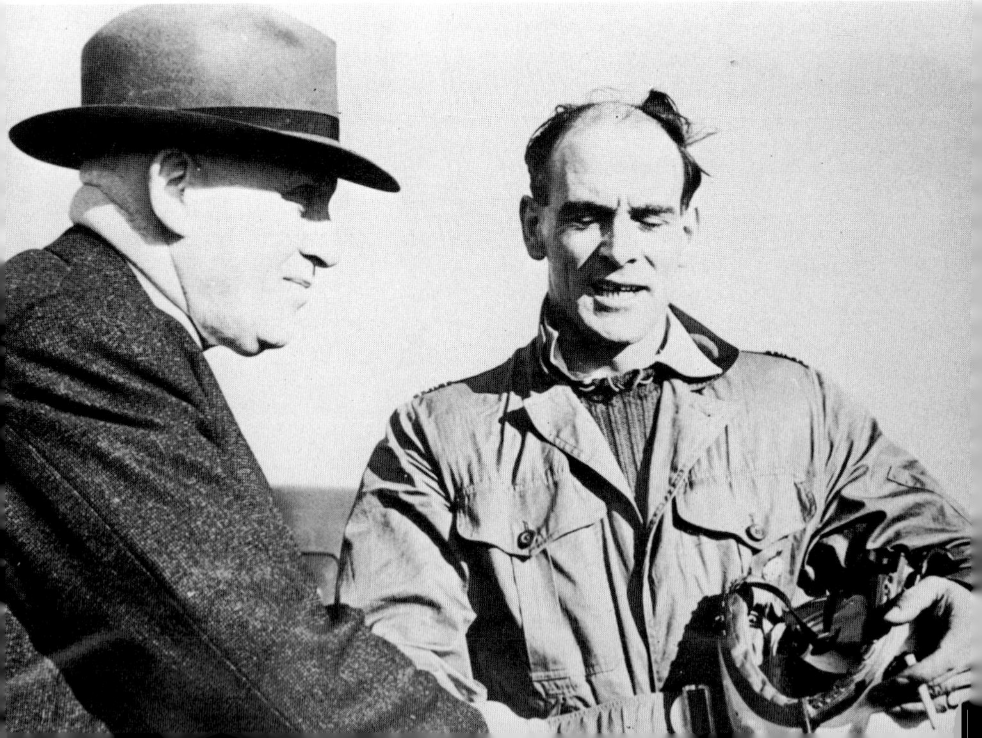

pressure-breathing system and tested it. In Bazett's system, counterpressure was applied to the chest by inflating bladders in a waistcoat, and oxygen was supplied under pressure from a bag worn around the trunk. Although there were possible hazards such as increased risk of fire, the likelihood that the oxygen inlet could freeze at altitude, and the general cumbrousness, the system was reasonably economical in its use of oxygen. Matthews' reaction, however, was that the altitude gain achieved was too small. His opinion was based on a pressure waistcoat, very similar to Bazett's, made by Baxter, Woodhouse and Taylor that the Lab had recently tested. This, however, had proved too complicated and caused undue circulatory disturbances; Stewart and Goldie both fainted in it after less than seven minutes. Then Matthews heard that Bazett was going to visit the UK. He immediately asked Whittingham to arrange for him to collaborate with, and advise, the Lab. Bazett came and stayed for over a year.

His period at the Lab was eventful, at least for his colleagues, as he insisted on playing a full part in the programme of experiments in the decompression chamber despite a serious heart condition. Indeed, on one occasion he was taken up to well over 50,000 feet by mistake. Bazett's suit and breathing system, after modification and improvement, worked consistently well in the decompression chamber, adding between 3,000 and 4,000 feet to the altitude tolerance. Flight tests were equally successful, Winfield taking it to above 44,000 feet, and Wing Commander Roland Falk of the RAE taking it to 46,000 feet. Falk reported that, 'Although the system of breathing in no way replaces a pressure cabin, it may prove of great value for test work and also possibly for use in fighters in the case of urgent operational necessity.'[31] The MAP agreed to obtain a hundred sets from Canada for further trials and to make six sets in the RAE as an interim measure, noting that 'Mr Cody was to make the straps'. (This bearer of a famous name was 'Colonel' Cody's son who still worked at the RAE.)

The system entered service early in 1944, mainly with the PRU squadrons. Its routine use raised the aircraft's ceiling satisfactorily, and the aircrew used it without problems. The Physiological Laboratory reported that, in terms of its simplicity, safety and applicability to British aircraft, the Bazett waistcoat was the most suitable form of pressure-breathing apparatus. Again, however, the introduction of pressure-cabin aircraft limited the waistcoat's use.

The first attempt to build a pressure-cabin aircraft had been at

Wright Field in the USA in 1921. The cabin was pressurized by a wind-driven pump, but control of the pressure was unsuccessful. While flying at 3,000 feet on the first flight, the pilot had experienced a cabin pressure equivalent to 7,000 feet below sea-level, the rapid pressurization resulting in the pilot suffering from acute earache and in the cabin air being heated to 65 °C![32] Development had been halted in 1922 and was not taken up again until much later.

The Physiological Laboratory was not directly involved in the development of pressure-cabin aircraft. Matthews and his team were, however, involved peripherally from time to time. The first occasion was in 1940, when some fairly esoteric experiments were carried out with the Instrument Department of the RAE on behalf of the Pressure Cabin Committee of the MAP to define the ventilation required in pressure cabins.

In 1942 the Lab produced a special type of double-hose mask for use in a pressure-cabin Spitfire being tested by the RAE. The canopy of the aircraft was exceptionally prone to misting, and it was thought that the expired air should be ducted away from the mask so that the moisture in the breath could not condense on the canopy. While helpful, the double-hose mask did not entirely solve the problem, but just over two years later the principle was again being used in modified G masks for the PRUs using pressure-cabin Spitfires.

The introduction of pressure-cabin aircraft had an enormous impact on oxygen equipment, which largely became relegated to emergency or 'get you down' use in other than military aviation. On the other hand they introduced new problems, not least of which was that of rapid decompression.

As soon as it had become apparent that pressure-cabin aircraft would be introduced, it became important to find out what would happen if the cabin lost its pressure suddenly. Theoretically a rapid change of pressure, resulting in a rapid expansion of gas held in the body, could have disastrous results. First, nitrogen bubbles would form in the blood to give rise to decompression sickness, and second, there was a possibility that the expansion of trapped gas in the body could burst the tissue enclosing it – for example, if the breath were held, the lungs could burst.

Unaware of the fact that rapid decompressions had been carried out by the von Diringshofens in Germany and by Heim in America in the 1930s, the Physiological Laboratory planned a careful series of experiments late in 1941. For the previous two years Professor de Burgh Daly in Edinburgh had, under the aegis of the FPRC, been carrying out experiments on rapid decompression in animals, and the time had now come to extend the work to man. The subjects sat in the small compartment of the decompression chamber while the large end was decompressed to a predetermined level. A hinged flap made of half-inch steel plate, and held shut by a 500-lb bomb release, was installed between the two compartments. On firing, it swung open, allowing air from the small compartment to be sucked into the large end until the pressure had equilibrated. The runs looked more impressive from outside the chamber than from inside. There was a loud bang and a cloud of water vapour condensed in the air. Inside the chamber, Winfield reported a feeling of air being blown out of the chest, but that was all. The first subjects, exposed to a relatively small pressure change (300 to 3,200 feet) were Winfield, Stewart and Parkinson. Further runs took the maximum altitude up to 45,000 feet. The experiments confirmed that, in healthy people breathing oxygen, rapid decompression posed few problems provided that adequate precautions were taken to avoid decompression sickness and hypoxia.[33]

It was this ever-present risk of sudden decompression which was to help keep the pressure suit research programme going at the Institute for many years after the war. Another reason was that, at very high altitude and very low outside pressures, achieving the necessary cockpit pressure incurred an unacceptable weight penalty; it became far more economical to pressurize just the man.

So in 1950 the Operational Requirements programme established by the Air Ministry called for research into the problems of using high-performance aircraft at very high altitude.[34] In addition to a study of the fundamental physiological difficulties, this implied development of equipment. Generally the concept for a suit was formulated in the RAE Mechanical Engineering (ME) Department, following which development was carried out in conjunction with industry, using firms such as Frankenstein of Manchester, Siebe Gorman and Baxter, Woodhouse and Taylor. The suits then came to the ME Department and to the IAM for testing, and here it was that experiments were done in the chamber and modifications were suggested. Thus, unlike in the early 1940s, the Lab did not have responsibility for the development of the suits.

The overall requirements were that the first priority was completion of the military task, and this usually meant staying at high altitude. Next, there was the need for the aircraft to remain airborne and to return to a friendly base safely; third, the equipment had to protect the airman during escape from his aircraft; and finally, the aircrew had to be able to survive thereafter. Although many types of pressure suit were evaluated at the RAE and the IAM during the 1950s, they were generally used on the same principles, differing mainly in details, material of manufacture and jointing of the limbs. There were exceptions of course. One rigid type of pressure suit tested at the RAE was so heavy that the pilot had to be assisted in and out of the aircraft by a crane![35]

It became evident early on that one of the problems that would bedevil development would be the difficulty of designing a suitable headpiece. It would be difficult to integrate the headpiece with the rest of the suit, difficult to move the neck when the suit was pressurized, and hard to balance the air pressure in the suit with that in the headpiece. One attempted cure of the last problem was to inflate the headpiece from an oxygen-fed waistcoat worn inside the suit, but no great success was achieved. The most comfortable type of helmet was the goldfish-bowl type, but this was heavy and a potential hazard on impact. The dangers of such a helmet were overcome by using a flexible, transparent material which could be folded and kept open when unpressurized but which closed automatically and inflated to a spherical shape when pressurized on exposure to altitude. Again, various types were assessed and, provided the pressure control system was adequate, proved relatively acceptable, although the open visor tended to be restrictively bulky. Misting was prevented by an air-ventilated 'gallery' along the edge of the visor and by incorporating a mask to duct away the man's moist expirate.

There were three main variants of full pressure suit tested at the IAM in the late 1950s and early 1960s. The first was an American suit made by B.F. Goodrich Aviation Products; the suit was light and comfortable and gave good mobility, but it could not meet the RAF operational requirement as a stay-up suit, and its thermal protection was insufficient. Next, two suits were designed jointly by the RAE and industry; one was made initially by Siebe Gorman and was called the Type B suit and the other was made by Frankenstein and was called the Type 51 suit. However, despite extensive testing, modification and retesting, neither suit was able to meet the Air Ministry requirements. This lack of progress in the development of pressure suits must have been very galling to the IAM team, which had devoted a considerable amount of time to the testing of the garments; but it must have been even more distressing to the RAE, for whom the IAM's contribution represented only the tip of the iceberg. One of the big disadvantages of all the garments made up to this point was that they were tailored to particular individuals, so that testing was limited to those individuals. What was needed was some way of making pressure garments fit more people more easily.

Although the development of full pressure suits had been led by the RAE, since the work involved mainly engineering, the IAM, with its wartime experience with Bazett's pressure waistcoat, had retained an active interest in partial pressure suits. It will be remembered that, in order to conserve consciousness above 40,000 feet, oxygen has to be breathed under pressure. However, limits have to be set because pressure breathing is tiring and causes blood to pool in the periphery of the body which predisposes to fainting, and it actually forces fluid from the blood into the tissues, reinforcing the likelihood of fainting. It was to overcome the fatigue caused by pressure breathing that Professor Bazett had developed his pressure-breathing waistcoat. Later the Americans were able to increase the breathing pressure tolerated by increasing the counterpressure coverage to the arms; in place of internal bladders, they adopted the 'capstan' system, which had previously been used on one of their early anti-g suits. (The capstan was a pneumatic tube running down the outside of a limb or down each side of the torso; when the tube was inflated, it pulled the fabric of the close-fitting suit even tighter against the body to give the necessary counterpressure.). In 1948 the United States Air Force (USAF) graciously donated one of their capstan suits to the British pressure suit research programme. At the time this acted as stimulus to British industry, which had not previously shown much enthusiasm for developing pressure-breathing equipment, mainly because no operational requirement officially existed until 1950. As a first stage, it was decided to make a similar suit whilst at the same time developing a new partial pressure helmet. It was decided that the general shape of the USAF facepiece was adequate but that the method of sealing it was not. In addition, an inner mask was incorporated to reduce the potential problem of misting of the visor. At this stage the visor was not designed as one that could be opened, although this was a declared intention for later. The new helmet, designated the Type A, did not itself meet the operational requirement in several respects, but it was good enough to test in the laboratory along with the suit and the inflation-control equipment developed for it.

During extensive testing in the ME Department and at the IAM, it was established that the American equipment gave protection during emergency descent from any altitude, provided that 40,000 feet was reached in 20 minutes and that it could also give limited protection while the aircraft stayed high, for example for up to one hour at 53,000 feet. However, the suit was individually sized, impossible to don unaided, uncomfortable when inflated, and hot to wear, and aircrew could not eat, drink or clear their ears in flight without removing the helmet. For all that, the emergency partial pressure suit offered significant advantages over the full pressure suit: there was less interference with sweat evaporation, mobility was not so seriously impaired, and entry into the suit did not necessitate gas-tight closure. Although the equipment was used in all high-altitude flying of the prototype Canberra, it was apparent that the capstan partial pressure suit was too complex, and it would be as expensive to make as a full pressure suit, whilst still not giving sufficient protection to allow altitude to be maintained in bomber or photo-reconnaissance aircraft in the event of loss of cabin pressure. Accepting that a full pressure suit would be operationally unacceptable, what could be done to provide protection? The first step was to change the rules – the partial pressure equipment would be used not to maintain altitude but just as a 'get you down' apparatus. The next step was to see how the current in-service equipment measured up to the new requirement.

The IAM found that with the American headpiece as used with the partial pressure capstan suit, with the pressure-breathing waistcoat as designed by Bazett and with an anti-g suit, subjects could withstand 5 seconds at 80,000 feet, followed by a descent to 40,000 feet at 15,000 feet per minute. The advantages of such a system would be found in comfort, mobility, sizing, fitting and training – all easier than with the capstan suit. However, experience with the American suit had indicated that the protection afforded by the Bazett waistcoat could almost certainly be increased by applying counterpressure to a greater area of the body. Therefore, over the next two years Mr H. Franks of the Ministry of Supply, the ME Department and Messrs P. Frankenstein & Sons developed a new pressure jerkin. It differed from the Bazett waistcoat in that coverage of the body was extended to include the lower neck, the shoulders, the groins and the crutch area. One early problem was that, when the garment was pressurized, the subject was forced forward, causing severe testicular pain – which was unlikely to be acceptable to aircrew! The difficulty was overcome by removing the appropriate part of the jerkin's bladder. In addition, it was found necessary to make the crutchpiece fixed in position, rather than as a flap, to prevent a hernia from 'blowing out' under high-pressure breathing; the unfortunate consequence was that the garment became more difficult to don. In the decompression chamber, the partial pressure helmet, jerkin and g-suit combination proved effective at simulated altitudes up to 70,000 feet for one minute, or lower altitudes for longer, followed by rapid descent to 40,000 feet without – and this was very important operationally – the need to pre-breathe a hundred per cent oxygen to prevent decompression sickness.

However, there was a requirement for even more protection with the planned development of the rocket plus jet Saunders-Roe P177 interceptor, which was designed to reach 80,000 feet but which could probably go as high as 100,000 feet. That protection was given by adding arm bladders to the pressure jerkin. The experimental work was carried out in two phases, first at the IAM, where pressure breathing to a level that would be required at 100,000 feet was tried without ascent to altitude, and then at the RCAF Institute of Aviation Medicine in Toronto where chamber runs were carried out in their higher-performance chambers. This time, to the ensemble of partial pressure helmet, jacket and g-suit were added pressure gloves, to prevent undue swelling of the hands when the tissue fluids 'boiled' above 63,000 feet. The experiments proved the acceptability of the equipment, even in subjects with little previous experience of pressure breathing, although intensive indoctrination was first needed. For good measure, John Ernsting from the IAM made a final simulated ascent to as high as the chamber would go, while wearing the equipment and without pre-oxygenation. He reached 140,000 feet, where he stayed for one minute before descending to 38,000 feet in 25 seconds. He experienced no undue discomfort and during his time at peak altitude was able to move his arms with 'comparative freedom'. An improved version of the jerkin with arms was tested at the IAM in July 1957, and subsequent versions, named the Type X and the Type Y, were tested at the Lab later in the same year. But the writing was already on the wall for protection to altitudes as high as 100,000 feet – the April 1957 Defence White Paper of Mr Duncan Sandys ruled out any fighter for the RAF, other than the Lightning, and the Operational Requirement for the Saunders-Roe P177 was cancelled.

For protection against lower altitudes where pressure breathing was still required, development of what was to be the Mark 1 pressure jerkin continued, the first garments being for the Javelin

Marks 7 and 8. However, as the jerkin came to cover more and more of the body, so the combined assembly of jerkin/g-suit had become heavy, hot and difficult to don. By the mid 1960s new techniques and new materials had become available, and Mr Franks, together with the RAE, Frankensteins and the IAM, produced an overall that combined both garments. It was lighter, easier to don and simpler in operation than the earlier combination of garments, but it was also still very hot to wear. Therefore a version was produced which incorporated an air-ventilated suit, and the new combined suit worked very satisfactorily in the Lab before being eventually introduced into service.

Whilst development of the pressure jerkin had been proceeding, so too had development of a completely British partial pressure helmet. Following the laboratory experience with the Type A, two companies vied with each other to make the definitive version – ML Aviation Ltd and Baxter, Woodhouse and Taylor Ltd. The Taylor partial pressure helmet was developed in close collaboration with the RAE and the IAM, eventually entering service in 1959 as the Type C, although its performance in the heat and the cold was never very satisfactory.

The ML helmet was initially less successful, and it never entered service with the RAF. However, it eventually went on to do as well as its rival, being chosen by the German Air Force for use in the Starfighter. Moreover, when a partial pressure helmet was needed for the test flying of Concorde, the Taylor helmet proved to be incompatible with the oxygen equipment installed in the aircraft, so the ML helmet was used. And it is now enjoying a new lease of life during the high-altitude test flying of the Air Defence Variant of the Tornado.

There was, however, an alternative to the partial pressure helmet. In the mid 1950s, much evaluation was done of the protection that could be offered by the use of the P/Q mask attached to the standard flying helmet. Theoretically, the protection was limited by the ability of the mask to withstand pressure, and by the time that the pressure differential could be tolerated across the neck and the ear-drums. With the mask and helmet alone, laboratory experiences showed that the ceiling was 50,000 feet but that this could be increased to 56,000 feet by adding pressure jerkin and g-suit, provided rapid descent followed to lower altitudes. Although the aircraft then in service could not descend quickly enough, the pressure jerkin/g-suit/P mask combination saw considerable RAF service in the V force and

Canberras.

Partial pressure clothing is very little used in service nowadays. First, pressure cabins have proved to be very reliable. Second, the shooting down of Gary Powers' U-2 aircraft by a Russian surface-to-air missile forced a re-evaluation of the policy of high-altitude penetration. Military aircraft now tend to fly at high speed and very low level in order to reduce their chances of being detected and subsequently brought down by missile. Although suitable full pressure clothing in this country never developed to the level of acceptability achieved in the United States, the partial pressure clothing that was developed offered several advantages in terms of cost, comfort and mobility in the cockpit. It remains to be seen whether recent advances in the 'look down, shoot down' capabilities of fighter aircraft will force strike/attack aircraft back up to high altitude, relying on electronics to prevent detection and on pressure clothing to protect the aircrew.

Not all the altitude research conducted at the IAM since the war has been devoted to oxygen systems and problems of decompression. For example, in the mid 1960s concern was expressed about the possible fire risk to aircrew exposed to either oxygen-rich or hyperbaric air environments. Clothed brass dummies and dead pigs were set on fire in the chambers at the IAM, and the experiments proved that a hundred per cent oxygen atmosphere could support a flash fire that would be fatal in five to twenty seconds. Hyperbaric air at five atmospheres posed a greater fire risk than air at one atmosphere, but even that was not as potentially dangerous as the pure oxygen environment.[36] The reports were given wide circulation, for there was considerable concern over the use of hundred per cent oxygen atmosphere in American spacecraft at that time. Unfortunately NASA was not able to change the system quickly enough to avoid the tragic flash fire in 1967 which killed astronauts Chaffee, Grissom and White during a static test of the Apollo capsule.

One of the problems on ascent to altitude is the expansion of body gases, with a consequent increase in the antisocial activity of passing flatus ('farting'). When, in the early 1960s, a drug company claimed to have produced a concoction which would prevent this, the IAM was very interested. The experiment that followed is still remembered in the Lab as one of the classics. At that time a large number of the doctors in the Institute lived in the Officers' Mess, and so advantage was taken of the captive population. Each evening the subjects had to sit down after dinner and eat a tin of curried baked beans. They were then forbidden to break wind until after they had been up in the decompression chamber the next morning, when the amount of gas they passed was recorded. Some days the subjects took the medicine, and other days they did not. The medicine did not prove in the slightest bit efficacious, but it became quite a common sight to see medical officers walking to work from the Mess, often with an extraordinary gait, as they tried not to pass flatus!

The Institute is often being called upon to advise participants in expeditions to esoteric parts of the globe, and also to help searchers after glory in their attempts to break records. The tradition had started with Wing Commander Struan Marshall in 1932, when he was an adviser to the Houston Mount Everest flights and tested the team's equipment in the RAE decompression chamber. At about the same time he was also advising the 1933 Everest expedition. The oxygen apparatus used was a continuous-flow device with a reservoir tube and a whistle, the latter at the suggestion of Sir Joseph Barcroft, to indicate that oxygen was flowing. The whistle, from a commercially available rubber duck called 'Adolphus', was incorporated in the apparatus by Marshall, but the noise was found to be intensely irritating and he removed it again, arguing that, 'If the climbers are unable to go on, they must go back and it is of no importance to them to know whether their failure is in spite of added oxygen or due to the fact that oxygen is not added.'[37]

The next time that the Medical Branch of the RAF was involved directly in oxygen equipment for climbers was in 1947 when a Captain R.S. Ross RAMC was attempting to obtain permission to climb Everest. Ross' expedition never materialized, but links between the Himalayan Committee of the Alpine Club, the Royal Geographical Society and the IAM had been forged and were to be of use later. Roxburgh in particular dispensed large quantities of advice, for example, to a firm that was interested in piping oxygen up Mount Everest in narrow stainless steel tubes! The IAM supplied equipment (which included three economizers) for the 1952 Expedition to Cho Oyu mountain in the Himalayas, but the main effort was directed towards the ultimately successful 1953 Everest Expedition, for which the Air Ministry supplied oxygen bottles, helmets, economizers and masks.

Record breakers aided by the IAM over the years have included Mr Julian Nott (world high-altitude hot-air ballooning records), the Army team which paraglided across the English Channel in 1980, and, in one less happy episode, the designing of equipment for a Mr Mike Field, who claimed a world glider altitude record but who was held by the British Gliding Association to have cheated. It is reassuring to know that his equipment would have got him there safely even if his glider did not. The Institute's attitude to such ventures is neatly encapsulated by the words of the present Commandant, Air Commodore Howard: 'A scientific organisation that loses the taste for the unusual and the freedom to indulge it will slowly desiccate. In this respect, the Institute has two cardinal assets: it possesses capital facilities that are unique in the United Kingdom, and it has a mandate to undertake work on behalf of approved civilian customers. In consequence, the piquancy of its research pudding is occasionally sharpened by an unconventional commission.' In 1977 the conduct of selection tests on potential Spacelab astronauts provided a substantial and profitable example of just such a commission.

1979 brought a briefer but more colourful encounter with the unusual when British Caledonian Airways decided that it would be fitting to mark the inauguration of their new weekly service to Guayaquil, Ecuador, with a ceremonial performance by its pipe band at the Ecuadorian airfield. However, the Airways' Principal Medical Officer (whose long association with the IAM had endowed him with physiological vigilance) realized that to play the bagpipes at a base altitude of 10,500 feet might not be without cardio-respiratory complications. The Institute was accordingly asked to provide specialist advice on the possible risks to the health of the pipers and the dignity of the airline.

The two musicians who had been selected to represent British Caledonian duly presented themselves at Farnborough, clad in full Highland regalia and bearing their instruments. They were exposed to simulated altitudes of 5,000 feet and 10,500 feet in the decompression chamber, and measurements of various respiratory parameters were made as they played a representative programme of marches, reels and strathspeys. They exhibited the moderate hypoxia and hyperventilation that inevitably affect those who indulge in physical exertion at altitude and, although the symptoms were not severe, the Institute felt obliged to recommend that the entertainment provided in Ecuador should be so planned that no episode would last for more than five minutes and that ample pauses for recovery should be scheduled. Moreover, the rarefied atmosphere had an unfortunate effect on the pitch of the bagpipes. Suitably forewarned, the pipers were able to re-tune their instruments, and the ceremony at Guayaquil took place with neither physiological nor melodic catastrophe!

Many other people approach the Institute for advice on breathing-equipment for a variety of tasks. While not everyone can be assisted, it is pleasing to know that the expertise and reputation built up by successive workers in the oxygen field at the IAM – men such as Matthews, Gilson, Roxburgh and Ernsting – is so well recognized outside the narrow confines of the Lab.

7 ...And Too Much Acceleration

In 1931 two Americans, Dearborn and Kirschbaum, had measured the accelerations achieved when fighter aircraft performed manoeuvres typical of dogfighting – manoeuvres such as loops, pull-outs from dives, turns of 180 degrees, barrel rolls and spins. All produced very considerable increases in g. For example, pulling out of a 175 m.p.h. dive could produce +9.3g, whilst pushing the nose of the aircraft down at 100 m.p.h. could produce a negative acceleration of nearly 2g. During a normal loop, accelerations greater than 1g could be sustained for nearly 10 seconds.

It was also at about this time that the pilots flying in the Schneider Trophy races were beginning to appreciate the physiological effects of too much acceleration. And if the consequences of blacking out were considered serious in a race, how much more serious would the consequences be in a life-or-death fight against an adversary who, perhaps, had some protection against blacking out? That was what worried Bryan Matthews. At the FPRC's second meeting he echoed contemporary physiological opinions: protection against g-forces, even if only to a small degree, would give superiority in battle over an opponent without protection. Contemporary military opinion, however, took a rather different view – as Air Vice-Marshal Richardson told the Committee, the Air Staff considered the speed of modern aircraft to be so great that dogfights would be virtually impossible; consequently, blacking out was unlikely to be a serious problem.[1]

It was, of course, the job of the FPRC to advise the Secretary of State for Air about what it regarded as urgent aviation medicine problems requiring immediate research and, on this matter of the likely operational significance of blacking out, the members of the Committee were firmly behind Matthews. Nevertheless, had it not been for one highly significant fact, it is quite possible that acceleration research would have remained near the bottom of the

Physiological Laboratory's priority list. That fact was that most of the research into effects of acceleration had been done, and was being done, by the Germans. Everyone knew this because the Germans had published the results of their work in the open scientific literature. What no one knew was how much more research they had carried out which had not been published. It does seem that the significance of this question had not entirely escaped the deliberations of 'higher authorities' within the RAF. Neither did it take much effort to deduce that, if the Germans were hiding something, it would, more than likely, relate to methods of protecting against acceleration. Since there had been hardly any work on that subject in this country, it was impossible to estimate the value, or operational significance, of the German research. There was, therefore, a real need for some sort of investigation.

If Matthews and the FPRC were successful in persuading the Air Staff that research into the physiological effects of acceleration was necessary, they were less so in persuading them to provide the equipment needed to carry out that research. For what Matthews and his team wanted was a centrifuge. Unfortunately centrifuges are expensive – the estimated cost in 1939 was £7,000 – and nobody had much experience of them anyway. The Americans had one, and it had been used by the father of American aviation medicine, Harold Armstrong, for what is now generally recognized as one of the classic studies of the effect of prolonged acceleration on man. Also, as Wing Commander Livingston had reported, the Germans had one, with a second under construction. However, there was no evidence that a centrifuge would be able to reproduce the rates of onset of acceleration encountered when 'pulling g' in an aircraft. Even if a suitable machine could be built, the war would probably be over before it was finished.

So Matthews did not get his centrifuge. He was to try again in 1943 and in 1945. On the second occasion it was the RAE that was unenthusiastic; on the final occasion he actually managed to extract a promise that money would be forthcoming, only to find that all the firms capable of tackling the job were still busy on war work. In fact, it was to be another ten years before the Institute of Aviation Medicine finally acquired a centrifuge.

With an acceleration research programme to get on with, but no centrifuge, there was only one thing to do – use aircraft. And this is what the Physiological Laboratory, and then the Institute, did, very successfully, for the next fifteen years. To begin with, the research got off to a somewhat shaky start with, as we have seen, a less than enthusiastic Struan Marshall in charge. But, with the arrival of Flying Officer Stewart just as the new decade was dawning, all was transformed.

On arriving at the Laboratory, Stewart was immediately given two tasks: to formulate a basis for the syndrome of blacking out and to produce a simple, reliable method of providing some degree of protection against acceleration. Renewed impetus had been given to the acceleration research programme by Matthews himself, quite inadvertently. He had acted as subject in one of the very first flights in the Laboratory's Battle aircraft and had adamantly claimed afterwards that, despite the high g 'pulled' during the flight, he had never blacked out; until, that is, he was shown photographs of himself slumped forwards, obviously completely unconscious!

During the first two years of the Lab's programme of acceleration research, Stewart was assisted by Squadron Leaders G.E. Watt and J.R. Tobin, both test pilots in the Experimental Flying Department of the RAE. Although it was generally Stewart himself who acted as experimental subject, the pilot's role was just as important, and just as dangerous. In particular it was vital that, even if the subject blacked out or lost consciousness, the pilot remained in full control of the aircraft. Hence Tobin and Watt both needed to have very high black-out thresholds. Occasionally they themselves acted as subjects. When the research was carried out using single-seater aircraft, then pilot and subject were one and the same. However, before Stewart and his team could do anything, they had to find out what g could be 'pulled' with the aircraft they had available, and also devise some means of measuring and recording the effects of that g on themselves. On the basis of Armstrong's classic study of the effects of prolonged acceleration on man which had been published only two years before,[2] Stewart decided that five seconds was long enough for sufficient useful data to be obtained. Preliminary experiments using the single-seat Gladiator flown by Squadron Leader Watt indicated that sustained g for this length of time was impossible in level flight but could be achieved in a diving spiral. Various modifications also had to be made to all the aircraft used in the Laboratory's flight research programme, in particular to make sure that there was no 'engine cutting' under high g loadings. The frequent application of prolonged g stresses also led to minor structural and engine failures. Since the aircraft which the Laboratory was loaned for its research activities were often in a poor state of maintenance anyway, the under-staffed RAE servicing engineers, although highly competent and keen to do their utmost to help, found it almost impossible to meet the demanding flying schedule imposed by Stewart. Indeed, so acute had the problems become by late 1940 that he considered discontinuing the experiments and suggested that the black-out programme should be transferred '... to some R.A.F. station where efficient organisation and maintenance of aircraft can be carried out'. Stewart went on to imply that inadequate maintenance could well lead to '... a more serious accident than any yet experienced ...'.[3]

Stewart's concern is readily understandable. Single-seat fighter aircraft during the war had a maximum 'g safety factor' of between +10 and +12g. For twin-seat aircraft the factor ranged from +7 to +10g, and for heavier, multi-engined aircraft, such as bombers, from about +5 to +7g. Maximum permissible negative g loadings, however, rarely exceeded –5g. Go beyond these limits, and the aircraft would disintegrate; in practice the upper limit was set at three-quarters of these maximum values. This still meant that fighter aircraft could 'pull' in excess of +6g – the pilot then weighing more than half a ton! Above +5g, movement of the limbs becomes extremely difficult, if not impossible. The increased weight drags the facial tissues downwards, creating a haggard, aged appearance. The trunk is 'concertina-ed', losing some two inches of height. Then there is the grey-out, black-out and sometimes complete loss of consciousness. However, provided consciousness is maintained, other sensory functions are not much impaired. Thus, in one experiment in which black-out was maintained for over ten seconds, oil of cloves vapour was delivered through a nasal catheter; the sense of smell was never lost. Neither was there any loss of hearing, and posture was maintained.

Another problem was the spatial disorientation which occurred when the aircraft resumed level flight, and the g decreased. This, which is best described as a forward 'tumbling' sensation, can be extremely disturbing, particularly in those with a sensitive vestibular apparatus, causing dizziness, nausea and profuse sweating. It is also potentially very dangerous, leading to illusory perceptions of the aircraft's attitude. However, in contrast to their predecessors in the Great War, the pilots of World War II had the important advantage of a fairly sophisticated cockpit instrumentation, which meant that they were no longer dependent upon their own, often misleading, senses.

Of the various measurements Stewart and his team needed to make, the most important was the g-force produced by a given manoeuvre. In fact, it was not so much the measurement of g which was the problem, for this was easily accomplished using a device called an accelerometer, but how to record the measurement. This had to be done automatically, especially if single-seat aircraft like the Gladiator were to be used. Two techniques were developed. The first involved having a thirty-five millimetre ciné camera with a two-inch lens located behind the pilot's head filming the accelerometer and other experimental instruments. The second, adopted for later work in Hurricanes and Spitfires where there was insufficient room in the cramped cockpits for mounting a camera, involved incorporating within the accelerometer a crude, but effective, paper-trace recording system.

The onset of grey-out was very difficult to determine. In the Gladiator it proved possible to photograph the pilot's face, so recording his reaction to the increased g-force, by positioning a mirror a front of the pilot. In the more cramped cockpit of the single-seat Hurricanes and Spitfires, however, the pilot himself had to note the g-level at which visual symptoms first appeared, and to facilitate this, Watt devised a new and extremely simple type of accelerometer which became known as the 'Watt accelerometer'. This was to prove invaluable for much experimental work and for educational purposes. For the experiments carried out in the two-seat Fairey Battle, and also later in a Boulton-Paul Defiant, a rather more scientific, although still essentially subjective technique was used for determining black-out. The end-point of vision was taken as the disappearance of black letters on a white card. When the letters could no longer be seen, the subject pressed a button attached to his Sutton restraint harness and held the button pressed until the letters could again be seen. This button illuminated a bulb which was seen by the recording camera.

One of the first investigations that Stewart carried out was a study of the effects of prolonged acceleration below the level at which visual symptoms first occurred. By diving in continuous spirals from heights of 20,000 feet, values of +3.5 to +4g could be maintained for 30 to 40 seconds, and values of 3g for much longer. Yet, apart from fatigue afterwards, there were no untoward physical symptoms. By gradually increasing the magnitude of the induced accleration, Stewart showed that between three and five seconds of sustained g were required to produce complete black-out; the value of g at which this occurred was called the 'g-threshold'. Stewart's own threshold actually increased during the first few months of 1940, which he attributed to a genuine physiological adaptation. Thereafter his threshold became fairly constant, any pronounced variations being explainable in terms of illness (such as a cold), after-effects of 'unaccustomed exercise' or after-effects of celebrations! Stewart's observations and experiences were reported back to the FPRC, often supported by impressive photographic evidence. As he well appreciated, it is always dangerous to draw conclusions from the essentially subjective impressions of just one man. Yet there is absolutely no doubt that these were also entirely typical of most fighter pilots. It also became apparent, following reports from the squadrons, that g thresholds varied widely between individuals, some being quite definitely 'g-resistant' and other 'g-sensitive'. The latter would not have been able to make such rapid turns as the former, and they were therefore at a considerable disadvantage when engaging in combat with a more g-resistant enemy. Some 5g appears to have been the average threshold value, although presumably the g-sensitive fighter pilots tended not to survive, this effectively raising the average. Attempts were made by Stewart and his colleagues to provide a means of predicting whether individuals had high or low g tolerance, but these were not successful.

By mid 1940, with the experimental methodology well established, Stewart concentrated his attention on the precise cause of the visual impairment associated with high acceleration. Several years before, Struan Marshall had attributed grey-out and black-out to 'anaemia of the eye', which, roughly translated, is a lack of oxygen to the eye. Armstrong's experiments in America supported Marshall's hypothesis, and Stewart's were to do so as well.

What Stewart did was to modify the camera system so that it provided a close-up of the subject's face, particularly his eyes. The necessary additional illumination was provided by an Aldis lamp which was operated by the subject, who then had to keep himself absolutely still to avoid blurring the photographs – and this with the aircraft, more likely than not, in a spiral dive to produce the g-load required! Under these incredibly difficult experimental conditions, the effects of various drugs, of hypoxia and even the mechanical effect of the increased g on the eyelids, were all examined. The most important findings were that the pupils of the eyes played no part in the visual impairment produced by increased g and that, even during black-out, light could be detected if the source was sufficiently intense – as when the Aldis lamp was switched on; furthermore, colour could also be appreciated. Failure of perception occurred only with unconsciousness. In other words, the blacked-out and supposedly non-receptive eye was, in fact, capable of responding to a light stimulus provided that the light was bright enough. This was an important finding, because it meant that the physiological basis of the loss of vision could not be a (temporary) destruction of the light-sensitive pigments in the retina of the eyes. Furthermore, since the brain still responded to stimuli received by the eye during black-out, neither was the loss of vision likely to be a result of pressure effects on the nerves leading from the eyes to the vision centres of the brain. The only logical hypothesis remaining was that the loss of vision was due, as Marshall had said, to an inadequate blood-supply being maintained in the eye.

Thus, even without a centrifuge, Stewart and his colleagues were able to contribute significantly towards the better understanding of the phenomenon of black-out. The cost was considerable, however, and not just in financial terms. Stewart, who was awarded the AFC in 1941 for his work, was to black out over two hundred times before the war was over, and sometimes he became completely unconscious. He has left a graphic account of one such episode which occurred on 9 May 1940, when, after a high-g manoeuvre in a Battle aircraft, he found himself lying on the floor of the cockpit. Whilst unconscious he had fallen out of his restraint harness, which on that occasion was just a gunner's waist-belt. Stewart's first reaction was one of intense fear for, in addition to disorientation and pain from bruised arms and face, he was aware of a clear fluid trickling over his skin. For one terrible moment he thought he had broken his skull and that the fluid was cerebro-spinal fluid from his brain. Then he realized it was just a nasal discharge; the level of the g-force had forced the fluid out of his sinuses![4]

The after-effects of blacking out were also very unpleasant, and even more so if consciousness had been completely lost. Stewart provided vivid accounts of the overwhelming feeling of lethargy and fatigue, the impaired memory and the inability to concentrate. This would lead to depression and a general unsociableness. After repeated episodes of blacking out, headaches were common; occasionally there was double vision, and almost always sleep was impaired.[5]

It is important to remember that these were not just the experiences of an isolated individual operating under conditions which were, even by wartime standards, exceptionally arduous and unusual. Fatigue, lethargy and all the other symptoms described by Stewart were familiar to most fighter pilots who 'pulled g' regularly. The situation would improve only with the introduction of the anti-g suit, the main purpose of which, at least then, was considered to be not the reduction of fatigue but the raising of the black-out threshold. Within days of his arrival at Farnborough, Stewart was trying to devise a simple method of achieving just this. By March 1940 Matthews was able to report to the FPRC that black-out thresholds could be increased by up to 1g by adopting a crouching posture in the aircraft seat. Since at this time the aircraft studies had been underway less than three months, with most of the flights actually taking place during that March, very rapid progress had obviously been made. In fact, it is clear from the Stewart's own writings that much about g-protection had been gleaned from the German reports, and there is no doubt that the early experiments were very similar to those carried out by the von Diringshofen brothers seven years earlier in Germany – deliberately so, to check the validity of the German work. It is also clear that the Germans believed the visual disturbances to be of circulatory origin and knew that g-tolerance could be improved by reducing the vertical distance between the heart and eyes (and, hence, the blood-pressure required to maintain the eye circulation). What is surprising is that, with this knowledge and with at least one working centrifuge, they failed to develop an anti-g suit during the war. Presumably the fact that the Germans were never found to be using anti-g suits explains, at least partially, why we in the UK never pursued our own anti-g suit programme, at least until much later in the war.

Recognition of the importance of adopting a crouching posture led to an education programme aimed at persuading Fighter Command of its value. Since the benefits were so immediately apparent, pilots did not take much persuading. Pilots were also encouraged to find out what their own g-threshold was, so that they could learn not to exceed it. This was where Squadron Leader Watt's simple accelerometer proved invaluable. And finally a film was made which showed the effects of high g-forces on the human body and of methods of minimizing these effects; this was circulated around the squadrons.

In addition to crouching, it was found that raising the legs also improved g-tolerance by approximately 1g. This was a result of effectively reducing the vertical distance between the legs and the heart, which meant that less blood pooled in the blood vessels of the legs, and more blood was returned to the heart. Auxiliary rudder pedals were fitted on to the existing rudder bars of Hurricanes and Spitfires so that the legs could be moved to a raised position for combat. By combining the pedals with a crouching posture, black-out thresholds could be raised by as much as 2g – not much less than that achieved by anti-g suits! No German aircraft were ever found with raised pedals, although it is certain that German pilots were fully aware of the benefits of crouching and that in some aircraft the seating position was designed with this in mind. In retrospect, the raising of the rudder pedals can be seen as the only concrete result of the Lab's g-research programme which was to be of any practical help to the pilots who were actually doing the fighting.

Since it was known that the adverse effects of increased g were a result of blood pooling in vessels whose relative orientation lay in the same (i.e. head-to-foot) direction as the g-force, and that reducing these vertical distances improved g-tolerance, quite clearly if these blood vessels could be taken out of the 'line of g', black-out thresholds should be much increased. Some years later this notion was to lead to the prone-position Meteor experiments; in the early 1940s, however, the fighter aircraft could not accommodate either a prone or a supine flying-seat. Reclining seats could be fitted, however, and late in 1940 Stewart carried out some experiments for the Gloster Aircraft Company. The seat-back angle was only 45°, but even so, with the feet raised, +6g could be sustained for 9 seconds, with hardly any impairment of vision; normally at this g-level, complete loss of consciousness would have occurred. However, this approach to the solution of the g-problem was not followed up. Neither was a suggestion, put to the FPRC in November 1939, that aircraft cockpits should be made rotatable, so that under increased g the pilot could be tilted either forwards or backwards out of the line of g!

Despite a wealth of evidence showing that they were ineffective in significantly raising g-thresholds, abdominal belts of various shapes and size were still available in 1940, and it was necessary to come to some firm decision whether or not to recommend them to aircrew. Therefore, in the summer of that year, the Physiological Laboratory undertook a full evaluation of the three principal types of belt then being marketed – elastic, pneumatic and hydrostatic. The belts were supposed to work by preventing blood from pooling in the abdomen. If they were to stand any chance of working, they had to fit as tightly as possible. So the elastic belts were tightened almost to the point of discomfort; yet they had no effect on the black-out threshold. The same result was obtained with the pneumatic, or Cadzow, belts (named after their inventor, Robert Cadzow). These had the advantage that discomfort could be minimized since the degree of pressure within the belt could be varied by means of valves.

The hydrostatic belts were similar, except they were filled with water (and not air) from a two-gallon tank at head-level. Not only was there no significant threshold gain, but there were also several problems with the belt. For example, when the subject was tightly strapped into his seat, insufficient water entered even under a loading of 6g. However, this difficulty was eventually overcome by modifications to the restraint harness. Another problem was the weight of the belt, which became intolerable under high-g conditions; also, after first exposure to g, the water tended to remain in the belt and not to return to the tank. And last, but by no means least, the water quickly became very cold.

Appreciating that belts alone were of little use, particularly in view of the discomfort they caused, Stewart experimented with hydrostatic leggings. These were of simple and crude construction, being tailor-made to fit just one person. The outer covering was of an inextensible rubberized fabric, and the leggings were designed so that pressure could be maintained only on the muscles of the calves and the thighs by bags containing water, and interconnected by rubber tubing. With this system a significant increase in the black-out threshold of 0.5g was achieved. However, the technique was never introduced into service – perhaps because by late 1940 the Physiological Laboratory team was aware of the work of Wilbur Franks in Canada; the first anti-g suit was soon to be available for testing by the RAF.

When the Allies landed at Oran in French North Africa late in 1942, the amphibious operation was supported by large numbers of carrier-based aircraft. It was afterwards reported that '... our planes performed feats of aerobatics deemed impossible without the pilots blacking-out'.[6] One fighter was seen to dive almost vertically for 3,000 feet and then pull out so sharply that the pilot should have lost consciousness; he did not but kept flying with complete control of his aircraft. Another pilot described how he turned inside an enemy fighter that he was engaging; when the enemy aircraft tried to follow, it was observed to spin out of control. The explanation for this, and many similar reports, was that the pilots of the British Fleet Air Arm were using a revolutionary new anti-g device, the Franks Flying Suit. It is with this suit that the g-suit story begins.

The best way to prevent blood-vessels from distending under g is to apply a counterpressure to the outside of the body. The Japanese had tried tightly binding the body below the heart with tape, but this did not work very well and it was also extremely uncomfortable. However, an alternative approach is to apply not external mechanical pressure but external hydrostatic pressure. This can be achieved, albeit somewhat impractically for a pilot, by immersing the body in a bath of water, the g-force then acting simultaneously on the water and on the blood within the cardiovascular system. The density of water and blood are very similar, so that the weight of both increases almost by the same amount under conditions of increasing g. An important limiting factor is the strength of the walls of the bath, which have to be inextensible and able to withstand the pressure.

The idea of using water to provide g-protection first came to Franks in 1938, when he noticed that small test-tubes could be prevented from breaking when being spun in a centrifuge if they were contained within larger, stronger tubes filled with water. At that time Dr Franks was employed by the University of Toronto, Canada, where he was conducting cancer research in the Banting and Best Department of Medical Research. His Head of Department was Professor Sir Frederick Banting who, with C.H. Best, had successfully identified and isolated the anti-diabetic hormone insulin nearly twenty years before. Banting, although a Canadian by birth, had a patriotic devotion to the British Empire and, foreseeing that another European war was inevitable, called in experts from the Canadian armed forces to explain to his team just what the outstanding military medicine problems were at that time. He was particularly impressed by one of these experts,[7] a Dr James, who spoke on behalf of the Royal Canadian Air Force about decompression sickness and black-out; it was these two problems which were to dominate the Department's activities over the next few years. And it was James who provided the link between the test-tubes immersed in water and the water-filled anti-g suit.

However, before Franks could start putting his ideas into practice, he had to resolve an all too familiar problem – money! As is so often the case with military organizations, the Royal Canadian Air Force wanted a solution to the g-problem but would rather avoid paying for it if it could (shades of Matthews' failure to obtain money for a centrifuge?). Discussions were held, fitfully, through 1938 and 1939 in an attempt to secure Air Force funding. Then, on 1 September 1939, Hitler invaded Poland, and Banting, galvanized into action, decided that, if the Air Force would not play, then he would try tapping the public conscience – which, on this occasion, was represented by the philanthropist Harry McClean. McClean proved incapable of resisting the combined appeals of Banting and Franks; in a very short time he had parted company with $5,000 – a considerable sum at that time. (It should also be pointed out that McClean was not alone in his generosity; throughout the war many donations were received from private citizens.) With the money Franks designed, to fit himself, a garment made of a non-stretch fabric containing water-filled bladders which fitted over the abdomen and lower extremities. However, to develop the system properly he needed to carry out flight testing, and at that time aircraft were in very short supply. The Air Force loaned him a vintage biplane and, fortunately, a very brave pilot who was prepared to push the aeroplane to the limits of its capabilities.[8] Before the structural engineers put a stop to their activities, Franks was able to show that his water-filled suit significantly raised his g-threshold. There were, however, many problems still to be resolved, and development work could not continue without a more suitable aircraft. But where to obtain one?

Even before war had broken out, Banting had been corresponding with eminent scientists in this country about how he and his colleagues might be able to help in the event of a conflict. Among those with whom he established a correspondence was Professor Bartlett, the Professor of Psychology at Cambridge and a member of the FPRC, and Professor Mellanby himself, the Committee's chairman. It is indicative of the obsession with secrecy that war brings that, despite all that Britain had to gain from these exchanges, informal interchange between members of the FPRC and Professor Banting and his team was banned. Surprisingly Whittingham, despite his abhorrence of red tape, was nevertheless always a powerful supporter of maintaining complete secrecy – about everything – which certainly irritated Matthews. On this particular occasion it caused a great deal of embarrassment on both sides of the Atlantic. Nevertheless, the FPRC went some way towards making amends by inviting Professor Banting to visit the UK. During his visit, made in the spring of 1940, he described Franks' work with the water-filled suit and explained how progress was being held back by the lack of a suitable aircraft. The RAF agreed to provide a Spitfire to further the test programme. This duly arrived in Canada, but at the same time as a signal saying that it was to be returned to the UK within the next few days – because of the Dunkirk situation. But not before an RAF Wing Commander called D'Arcy A. Greig, who happened to be in Canada at the time, had been invited to carry out a few tests on a suit Franks made especially for him.

Greig flew several test flights in the few days that were available, and although he found the suit cumbersome and uncomfortable, it most definitely worked.[9] On one occasion the acceleration developed during recovery from a dive was in excess of 8g – and he did not black out. He strongly recommended that further development work should be carried out. At this point, however, there were no offers of help from the British, and Franks concluded that, if work was to continue and if no aircraft were to be made available, then he must have a centrifuge. Professor Banting successfully persuaded the Canadian government to provide $25,000 to fund the project, and a centrifuge was built in Toronto at what would become the Canadian Institute of Aviation Medicine. However, it was not commissioned until early 1942, and in the meantime the Canadian Air Force agreed to continue with an aircraft testing programme. In the spring of 1941 Franks himself, now a Flight Lieutenant in the Royal Canadian Air Force, came over to the UK to demonstrate his suit and assist in its development. Flight tests were carried out at the Physiological Laboratory by Stewart and his team. The tests had been preceded by tragedy, however. In February 1941 Banting had lost his life in an aeroplane accident over Newfoundland whilst travelling to England to discuss the progress of the Anglo-Canadian medical research programme; high on his list of priorities had been the further development of the Franks suit within the UK. A courageous and brilliant man, and a world celebrity, his loss was keenly felt, no less in this country than in Canada.

By the time the Physiological Laboratory became involved in the flight testing of the suit, Franks had been working on it for well over a year. The problems with which he was grappling mainly concerned the distribution of the water-filled bladders, how much water they should contain and the best fabrics to use. Basically there was an inner lining of rayon to which rubber bladders were attached. These bladders were part of a rubber interlining supported by straps over the shoulders. The problem was to locate them so that the contained water applied the necessary counterpressure in the right places but did not restrict movement. There were none over the calves, because pressure here caused considerable discomfort; they were positioned over the thighs and trunk, and also over the feet, where later they were to cause problems. The greatest difficulties arose, however, with the outer layer. This had to be inextensible, yet flexible, and fit tightly around the body; in other words, individual sizing was necessary. With the early prototype suits this was achieved by actually tailoring each suit on the subject, the canvas material used being secured with pins and paper-clips. Zip-fasteners then replaced the clips. It was important to fit the canvas outer layer with the subjects in a position which allowed the tightest possible fit to be obtained. To facilitate movement, the zippers, which were obviously fastened prior to flight, could be loosened and the complete assembly could be worn under a uniform.

The laboratory flight trials were completed in July 1941, and shortly afterwards two operational squadrons carried out a preliminary service trial. The reports from all the participating pilots were favourable, the only real complaint being that the suits were hot to wear, causing profuse sweating. There was no doubt that black-out thresholds were raised, sometimes by as much as 3g and that, furthermore, the fatigue associated with high g manoeuvres was considerably reduced.

A very significant benefit which accrued from the 1941 trials was the experience gained by the Physiological Laboratory in actually making the anti-g suits. Franks himself, who was to remain at the Laboratory for a full year, had extensively modified the design of the suit and the technique used to manufacture the latex rubber bladders. Consequently by September of that year the Laboratory was able to recommend that a contract be placed for the manufacture of the suits. This was negotiated with the Dunlop Rubber Company by the MAP; a representative of Dunlop's, a Mr W. Gorham, had been called in by the Physiological Laboratory to help Franks earlier in the year, and so the firm was well aware of the potential manufacturing problems. These were considerable, but their solution was aided by the attachment of Franks to the production team as the senior service representative. So, by the end of the year fifty suits, made in three sizes, were ready for trial. However, whilst the suits were being made, the Canadian centrifuge entered service, and several basic flaws in the suit design became apparent which had not been revealed in the aircraft trials. Most important was that the three-size range was inadequate, a tight fit being of crucial importance. In the flight trials Franks had sized each suit to the individual pilot's specification, and so a tight fit was ensured; not so with just three pre-determined sizes. Consequently the Mark I Franks Flying Suit, as it was now officially known, not only never entered service but was actually destroyed as being useless!

During the early months of 1942 various modifications were made to the original specification and tested both in flight by the Physiological Laboratory and on the Canadian centrifuge. Alterations were frequent, and this was an exasperating time for everyone involved in the programme, not least for the Dunlop Rubber Company. As a result of body measurements taken from 750 aircrew, a seven-size range was agreed, and full production of the Mark II Franks Flying Suit began in the middle of the year. Flight trials revealed two problems – the feet tended to slide off the rudder bar under high g, and there was also a general loss of sensation through the boots because of the water-filled lining. The boots were discarded, and the Mark II Franks Flying Suit became the Mark III.

From this point on, the story becomes less clear. At least eight thousand and possibly more suits were eventually manufactured, but few, if any, appear to have been used in aircraft operations. Franks, by this time a Squadron Leader, was in charge of what became an extended trials programme, for, officially, the Franks Flying Suit never entered service. The problem was that by 1942 there were clear signs that an alternative to the Franks suit, based on air-filled rather than water-filled bladders, might provide a simpler solution. This notion of simplicity is important, because the Franks suit was a complicated and therefore expensive piece of kit. It was fine in the air, doing its job well, but only provided that exactly the right amount of water was used; on the ground it was hot, bulky and cumbersome and had to be filled before use and emptied after.

The suit was only little used by squadrons of RAF Fighter Command, mainly because of a fear that the large gain in black-out threshold achieved might tempt the pilots to exceed the structural limitations of their aircraft. However, the Navy appeared to have no such qualms; the Mark III suit was issued for trial to the Fleet Air Arm and, as we have seen, used in operations against the enemy in French North Africa. By July 1943 some 150 Royal Naval pilots had used the suit, and it was generally agreed that it was a great advantage. Another factor which certainly did not help getting the Franks suit into service was the continued obsession with secrecy.

The Fleet Air Arm, despite the successful action at Oran, was now forbidden to use the suit over enemy territory – which, at this stage of the war, made it pretty redundant![10] Secrecy restricted the RAF units which could be issued with the suit to a mere handful, and prevented the dissemination of information regarding the suit's undoubted value. For example, the Physiological Laboratory, despite the fact that it had been instrumental in developing, producing and testing the suits, found it very difficult to secure copies of the Fleet Air Arm's trial reports. Matthews expressed the view that the secrecy restrictions were killing enthusiasm. The veil of secrecy was partially lifted in 1944, when the suit was finally passed for operations. But, the ultimate irony, it was no longer needed! Results from the later trials all suggested that, whilst the suit worked well, the advantages it offered were really not necessary for the type of combat operations then being flown.[11] The truth was that g- protection was needed most during the Battle of Britain, and thereafter the requirement for protection steadily diminished.

The idea for the air-operated anti-g suits also came from abroad – from Australia. It was conceived by Frank Stanley Cotton, a Research Professor of Physiology at the University of Sydney. Although basically an exercise physiologist with a keen interest in sport, Cotton was also concerned with the physiological effects of gravity, and his ideas on means of protecting fighter aircrew attracted the interest of the Royal Australian Air Force (RAAF) – so much so, in fact, that by 1942 he had acquired a centrifuge, installed at the University by the Air Force, to test his suit, development of which had begun late in 1940.

This suit, which Cotton called a 'pneumo-dynamic suit', was a two-piece gradient pressure-garment made, like the Franks suit, from rubber and an outer layer of inextensible fabric. In order to simulate the increasing blood-pressure gradient from the waist to the feet (accomplished simply and automatically by the water in the Franks Flying Suit), the suit was divided into a series of six overlapping bladders which extended from ankles to thighs, these being filled with air from a high-pressure reservoir through a reducing valve. Six automatic valves gave pressures from fifty-five to eighty-five millimetres of mercury per g with the pressure gradient increasing from the thighs down. To reach this stage of development took Cotton about one year, and by the end of 1941 his suit was ready for aircraft trials with the RAAF. A suit was also sent to the RAF Physiological Laboratory for evaluation. Stewart was unenthusiastic,[12] not because it failed to provide g-protection – it did, perhaps more than the Franks Flying Suit – but because the latter was already at an advanced stage of development, and there could be no justification for pursuing two independent approaches to a problem which was already, from an operational point of view, diminishing in importance. Stewart wrote that 'the pneumo-dynamic suit has no possible application at the present moment', although he acknowledged the concept was both good and sound and that it should be pursued further – but by the RAAF and not by the RAF. In fact, the suit did have several very serious disadvantages: first, it was hot and, like the Franks suit, heavy, cumbersome and uncomfortable; second, the suit's pressure-supply system was complex and required the installation of heavy and elaborate equipment into the aircraft cockpit – the suit and supply system weighed over fifty pounds. Also, the air-pumps operated from the aircraft engines. Therefore, not only did they take power from the engines but also their performance fell with increasing altitude. Both of these problems were later overcome by replacing the air-pumps with a carbon dioxide inflation system. Nevertheless, from a historical viewpoint, it was most unfortunate that the development of what was probably the world's first air-operated anti-g suit should have begun a year after Franks had started work on his hydrostatic suit and, more significantly, after the RAF had placed a contract for manufacture of the suit. For it was to be with the air-operated suit that the future lay.

Cotton must have been disappointed with the rejection of his suit by Stewart and his team at Farnborough. Nevertheless, the RAAF continued to support him, mainly as a result of the favourable outcome of trials conducted in mid 1942. A contract was placed with an Australian firm, and by late 1943 the Cotton pneumo-dynamic gradient-pressure anti-g suit was being worn by Spitfire pilots flying from Darwin. Even then, however, the suits were never properly tested under actual combat conditions.[13] Although they were excellent in dogfighting manoeuvres, the pilots were not permitted to dogfight because the performance of their ageing Spitfire aircraft was inferior to that of the Japanese aircraft. Anyway, by late 1943 enemy fighters over Darwin had become unusual.

In complete contrast to the ambivalent British attitude towards g-protection, the Americans, after Pearl Harbor, concentrated much of their attention on this particular problem. From mid 1942 to the end of the war the anti-g suit story becomes increasingly American, and the Physiological Laboratory at Farnborough was involved in testing and evaluating the various types of suit as they became available. The Americans started off with one big advantage – familiarity with both the Franks Flying Suit and the Cotton pneumo-dynamic suit. As a result of extensive centrifuge studies, it was established that air-pressure was just as effective as water in providing g-protection, that a gradient pressure offered no advantage over a single pressure and that the amount of protection afforded was determined by both the bladder size and the inflation pressure.

By containing the bladders within relatively inextensible fabric, pressure is exerted on the underlying skin both directly and indirectly as the inflating bladders tension the fabric surrounding the legs and abdomen. These discoveries and developments led to the development of anti-g suits which were, in all important respects, the same as those in use today. Modifications have been made from time to time, usually for the same reasons – to improve the mobility of the wearer, reduce the heat load and generally try to make what has to be a tight-fitting garment as comfortable as possible.

The first of the American single-pressure suits was made by the Spencer-Berger Company, and it was very well received in both America and Britain. According to Davidson, the suit and inflation system represented 'the most practical anti-g outfit tested so far, and shows a great advance on previous endeavours in this field'.[14] The g-valve which controlled the rate of inflation, and the pressure of inflation of the bladders, was particularly singled out for praise. In the future, refinement of g-valve function would be a continuing objective of acceleration research.

It was quickly appreciated, both at Farnborough and in America, that the single-pressure, or G_2 suit (the G_1 had been an imitation of Cotton's gradient pressure-suit), could be further simplified by locating the air bladders in a skeleton type of suit, thereby eliminating the full coverall. The result was a suit weighing less than three pounds, which was comfortable to wear at all times and, most important of all, a lot cooler. At Farnborough the G_2 suit formed the basis of the RAF Type 1 anti-g suit. Essentially this comprised trousers containing bladders connected by rubber tubing. Comfort problems led to the use of softer rubber for the tubing in what became the Type 2 suit. The g-valve was American, produced by the Spencer-Berger firm, and pressurization was provided by a pump powered from the aircraft engine. A rather simpler scheme for inflation of the suit however, was the system devised by Cadzow for his (unsuccessful) pneumatic belt. The pilot sat on an air-filled cushion and, as his weight increased as he 'pulled g', so the cushion supplied an air-pressure to the suit which was directly proportional to the magnitude of the g-force. This principle was eventually to be adopted for all British anti-g devices, although, instead of a cushion, a loaded spring regulated the pressure delivered through the anti-g valve.

Despite all the work by Stewart and his team, the war was over before the RAF Types 1 and 2 anti-g suits became generally available, and no anti-g suit saw operational service with the RAF during the war. Writing shortly afterwards, Stewart noted that '... so far as the R.A.F. was concerned, blacking-out did not provide any limitation to any form of operational activity ...'[15] – and this from the man who had been responsible for the RAF's entire acceleration research programme! The American experience was rather different, however. As early as the summer of 1944, when anti-g suits had been available for only a few months, the Americans considered that they had 'proven their tactical usefulness'. A year later, statistics were made available showing that anti-g suits had greatly reduced the incidence of grey-out and black-out and that consequently tighter turns could be made. Fatigue was reduced and, most significantly, there was a direct relationship between the use of the suits and the number of enemy aircraft shot down in air-to-air combat.[16] In the final analysis, therefore, perhaps Stewart was mistaken and Matthews right – had anti-g suits been available, some operational activities might have been carried out more effectively; only a comparative study with and without the suits would have provided the answer, and this the British, in contrast to the Americans, did not carry out. Many years later, Group Captain Ruffell-Smith observed that the successful British fighter pilots were not interested in anti-g suits because they had a high g-tolerance anyway; those who were not successful were shot down!

The RAF's lack of enthusiasm for anti-g suits continued for some years after the war. Indeed, they did not become an integral part of the fighter pilot's flying clothing assembly until 1954, when the Hawker Hunter aircraft was introduced into service. The reason for this lies with the types of fighter aircraft which were then being flown by the RAF. These were the Gloster Meteor, which was the only British jet aircraft to fly operationally in World War II, and, introduced soon after the war, the de Havilland Vampire. Because both were relatively low-performance aircraft and because flying training no longer had to meet the demanding exigencies of wartime, there was little need for g-suits. Also, when the early single pressure-suits had been given an extensive service trial in 1945, they had been viewed with some scepticism by the pilots concerned. It should come as no surprise, therefore, that little research into anti-g devices was conducted at the IAM in the immediate post-war period. As Stewart pointed out, 'The Operational Requirements Branch do not consider that simple devices such as anti-g suits are of value on modern aircraft ....'[17] By then he was a Wing Commander and Head of the RAF Institute of Aviation Medicine. Whether this echo from the past reflected what Stewart himself believed, or whether he was just citing the 'official line', is not clear. Certainly at that time his research interest was directed more towards defining tolerable limits for ejection than towards anti-g suits.

To be fair, in 1948 it was not too difficult to justify the 'official line'. The war was over, and with it any need for pilots to 'pull' the high-g manoeuvres of dogfighting and dive-bombing. Furthermore, the economic prospect facing the country was bleak; this was a time of ration books, food- and fuel-shortages and unemployment as the Armed Forces demobilized – hardly an atmosphere conducive towards research of any sort, and particularly military research. But all this was about to change. Radical and far-reaching decisions were being taken which would change the face not just of Britain but of all western Europe. The Marshall Plan transformed economic climate, whilst the Berlin Blockade abruptly transformed the euphoria of peace into a grim realization that international relations were really little better than they had been ten years before. Both the Marshall Plan and the decision to airlift supplies to Berlin were good news for the IAM. Any doubt that Britain no longer needed an efficient and effective Air Force was dispelled, and there was also the hope that it might now be able to afford one! That Britain did not have an effective Air Force was demonstrated forcibly just a couple of years later, with the abysmal performance of the Meteor and Vampire in the Korean War. So hopeless were they that Britain was forced to make a hurried purchase of Sabres from Canada. Furthermore, the Korean War quickly proved that the day of the dogfight was most certainly not over and that the high-g manoeuvres typical of dogfighting would be performed by much faster, supersonic, jet aircraft. G-protection had become, and was to remain, a matter of crucial importance.

There were two types of anti-g suit available for RAF pilots at that time, both manufactured by the Dunlop Rubber Company. The Type 2 was still being used, but it had been joined by the Type 3, which was a copy of an American skeleton-type and, in contrast to the Type 2, was designed to be worn over the pilot's flying clothing. However, by 1951 both had been in service for nearly six years, and during that time aircraft had changed from subsonic to transonic and supersonic. So that year, stimulated by events in the Far East, a major re-appraisal of anti-g suits was undertaken jointly by the IAM and the Central Fighter Establishment, with the object of developing an improved anti-g suit for use in the new generation of fighter aircraft – specifically, in fact, for the Hunter and the recently acquired Sabres. The Types 2 and 3 were now known, somewhat confusingly, as the Marks 1 and 2 respectively. The disparity arises because the original Type 1 had never been produced as an official item of aircrew clothing, and the term 'Mark' is restricted, at least in theory, to production versions, whilst 'Type' refers to pre-production prototypes. In practice, the terms tend to be used interchangeably in much of the official literature relating to flying clothing.

It was quickly discovered that the suits, when inflated, were very uncomfortable, pinching the skin and compressing the lower ribs. Furthermore, the double air-entry system of the Mark 2 was incompatible with the g-valves used in American aircraft. In the space of three months the suit had been modified by replacing the two abdominal bladders with one, and re-trialled as the Mark 3. Unfortunately it was then found that restrictions at the knees and waist made walking uncomfortable and climbing into the cockpit difficult. So it was back to the drawing-board. What eventually emerged, following extensive liaison between the IAM and Dunlop Special Products, was the Mark 4, which was essentially just a cut-away version of the Mark 3. All unnecessary covering material had been removed so that the crutch, knees and back were uncovered. In subsequent trials with the RAF and the Navy, the new anti-g suit was well received, and shortly afterwards the Marks 1 and 2 were officially withdrawn in favour of the Mark 4 and the Mark 5, identical to the 4 except that the air-inlet hose for suit inflation was on the opposite side to cater for other types of aircraft.

During the early 1960s a requirement arose for an anti-g suit which would integrate better with the Lightning AEA. Also, the Marks 4 and 5 were proving unsatisfactory in some respects. Particularly when worn during operations in the Middle and Far East (those were the days when Britain still had extensive defence commitments outside Europe), the suits were hot and uncomfortable. In addition, the heavy rubber bladders were not proving very robust, and a new material for them was needed.

So in 1962 Frankenstein, in association with Squadron Leader (now Group Captain) Tony Nicholson of the IAM, undertook a development programme to investigate suitable fabrics for the next generation of anti-g suits. The outcome of this programme was a garment of lightweight terylene plain weave, with the heavy rubber bladders of the Marks 4 and 5 replaced by bladders of lightweight neoprene-impregnated nylon fabric. Early prototypes, including one version with detachable bladders (to facilitate laundering), were evaluated on the IAM centrifuge, but once the basic design had been agreed, and it had been shown that the proposed new suit provided adequate g-protection, the opinions of operational aircrew were sought. Particularly important was that the garment should prove acceptable to aircrew operating in hot climates. Many minor modifications were made before Frankenstein went ahead and produced the Marks 6 and 7 anti-g suit. The success of this extremely thorough and well-planned development programme, which was essentially complete by 1965, is demonstrated by the fact that the Marks 6 and 7 are still the standard-issue internally worn anti-g suits of the RAF.

To bring the g-suit story to a close, brief mention should be made of the work carried out at the IAM between 1970 and 1975 on external anti-g suits. These represent an attempt to get over the old problems of discomfort, encumbrance and heat load when the suit is worn for long periods on the ground. The research programme was prompted by British RAF aircrews in Germany noticing that the Americans had externally worn anti-g suits, so why couldn't they! Harrier pilots were particularly vociferous in their complaints, since they are frequently engaged in operations away from their base, where dressing facilities are often poor; they are obliged, therefore, to wear the same clothing for far longer than other aircrew. So centrifuge studies were conducted with an external anti-g suit employing the same bladder system as the Marks 6 and 7. Provided that only thin clothing, such as the standard flying coverall, was worn beneath the suit, then there was no demonstrable reduction in the amount of g-protection provided. There was, however, a significant degradation if thick clothing, such as a cold-weather coverall, was worn. Consequently, whilst the external anti-g suit is now in full service use, it is only worn over the minimum of flying clothing if high levels of acceleration are expected. Nevertheless, the external anti-g suit does represent an almost unique item of aircrew clothing, for one very good reason – it seems to be universally popular!

Although the area covered by the bladders of the anti-g suit, and the amount of pressure exerted, both determine the degree of protection provided against black-out, during combat manoeuvres 'g' can be 'pulled' extremely quickly, and so the bladders have to be inflated just as quickly if the applied pressure is to be effective in enabling blood-flow to the eyes and brain to be maintained. The device that provides the right pressure at the right time is the anti-g valve. Whilst g-valve design is more the province of engineers than of doctors and physiologists, the design specifications are determined by physiological considerations, and so each new type has to be extensively tested under realistic operational conditions. Indeed, the main reason why both g-valves and anti-g suits were to prove safe and reliable in service, particularly when compared with the oxygen-supply systems of this period, was the very intensive ground and flight testing carried out, and also the meticulous quality control on the production line.[18] Although preliminary evaluations could be carried out on a small centrifuge that the RAE possessed, with the valve mounted on a dummy, most testing was carried out in aircraft. Three men in particular were involved in this work: Mr G.R. Allen, an RAE engineer, Squadron Leader (later Group Captain) J. Howitt, an IAM doctor and pilot, and Surgeon Lieutenant (now Surgeon Vice-Admiral Sir John) Rawlins, also of the IAM. Each of these men was to make significant contributions to aviation medicine over the next two decades: Allen, with his work on oxygen systems, air-ventilated suits and integrated AEAs; Howitt, with his work for both the RAF and the Civil Aviation Authority on in-flight physiological monitoring; and Rawlins with his work on underwater ejection.

As Howitt later recalled, these flight tests of anti-g valves demanded manoeuvres pulling more 'g' than was being experienced by any other pilots in the UK at that time. Each prototype had to be tested over a range from 1 to 8g, and the appropriate g-level had to be sustained whilst note was made of the precise g-level and the pressure in the anti-g suit. So difficult was it to maintain the acceleration and look at the instruments that eventually a camera was fixed behind Howitt's head to record the necessary data – just as in Stewart's experiments ten years before. Squadron Leader Howitt first became involved in g-suit and g-valve flight testing in 1948, when the Institute's aircraft was a Mark 9 Spitfire. Ironically this Mark of Spitfire was rather less tolerant of high-g loads than other Marks and certainly resented 8g turns – the wings tended to buckle! Perhaps it was just as well that the other IAM pilot at that time, Wing Commander Ruffell-Smith, 'wrote the aircraft off' when forced to land with a retracted undercarriage. The Spitfire 21, which replaced the 9, was rated to a very high g-level. Subsequently, until the IAM centrifuge came into operation in 1955, Meteor and Vampire aircraft were used for the trials. Then flight trials were needed only as a final test stage in the development programme.

The object of the flight trials was to make sure that, at any g-level, the bladders of the anti-g trousers were filled with gas at the right pressure at the right time. Precisely when, and how quickly, the anti-g suit should be inflated have always been difficult problems to resolve. Too early is wasteful of gas, and too late can mean black-out. Too quickly, and the abdominal bladder can give a severe 'punch to the stomach', which can be not only disconcerting but also dangerously distracting if it occurs at a low level of g. Too slowly, and vision starts to fade before the bladders start to inflate. And related to the problem of rate of inflation is the question of at what g-level to begin inflation. Both of these issues have been the subject of an intensive research effort at the IAM during the 1960s and 1970s. Without the centrifuge, this research would have been impossible, as the alternative, aircraft testing, would have been prohibitively expensive.

This impressive machine, which took five years to build, comprises a horizontal arm, 60 feet in diameter, at each end of which is mounted a car, or 'gondola', weighing 1,150 pounds. The gondolas are stressed to withstand 120g, or four times the upper operational limit, and swing out passively during rotation of the arm, so that the vertical axis of the gondola is in line with the resultant acceleration. They can also be detached from the ends of the arm and mounted at radii of 25, 20, 15 and 10 feet, so allowing the effects of different angular accelerations, at a given centrifugal acceleration, to be studied. Or, they can be removed completely and replaced by 'end-barriers'. These are fixed, open-ended compartments consisting of just a floor, with 'Dunlopillo'-padded end and side walls. The arm of the centrifuge is supported by a 12-ton fly-wheel, which is attached directly to the shaft of a vertically mounted electric motor. This 1,350 h.p. motor can provide a maximum 30g acceleration in 9 seconds, equivalent to a speed of 115 m.p.h., whilst a regenerative braking-system can bring the arm to rest in the same time.

In a typical 'run' the subject sits (or lies) in the gondola, strapped firmly and securely into a seat. Measurements can be made during centrifugation of a variety of physiological variables, such as heart and respiration rate, blood-pressure and even the amount of blood going to specific organs of the body such as the lungs. Most commonly, however, it is the grey-out or black-out thresholds which are being determined, and this is done using peripherally and centrally located signal lights. The subject is required to fix his gaze on the central light and to keep extinguishing the peripheral lights by pressing a button. Once cancelled, they are switched on again, and once more have to be extinguished by the subject. If the subject 'greys out', he can no longer see the peripheral lights and so no longer presses his button to cancel them. At this point, if the black-out threshold is also required, the process is repeated with the central light. In practice it may take several 'runs' on the centrifuge before the thresholds are identified – particularly if the subject has a high g-tolerance. For some subjects this is a nauseating and distressing business, whilst for others it is exhilarating and exciting.

During all experiments involving human subjects, an observer is seated near to the centre of rotation. He has responsibility for the safety of the subject. In the early days only the observer could see the subject and note his reactions to g, but now TV monitors in control and observation rooms provide a full-colour close-up of the subject. Even today, however, in the most straightforward determination of grey-out threshold, the observer is still a vitally important person and must always be prepared for the unexpected. What he particularly watches out for is the subject completely losing consciousness. A number of individuals, for reasons that are not entirely clear, tend to have fits of varying degrees of severity as they recover from unconsciousness. This can be extremely distressing to all concerned and is avoided if at all possible by starting determination of g-tolerance at a low level and then working up to the threshold value. The average relaxed grey-out threshold is 4.1g and the average black-out threshold 4.7g. Anti-g suits raise these thresholds by, at the most, some 25 per cent; today's aircraft are capable of sustained turn rates which produce accelerations well above human tolerance, even with anti-g trousers. Furthermore, anti-g suits provide no protection against negative acceleration – which perhaps is so rarely experienced because pilots usually try to avoid negative-g manoeuvres. Then there is the discomfort and the increased heat load, as already mentioned. In other words, anti-g suits represent a far from ideal solution to the problem of g-protection. An alternative approach, at least theoretically, is for pilots to adopt a horizontal position within the aircraft, so converting headward acceleration into transverse (i.e. across-the-body) acceleration. The Germans carried out some experiments using modified gliders, one of which fell into British hands after the war. There was even a rumour that Heinkel aircraft were being built with prone positions for both pilot and observer, and this German research had prompted a preliminary study by Stewart, in 1941, of the possibilities of prone-position flying.[19] However, this had revealed two apparently insuperable difficulties; first, the visual field was restricted – a very serious handicap when you are on the look-out for an enemy, and second, lying face down on the couch was very uncomfortable. Primarily for these reasons, plans for design of a practical installation for aircraft and for flight trials were abandoned (although the Italians did develop a single prototype prone-position fighter, the Savoia-Marchetti SM 93, which was flown in 1944).

They were soon to be resurrected, however. The Germans prone-position glider was taken to the RAE where, in 1946, it was given a thorough examination and flight trial by staff from both the RAE and the IAM. It became clear that the Germans had spent considerable time working on the problem and that prone-position flying probably was regarded by them as a practical proposition. Certainly the matter seemed worthy of further investigation, particularly as the semi-kneeling position which had to be adopted in the glider was found to be surprisingly comfortable both in flight and in ground trials. Unfortunately, at this time blacking out was, as we have seen, no longer considered to be an important operational problem, and so further developments had to await a more favourable opportunity. As it happened, it was not to be greatly superior g-tolerance afforded by the prone position which reawakened 'official interest' but the possibility that, for extremely high-performance aircraft, a very small frontal area, with no 'bulge' for the cockpit canopy, might be necessary; this would, inevitably, mean a prone-position seat.[20] The Gloster Aircraft Company Ltd took up this idea in the late 1940s when they were contracted by the Ministry of Supply to build a rocket-propelled fighter aircraft. Consequently the Institute was instructed to carry out research into likely physiological and other human factor problems.

The first requirement was to obtain an aircraft. As it happened, the Air Ministry had a trainer surplus to requirements and agreed to loan it to the IAM. This aircraft was the RS3 Desford, one of only two aircraft ever built by Reid & Sigrist Ltd, a firm specializing in the manufacture of instruments, which had established an aircraft department at Desford in 1938. The Desford was a two-seat pilot-trainer suitable for the complete novice. With a maximum speed of 162 miles per hour, it was far removed from the rocket-powered fighter for which the prone position was being investigated. Indeed, it is difficult to imagine why the Institute should have considered the aircraft suitable for their requirements. Perhaps it was because the Air Ministry had a vested interest, intending it to be used for training pilots in prone-position flying.

First of all the Desford had to be converted for prone-position flying. The conversion was carried out, to IAM specification, by Reid & Sigrist. Substantial modifications were needed, and these were to take two years. The cockpit had to be extended to accommodate a couch, and much of the instrumentation and control system had to be re-arranged. So changed was the Desford that it was re-designated the RS4 Bobsleigh.

When the Desford eventually did arrive at Farnborough, one of the first to fly it was Wing Commander Ruffell-Smith. Several problems quickly became apparent. The principal one concerned the layout of the instrument panel – a subject on which Ruffell-Smith was an expert. Not only were the pilot's eyes too close to the instruments but also, because his head was relatively fixed, it was difficult to see them all. Any attempt to move the head caused the neck to ache, despite the provision of a chin rest. When rough air was encountered and the going got bumpy, flying the aircraft became virtually impossible.[21]

In any event, the Desford was totally incapable of providing any information about the increased protection to acceleration provided by the prone position, and it was this aspect which primarily interested the IAM. The aircraft also had a low-altitude ceiling, and so none of the potential difficulties of high-altitude flying in the prone position could be investigated – such as the use of pressure suits or pressure breathing. As Group Captain Stewart observed, what was needed was a fast jet; a Meteor, suitably modified, would be ideal, so a formal application was made for just such an aircraft.

Tied as the prone-position research programme was to the

proposed Gloster Rocket Fighter, a contract was agreed between the Ministry of Supply and W.G. Armstrong Whitworth Aircraft Ltd, who were manufacturing Meteors under licence on behalf of the Gloster Aircraft Company, for the necessary modifications to be made to a Meteor 8, and all seemed set fair for flight experiments in the summer of 1953. Then the Gloster project was cancelled, and the Ministry suspended the contract. Fortunately the conversion programme was so far advanced that Armstrong Whitworth decided that the aircraft should be completed so that research into the implications of the prone piloting of jet aircraft could still be undertaken. The firm's motives were not totally altruistic; aircraft designers were still musing over the possibilities of prone piloting, and to be first in the field could only have been advantageous. So it came about that on 31 August 1954 a very strange Meteor aircraft was delivered to the Flight Section of the RAF Institute of Aviation Medicine. The nose had been modified to take a prone pilot, with a normally seated pilot behind, just as in the Desford. All controls had been made power-assisted to reduce the physical load on the pilot, and, compared with the Desford, the layout of the instruments was much improved. The couch was of foam rubber covered with leather, on a tubular steel frame. At the head-end was a V-shaped chin-rest, and on either side the couch was moulded to the pilot's shoulders. Adjustments to the couch could be made to vary eye level, thigh and leg angle and position, and foot position.

Actually installing oneself in the prone-position cockpit was not too difficult, although assistance was sometimes necessary to place the feet on the organ-type rudder pedals. However, once strapped in, it was impossible to move the arms from the padded side-rests or to move the head upwards or sideways. The pilot had virtually no muscle power available – hence the need for the power-assisted controls. If the discomfort of being trussed up in this manner for an hour or more was not enough, the aircraft was not pressurized, and the draughty nose-wheel bay formed part of the front cockpit, which made it 'unbelievably cold'. Yet it was far from being all bad. The trial team found no difficulty in piloting the aircraft, and in smooth air the prone position was described as 'a most comfortable and relaxing position for flying'.[22] Taxying, take-off and landing presented few problems, although the restricted sideways vision was irritating. The restricted vision became a serious problem, however, when navigating across country; even simply folding a map became a major undertaking. This led to an attempt by Squadron Leader (later

Group Captain) Tom Whiteside, soon to become the Institute's acknowledged expert on all problems of applied vision, and Wing Commander Ruffell-Smith to devise a moving map driven at the (scaled) speed of the aircraft. The worst problem of all was, as in the Desford, the effect of turbulence, which produced intense discomfort. So serious was this that piloting at low level was totally impossible; the chin continually banged on the chin-rest, making navigation even more difficult. On the other hand, g-tolerance was very considerably enhanced, to a point which exceeded the 6½g structural limitation of the aircraft – perhaps a dubious asset!

In all, ninety-nine sorties, lasting a total of fifty-five hours, had been flown when the trial finished in July 1955. And the end of the trial marks the end of the prone-position story, at least in the UK. Both the Desford and the Meteor flights had shown the prone position to be perfectly feasible, but the overall conclusion was that it should be adopted only if the aerodynamic advantages were overriding; as subsequent developments in supersonic flight have shown, they are not. Indeed, with hindsight it seems strange that the aerodynamic advantages of the prone position could ever have been seen as so overwhelming as to outweigh all the ergonomic disadvantages. Even more strange, perhaps, is that the two basic disadvantages, namely the discomfort and the reduced visual field, were exactly those identified by Stewart, using a mock-up of a prone-position cockpit, back in 1941.

This brings us to the final chapter of the g-protection story – reclined seats. If the prone position makes piloting an aircraft more difficult, then the supine position makes it impossible, at least without sophisticated, indirect visual aids. However, a degree of supination may be acceptable, and, as Stewart had found in 1940 when investigating a seat inclined at 45° to the vertical in a prototype Gloster aircraft, the gain in terms of increased g-threshold can be considerable. to quote Stewart: 'The most noteworthy effect ... was a marked degree of confidence and well being at values of g where complete black-outs had usually been experienced.'[23] The idea was investigated further by the Americans in the early 1950s, who actually carried out some flight tests in a F7F Tigercat aircraft modified to take a reclinable seat, and successfully demonstrated the feasibility of the concept. After that, however, little more work was done, and it was not until the 1970s that studies resumed on both sides of the Atlantic. The stimulus has undoubtedly been the inability of the anti-g suits to provide adequate protection against the high acceleration modern jet fighters can achieve and sustain. In the UK this work has been carried out at the IAM by Group Captain D.H. Glaister, in association with Squadron Leader B.J. Lisher. Attention has been focused on the relationship between the seat-back angle and the relaxed grey-out threshold. The main finding has been that the grey-out increases roughly in proportion to the seat-back angle. However, because forward vision is increasingly impaired as the seat angle moves further from the vertical, the maximum acceptable reclination is about 65° to the vertical.

Like the work on anti-g valves, the reclined-seat studies would not have been feasible – or at least would have been prohibitively expensive – without the centrifuge. So, too, would have been many of the other acceleration research programmes carried out over the last twenty-five years. Most notable of these have been the continuation and extension by Peter Howard of Stewart's work on the origin and nature of black-out, and the studies of the effects of acceleration on lung function by David Glaister. Some of Howard's experiments involved suspending subjects inside-down in the gondola whilst the centrifuge was rotating, so producing negative g. In others he actually measured, whilst the subject was spinning on the centrifuge, the amount of blood pumped out by the heart – the cardiac output. To do this he used what is known as the 'Fick Principle', which involves measuring the amount of oxygen consumed by the subjects, the oxygen content of arterial blood, and the oxygen content of venous blood. The first two measurements are fairly easily made, but the last involved inserting a catheter into the heart itself, in order to obtain samples of venous blood. Because, for safety reasons, the subject had to be accompanied by an observer, the gondolas were removed and the end barriers used for the experiments. Measurements were made on only two subjects, but these demonstrated that, contrary to some contemporary thinking, the output of the heart was reduced by the application of positive acceleration. Commenting afterwards on these heroic experiments, Howard admitted that, 'The conditions under which the experiments were performed were hardly conducive to the peace of mind of the subject.' It was perhaps appropriate that they should represent the culmination of his researches in this field!

David Glaister, by developing some highly sophisticated radioisotope techniques for use on the centrifuge, has shown that acceleration does impair lung function and that, if acceleration is combined with breathing pure oxygen, partial collapse of the lung can occur, causing pain and breathing difficulties. Apart from its obvious application to flying high-performance aircraft, Glaister's work has also led to a better understanding of lung function in certain diseases – the first step to finding a cure.

8 Down to Earth

The safest way down to earth from a disabled or out-of-control aircraft has always been by parachute. Unfortunately, as we have seen, during the First World War officialdom was seemingly oblivious of the parachute's great potential for saving lives, and undoubtedly some airmen must have died unnecessarily as a result. What is even more astounding is that nothing much was done for several years after the war; it was 1926 before the Irvin parachute was introduced into the RAF. Leslie Irving, the inventor, was an American who had spent much of the First World War designing and making parachutes, although it was not until 1919 that he received his first 'official' order – for three hundred from the US Army. Thereafter, however, success was assured, and his manually operated free-fall parachute was eventually adopted by many countries besides Britain. The adoption of the American parachute was, nevertheless, a serious blow to two Englishmen who for quite some time had been championing the parachute's cause against entrenched official hostility. True, Everard Calthorp's 'Guardian Angel', being of the attached type, stood little chance once the advantages and greater safety of the rip-cord free-fall type had been conclusively proven. Yet Colonel H.E.S. Holt's free-fall 'Autochute' was very similar to the Irvin chute, and it was British! The crucial factor was that the latter had proven its value during seven years of use in America.

As it happened, the Irvin parachute did soon become British. Leslie Irving settled in England and built a factory at Letchworth in Hertfordshire, where all his parachutes were manufactured. The business thrives today as Irvin Great Britain Ltd. By the early 1930s, however, two new and genuinely British names appeared on the parachute scene – James Gregory and Raymond Quilter. Quickly joining forces, these two powerful extroverts, with a common love of parachuting, claimed that the Irvin parachute was capable of considerable improvement. To prove their claim they formed, in

1934, the GQ Company and started producing parachutes. Making them was one thing, but selling them to an Air Ministry which was perfectly content with the ones it had was quite another! However, their opportunity was to come in 1940.

By that time paratroop training had begun at Ringway Airport, Manchester, and it was then, because of the large number of soldiers being trained, that it was noticed that an unacceptably high number of the Irvin parachutes were failing to open. The GQ Company was consulted and came up with a solution. In effect, the Irvin canopy was retained, but the packing system was completely redesigned, and the resulting parachute became known as the X-type. It was used with great success throughout the war. The accident rate at the Ringway Training Centre, which initially had been a horrific one in every hundred or so, had been reduced sixty-fold by 1942, and one thousand-fold three years later. It could doubtless have been reduced even further had trainee parachutists been provided with a reserve parachute as was done in America and Canada. The war would be long over before this eminently sensible idea was adopted by the British. It was argued that a reserve parachute was bad for morale, as the pupils might think that the parachute was likely to fail![1]

The X-type evolved as a result of incontrovertible evidence of the shortcomings of the Irvin parachute. No such evidence was available with regard to the parachutes used by Bomber and Fighter Commands. For the former, the B-5 was developed to be worn continuously in bomber aircraft, and it was accepted into service in large numbers following a single test drop at Henlow. Yet later tests showed it to be highly unsatisfactory in several respects. For the latter, no trials were ever conducted of the pilot-type parachutes, although one in every two or three thousand failed to open properly. There seems to have been a certain lack of vigour in the Air Ministry attitude towards parachutes!

Since the war, research into the mechanics of parachuting has resulted in larger, more elaborate and much safer parachutes. This is just as well, as escape from aircraft these days may be necessary at far higher altitudes and at far greater speeds than any experienced during World War II. At very high altitudes the main problem, hypoxia and cold apart, is the tremendous opening shock as the parachute deploys. Indeed, so great is the risk of causing damage to the parachute, and to the man, that above a certain altitude, usually between 10,000 and 20,000 feet, free-fall is adopted, with automatic release of the parachute rip-cord at the appropriate altitude by a pressure-sensitive mechanism. Free-fall, however, presents its own problems, spinning and tumbling, which can be so severe as to force blood into the limbs and away from the heart, resulting in ruptured blood-vessels, unconsciousness and even death. The solution has been to deploy, before the main parachute, a much smaller 'drogue' parachute, which stabilizes the man and holds him upright as he descends. As we shall see, this principle was adopted very early on by the Martin-Baker Aircraft Company in the design of ejection seats.

During World War II most aircrew wore, or had ready access to, parachutes. However, with the introduction of first jet fighter aircraft, and later jet bomber aircraft, speeds became so great that bale-out either over the side of the cockpit or through a hatch became virtually impossible. In fact, as information compiled from German sources showed, once aircraft speeds exceeded 200 m.p.h. the chances of making a successful escape were less than even. The only solution was to eject the aircraft seat, with its occupant, from the aircraft by means of an explosive device fitted to the seat. But this seemingly simple idea was fraught with difficulties, not least of which was the effect on the man of the very high rates of acceleration needed to throw the seat sufficiently far upwards to clear the aircraft structure.

The Germans appear to have been the first to study the problem in any detail. An untested catapult-type ejection seat was built in 1939 by the German firm Junkers, and during the course of the war seats were also built by Dornier and Focke-Wolf. The very first successful live ejection was, almost certainly, by the German test pilot Schenk, who was forced to abandon his aircraft after encountering icing problems on 13 January 1942. Subsequently about sixty ejections were made by pilots of the Luftwaffe, although how many of these were successful is not known.

Although the feasibility of seat ejection had also been under consideration in Britain, it was only in April 1944, following an accident when an RAF test pilot had been killed trying to escape from an early version of the Gloster Meteor, that the problem was examined in any detail. Later in the year two firms, the Martin-Baker Aircraft Company Ltd and M.L. Aviation Ltd, were invited by the MAP 'to investigate the practicability of providing fighter aircraft with a means of assisted escape for the pilot'.[2] Unfortunately M.L. Aviation's foray into assisted escape systems proved to be brief and traumatic, with a fatality on the first live ejection in 1947. In complete contrast, Martin-Baker, following their successful first live ejection, went on so to dominate the development of aircraft ejection seats that at least one authority, in apparent ignorance of the German work, cites James Martin, founder of the company, as being the inventor of the ejection seat.[3] Whilst this is not true, since 1947 the history of the ejection seat in the UK and the history of the Martin-Baker Aircraft Company have been virtually one and the same.

The MAP's invitation to Martin-Baker to develop an ejection seat had not been merely fortuitous, as the company was already doing much first-class work for the Ministry, especially in the field of explosives, a subject on which James (later Sir James) Martin himself was an expert. The firm had also been able to help the RAF with a problem it was having with the automatic jettisoning of the canopies of Spitfire aircraft – this being the sole provision made to enable pilots to escape; the canopy-release mechanism was failing to displace the canopy from the aircraft. Within a couple of weeks James Martin had developed a reliable mechanical device which unfastened the canopy from the fuselage, allowing it to be taken away by the slipstream. No more problems with automatic jettisoning were experienced.[4]

Preliminary experiments to try to determine the physiological consequences of abrupt accelerations began at the Physiological Laboratory late in 1944. Using the RAE rocket track, with subjects carried in a supinated seat mounted on the rocket-propelled trolley, Bill Stewart was able to produce peak accelerations of 12g in the first tenth of a second as the trolley was decelerated from a speed of 44 m.p.h. over a distance of 6 feet. The following year, however, the research programme was transferred to Martin-Baker's factory at Denham, and here a different technique was used to produce the desired abrupt accelerations, or 'jolts', as they are more descriptively known. A vertical test rig sixteen feet high was built in the form of a tripod, with one of the legs having guide-rails in which the ejection seat was located. The seat was fired up the rails by an explosive cartridge in a gun which consisted of two telescopic tubes, a series of ratchets in the rails preventing the seat from descending once it had reached the top of its travel. After some dummy trials one of the company's experimental fitters, Mr Bernard Lynch, experienced the first 'live ride', without mishap. In subsequent tests the explosive power of the cartridge was gradually increased, so that eventually the seat reached a height of 10 feet, compared with the 4 feet 8 inches of the first test. However, in reaching 10 feet, the rate of acceleration had been about 700g per second, and the volunteer subject, who unfortunately happened to be a reporter, suffered a compression fracture of the spine. Valuable lessons had been learned from the many test firings, however, and it became clear that three specific conditions had to be fulfilled if injuries to the back were not to occur. First, the peak acceleration should be no greater than 21g, and this peak should be sustained for no longer than one tenth of a second. Second, the imposed acceleration should not exceed 300g per second. And third, during the acceleration the subject should be firmly strapped upright so that adjacent spinal vertebrae were square to each other. These three factors are still basic design criteria for ejection seats. In later years, when the RAF was experiencing a much higher incidence of spinal fractures following ejection than their flying colleagues in the Royal Navy, the importance of the third factor was clearly demonstrated. Because for deck-landing and catapult launchings from aircraft carriers it was imperative that the pilot be firmly restrained, Navy pilots, when they were forced to eject, were better able to withstand the accelerative forces than the RAF pilots, many of whom undoubtedly wore their safety harnesses too loose or even incorrectly fitted.

The accident to the reporter prompted a redesign of the seat. To ensure that the rate of g onset was not excessively high, a two-cartridge gun was developed, one cartridge firing before the other, thus allowing the pressure generated in the ejection gun to build up more gradually. However, since the total pressure was actually increased, the seat started to overshoot the rails, and so a second rig, sixty-five feet high, had to be built before another 'live' shot could be made. By August 1945 the rig was complete, and Bernard Lynch again volunteered to be the first subject, being propelled to a height of twenty-six feet without injury. From about this point onwards, the research effort was directed mainly towards defining more precisely the physiological limits of jolt and the peak acceleration tolerable.

Most of the early physiological assessments of tolerance to the accelerations produced by ejection seats were purely subjective. Consequently the most useful subjects were those combining experience of short-duration accelerations with a physiological or medical background, which is why the IAM had always been involved in the ejection-seat research programme. In the early days at Martin-Baker's factory the IAM provided many of the subjects. Stewart was a 'regular', and newcomers to the Lab, like Tony Barwood, all 'had a go'. By mid-1947, however, most of the physiological work was being carried out at the RAE using a 110-foot vertical rig, built by Martin-Baker. The RAE needed its own rig because Mr Martin was not prepared (and the company maintains this policy still) to accept contract monitoring by 'the Ministry'. Squadron Leader (later Wing Commander) Freddie Latham took over the ejection work from Bill Stewart at about the time the RAE rig was commissioned, and was himself regularly 'fired'. In 1953 the rig was increased in length to 160 feet, increasing the maximum seat velocity attainable from 60 to 80 feet per second.

Physiological assessments have become more objective over the years, with emphasis being placed on ciné photography and on recording accelerometers attached at strategic points on clothing, equipment and seat. These provide a direct measure of both the rate of onset of the acceleration and the peak value of the g induced. Latham was particularly interested in the mechanical loads on the skeleton during ejection, and how these loads could be minimized by appropriate body alignment and restraint. He was able to show that the greater loads are consistently experienced at the base of the spine, in the lumbar region, which is exactly where many of the all too common compression fractures generally occur on ejection.

Although not really aviation medicine, the foregoing account would be incomplete without at least some mention of how British ejection seats have developed between 1945 and the present. In September 1945 Martin-Baker had received a contract from the MAP for the manufacture of two pilots' ejection seats. By this time the company had already carried out the first aircraft ejection in Great Britain when, on 10 May 1945, a seat loaded with sandbags had been ejected successfully from a Defiant aircraft. Once the double-cartridge ejection gun had fired the seat clear of the aircraft, a small stabilizing and retarding drogue parachute deployed, which itself then deployed a twenty-four-foot parachute which returned the seat safely to earth. Consequently the company was well prepared to proceed with installation of a prototype ejection seat in a Meteor III. After making the necessary modifications to the aircraft, several high-speed ejections were carried out using dummies. Then, on 24 July 1946, in the first live ejection outside Germany, Bernard Lynch ejected himself from the Meteor at 320 miles per hour and at an altitude of 8,000 feet. The system worked faultlessly, and, after releasing himself from the seat, he made a perfect landing. For the record, Lynch went on to make thirty more airborne test ejections and survived to enjoy a well-earned retirement many years later.

To allow for production on a quantity basis, the prototype seat was completely redesigned, and by June 1947 the Air Staff had decided to adopt what was to be the Mark 1 seat for installation in all new service jet aircraft. The first of fifty emergency ejections with the seat was made on 30 May 1949, when J.O. Lancaster, a test pilot with Armstrong Whitworth, ejected himself from a prototype Flying Wing that went out of control at 3,000 feet. Unfortunately, however, the seat did not prove so successful at low altitudes, as there was just too much for the pilot to do in too short a time. Indeed, it could not even be regarded as very successful at moderately low altitudes of 1,500 to 3,000 feet, where pilots were normally able to bail out manually without much risk, provided the speed was low enough. Furthermore, because the pilot had to unfasten the seat harness himself, he was unlikely to survive if he lost consciousness during the ejection. The company's response was to develop the world's first fully automatic aircraft escape system, which by 1953 was already entering service with the RAF as the Mark 2 Martin-Baker ejection seat; safe ejections were now possible from 500 feet.

Although the new automatic seat was generally successful, problems still arose at very low altitudes and very high speeds. Also, aircraft like the Javelin and the V-bombers were being introduced in the mid-1950s, and these had both high fin projections and high operating speeds. It was therefore necessary to increase the height attained during ejection in order to avoid collision with the fin – which at the same time improved the chance of successful ejection at low altitudes. The extra height was gained in the Mark 3 seat by increasing the stroke of the ejection gun, giving an ejection velocity of eighty feet per second, compared with the previous sixty feet per second. Also, since in both the Mark 1 and 2 seats problems had been experienced with leg flailing caused by wind blast, a leg-restraining system was incorporated, which operated automatically on ejection to hold the legs firmly against the seat. Finally improvements to the drogue system reduced the delay between ejection and the deployment of the main parachute from 5 to 3 seconds, and then to $1\frac{1}{2}$ seconds. This allowed the first live ground-level ejection to be attempted, which it was, successfully, by Squadron Leader J. Fifield, from a Meteor 7, on 3 September 1955.

Following the Mark 3 came the Marks 4 and 5, new designs of a seat which also eliminated the need for a separate seat harness. However, the performance of cartridge-operated ejections seats was approaching its limit. The major problem was that a forward speed of at least 100 m.p.h. was needed to give the seat a long enough flight time for full deployment of the main parachute. With prototype vertical take-off and landing (VTOL) aircraft already being put through their paces, escape would undoubtedly soon be necessary at speeds well below 100 m.p.h., and even from aircraft with no forward speed during the critical moments of vertical ascent and descent. So, with the power of the cartridges already pushed to their limit and with the stroke of the ejection guns as long as practically feasible, there was only one alternative left – rockets.

By March 1962 Martin-Baker had developed a rocket-assisted ejection seat which proved successful in tests on a specially designed rig and, using dummies, from aircraft both in the air and on the ground. A demonstration had even been given at the Paris Air Show the year before. What was needed now was a live test in the air, and the man who volunteered to carry out the test was Squadron Leader Peter Howard. Howard was well qualified for the job. In addition to his extensive experience of more prolonged accelerations, he had often been a subject on the ejection test-rigs, both at the RAE and at the company's factory. He was also a qualified parachutist. So on 13 March 1962 he fired himself from the back of a modified Meteor 7 – so modified, in fact, that it was referred to by the test team as the Meteor $7\frac{1}{2}$! The altitude was 250 feet, and the airspeed 290 m.p.h. The Mark 4 seat left the aircraft at a velocity of 80 feet per second, the 3,600 pounds of thrust over less than one fifth of a second giving a peak force of 16g. What it felt like is best described in the subject's own words:

> The first sensation was of the wind and turbulence acting on my face and arms, and to a lesser extent on my chest. I was conscious at this time that I was still being pushed upwards by the rocket, although there was at no time any of the violent jolt usually associated with ejection seats. The flame from the rocket was clearly visible between my feet, which indicates that, in spite of my efforts, my head had been thrown forward early in the sequence. This was confirmed by the development of a slightly stiff neck the next day.[5]

A stiff neck apart, the world's first rocket-assisted ejection from an aircraft in flight was remarkable for its comfort. As Peter Howard later commented, 'The greatest hazard of the whole venture was the risk of landing on top of Mr Martin's car!' But that, of course, was only apparent after the event. The risks had been considerable, as they are in any 'first', but so was the reward; the safety of rocket-assisted ejection seats had been proven. Rocket packs were fitted retrospectively to the Marks 4 and 5 seats, creating the Marks 6 and 7 respectively. A highly advanced rocket seat, the Mark 8, was developed for the TSR2, and although cancellation of the aircraft meant that the seat never entered service, many of its features were incorporated in the Marks 9 and 10. The former, which was fitted in Jaguar and Harrier aircraft, had superior performance and comfort (early ejection seats were notorious for their discomfort and for the backache they produced). The Mark 10 seat is used in Hawk, Tornado and Sea Harrier aircraft. Just as the development of the rocket seat can be seen as a major advance in ejection-seat technology, so can the seats which have evolved from the abortive Mark 8. The Mark 10, for example, provides for ejections from zero to 720 m.p.h., at zero altitude up to 50,000 feet. Full parachute deployment can be effected within 2½ seconds, and, as a result of the development of a new type of aeroconical parachute, deceleration on parachute opening is far smoother and more reliable. And further improvements are still being sought and attained. The next generation of seats will deploy the parachute in less than a second after the initiation of ejection!

If the problems of ejecting a man from an aircraft flying, perhaps out of control, at speeds of up to 720 m.p.h., seem bad enough, then at least equally so are those of ejecting him from a stationary aircraft, but one which is submerged beneath the sea. When fast jets were first introduced into the Navy there were many appalling accidents associated with operations from aircraft-carriers, because of the extremely restricted take-off and landing area. Although during the six year period 1954 to 1960 only twelve per cent of major accidents involved aircraft actually entering the sea, over half of those that did were fatal, a fraction which represented one third of the total fatalities. During the late 1950s and early 1960s the IAM was directly involved in a series of investigations, the object of which was to make these accidents more survivable by developing a technique for ejecting underwater. That a Royal Air Force establishment should be so involved in an essentially Naval problem may seem surprising. It came about because of the close liaison between the Air Force and Navy Medical Branches that had been maintained ever since the attachment of a senior Navy medical officer to the Physiological Laboratory staff during the war, a direct liaison which continues to this day. The Navy man at the IAM who took charge of the underwater ejection programme was Surgeon Lieutenant Commander John Rawlins, whom we have met before, working on anti-g suits.

Until 13 October 1954, when a young pilot successfully ejected himself from his Wyvern aircraft, which had submerged after engine failure during a catapult launch, it had been believed that the use of the ejection seat underwater was impossible.[6] It was this incident, more than anything else, that established the need for an investigation into the general feasibility and limitations of ejection-seat escape from submerged aircraft. Underwater ejection presents several unique problems, but possibly the most important is what to do about the canopy. Before the advent of jet aircraft, take-off and landing were carried out with the cockpit open; jet aircraft had sealed pressure-cabins, which raised the possibility that when submerged the pressure of the water might prevent jettisoning of the canopy. Indeed, the Navy pilot who made that first successful underwater ejection did so by ejecting through the canopy – he had to, as the canopy would not budge! Clearly what was needed was a comprehensive evaluation of a hatch-jettisoning system underwater, and so Rawlins set up a trial at the Admiralty Hydro-Ballistics Establishment at Glen Fruin, in Scotland.[7] Here there was a tank, 120 feet long and 40 feet deep, which would easily accommodate the fuselage of the prototype Sea Vixen aircraft it was planned to use. Additionally, the tank had one side which was completely glazed, and the water was specially filtered to provide optimum conditions for photography.

Preliminary calculations had indicated that, with a water-tight cockpit, a pressure head of only four feet would be sufficient to prevent the canopy from jettisoning. However, this was a theoretical eventuality only, since water would enter through the inward relief valve of the cabin-pressurization system. This meant that the pressure within the cockpit would rise as the inrush of water compressed the trapped air. Eventually the pressure difference between inside and outside would reduce sufficiently to allow the jettisoning system to operate. The important questions for any man inside the cockpit were how long this would take and at what depth the canopy would jettison. The answers depended upon the sink rate, which in turn depended upon the attitude of the aircraft in the water, and the rate at which water entered the cockpit. A series of remote firings of the canopy underwater proved that it did come cleanly away from the fuselage, although at ten feet and below there was a delay of several seconds between initiating firing and the canopy actually being jettisoned, whilst the pressure differential narrowed.

Although the main objective of the trial had been to determine the behaviour of underwater canopy-jettisoning systems, it seemed a shame not to use the experimental set-up to look closely at other factors which affected the chances of escape and to develop techniques for future studies. This, however, implied jettisoning the canopy with a man sitting in the cockpit, a singularly hazardous undertaking. For example, it was known that the commonest cause of failure to escape from submerged aircraft was the inability to clear the cockpit in time to escape drowning. Then there were worries about the effects of sudden changes in pressure on lungs and ear-drums. The effect of the sudden inrush of cold water through the relief valve also had to be considered; the valve had an area of twenty square inches, quite sufficient to produce a powerful blast of water. And what would happen if the outside water pressure collapsed the fuselage? The subject could be trapped. Then, to cap it all, doubt was expressed concerning the efficiency of the lifting-gear used to lower and raise the fuselage. Naturally, every possible precaution was taken. Subjects wore a self-contained breathing-set, and a special waterproof intercommunication set was designed and constructed at the RAE. Three divers were in attendance throughout each test, and nets were fastened beneath the canopy to catch the pieces in the event of an implosion.

The first live run was on 19 September 1956, and in the best IAM tradition the trials officer, John Rawlins, was in the 'hot seat'. Fortunately everything went smoothly, the most disconcerting experience being the inrush of water, which swept him against the side of the cockpit. The Sea Vixen had a double cockpit, and in this first experiment the front canopy had been left open for safety reasons. Consequently the inrush of water was much greater than in later runs with both canopies closed – a powerful argument in favour of not jettisoning the canopy before hitting the sea in any ditching. Successful canopy jettisoning was always achieved, down to a depth of twenty-eight feet, provided that the aircraft was in a normal (upright, horizontal) attitude. Rather more difficulty was experienced, however, when the aircraft was inverted. Anyway, at least the feasibility of underwater canopy jettisoning had been proven. The next stage was to look at methods of ejecting the seat.

Some preliminary experiments were carried out at the RAE, using the tank which had been built for fatigue-testing the fuselage of a Comet aircraft, following the two disastrous in-flight structural failures in 1954. After a number of dummy ejections had successfully been carried out, it was time once again for a live subject to have a go. And again it was to be John Rawlins. For this first (voluntary!) live underwater ejection, a Martin-Baker seat was installed, with all the necessary recording apparatus, at the bottom of the seventeen-foot tank, before filling the latter with water. Because it would take a while to fill the tank, Rawlins was provided with a breathing-apparatus, of limited endurance, which would allow him to breathe whilst this was being accomplished. Unfortunately the tank filled far more slowly than expected, and an emergency call had to be put through to the fire brigade to come and add their bit of water. This, of course, did nothing to help the equanimity of the subject, who recollects the seemingly interminable wait for the tap on his shoulder from the safety diver, which would be the signal for him to pull the firing-handle. The safety diver was Surgeon Lieutenant (later Surgeon Captain) 'Sandy' Davidson, who was subsequently to be much involved in the underwater ejection programme. It turned out to be fortunate that it was Davidson, an expert diver totally familiar with the potential dangers of the experiments, who was with Rawlins, for, when the tap on his shoulder came, Rawlins nearly forgot to breathe out, until forcefully reminded by his colleague. A rapid acceleration up through seventeen feet of water with lungs full of air could have been very nasty, for the air would have expanded, tearing and rupturing the delicate lung tissues. All went well, however; Rawlins' main recollection was a very distinct double explosion – the second being a reflection off the walls of the tank – and then finding himself floating on the surface.

After a few more ejections, the team moved back, early in 1957, to the deeper tank at Glen Fruin. Rawlins was joined by an American Naval Commander (later Professor), Ed Beckman, who had been posted into the IAM as an exchange officer. Beckman had been attached to the centrifuge section, where Peter Howard was conducting experiments to improve techniques for determining grey-out thresholds. As Rawlins later recalled, Ed Beckman found all this deadly dull and wanted to be where the action was. Had he waited a while longer, he might have found himself a subject for the negative-g experiments which, one suspects, he would have found rather less dull. Or perhaps he knew what was coming and didn't want to wait! In the event he was obliged to undergo something almost as unpleasant before he could join Rawlins – to be the first foreigner on a course of diving instruction at HMS *Vernon*.

The object of the second Glen Fruin trial was to examine, in detail, the physical forces which acted on the pilot when ejecting under water. By this time the recording system and associated experimental procedures had become fairly sophisticated, and precise determinations could be made of accelerations and pressures as first dummies and later subjects were propelled upward through the water at velocities that increased progressively as the explosive power of the cartridges was increased. To get an idea of human tolerances to drag through water, some preliminary studies had been carried out in which subjects were towed through water, whilst hanging on to an iron bar trapeze, at speeds up to 30 m.p.h. In other studies, subjects were exposed to ejection blast without actually ejecting, and the magnitude of the pressures experienced was recorded. Then three subjects were ejected underwater using the full explosive power of the cartridges. All the results were consistent with the concept that underwater escape was perfectly feasible with the standard ejection seat and cartridge charge then in use, provided that the ejection mechanism was adequately waterproofed. In addition, using dummies, it was shown that, in aircraft with frangible canopies, ejection through the canopy was probably preferable to waiting for the canopy to jettison. However, not all Naval aircraft did have frangible canopies, and this meant that each type would have to be evaluated separately. More trials were needed.

The first of these was again at Glen Fruin, where the problems of escape from the Scimitar aircraft were examined. In this trial attention was focused on the question of what procedure a pilot should follow to extricate himself from his seat after ejection. In the air the seat harness is, at the appropriate time, automatically released, and the retardation produced by the drogue parachute attached to the seat slows it down, but not the man. So, in effect, the man is 'pulled' out of the seat by his own momentum and, as this happens, a line back to the drogue from the man deploys the main parachute. Underwater there is no momentum to separate the man from his seat, so he has to push himself free but first disconnect himself from his parachute harness, as otherwise the parachute would deploy and, acting as an immense drogue, prevent him from reaching the surface. The major discovery of the trial was that this operation was very difficult to perform in a seat which is sinking through the water. Wet gloves slipped on the harness-release mechanism, and the rising water pressure as the seat sank caused intense pain in the ears. It was also found that, in the Scimitar, ejection through the canopy would be most unwise. All this pointed towards a need for a fully automatic underwater ejection system.

This was further demonstrated in the next trial at Glen Fruin, the first part of what was to be a comprehensive and prolonged study of underwater escape from the Sea Vixen aircraft. As often seemed to be the case, the experiments were undertaken at the coldest time of the year, when water temperatures were about 4 °C. Experiments showed that it was impossible to jettison the Sea Vixen canopies underwater. In one test the explosive jacks lifted the observer's canopy up slightly, but then it slammed back, 'making an impressive dent in the top of the ejection seat' – but not, fortunately, in the head of the subject. So escape from the Sea Vixen had to be achieved from a submerged fuselage with a totally immersed pilot breathing on the aircraft oxygen system. As a safety precaution, however, there was a back-up air supply – simply a hose supply line which, although providing air, did not provide cover for the face. The first test was especially memorable: '... a torrent of water at 4°C pouring onto the face produced mental and physical paralysis for a space of some 7 seconds'. This paralysis, at a time when every second was vital, was a very real problem for aircrew ditching in cold water. So, too, was the great difficulty in seeing underwater; vision was virtually zero, and so the subject had to rely on feel alone to carry through the escape routine. Cold and blackness combined to produce a truly nightmarish quality to the entire procedure, as illustrated by Rawlins' own account of one experiment carried out on 17 December 1959.

> The fuselage submerged and horribly cold water poured over my face obscuring my vision. For a moment all seemed well, and then, as the water rose above my head, breathing became progressively more difficult. Thinking it must be due to the high position of the regulator I reached across to press the emergency oxygen button which I could just manage in the dry, and found that owing to my size, the quantity of underwear I had on and the stiffening-up of the immersion suit when wet, I could no longer reach it. Meanwhile the oxygen supply failed altogether. We had had trouble with the expiratory valve sticking so I blew hard to clear it. This, of course, lost me the remainder of the air in my lungs, the mask was drawn in on my face as the fuselage descended, and I could get nothing more. With a desperate effort I reached the

> emergency button and pushed, but nothing happened, so I gave a 'thumbs-down' signal to the stand-by divers to get the fuselage up. It promptly subsided further and I thought 'the crane brakes have gone'. Repeated 'thumbs-down' signals were given and the fuselage now started to move towards the surface but breathing being impossible the movement seemed very slow and I at once turned the harness release to bale out but the straps remained in place. Panic now occurred. By now the crane driver had got the fuselage out of the water but I was inside and still submerged beneath the water in the fuselage. I could see the surface just above my head and was making frantic efforts to stretch up to it. I forgot entirely about the air supply hose dangling a few inches away. Finally they surfaced me by tilting the fuselage and I pulled off my mask. A very unnerved subject emerged.

In the second phase of the Sea Vixen underwater escape trial, live ejections were carried out. Martin-Baker had been persuaded to modify an ejection gun for use with compressed air, something Rawlins had been convinced was necessary ever since the very first experiments. Also, with the frightening experiences of the first phase well behind them, the team was, in July 1960, working in 'near perfect co-ordination', and test techniques were greatly improved. So confident was the team that a senior representative of the aircraft manufacturer, de Havilland, was allowed to be the first to eject with the new compressed-air seat. Although the ejection went off faultlessly, the poor man was nearly asphyxiated when, on being pulled out of the water after John Rawlins had released him from the seat, his oxygen line snagged on the side. Although he had no air for only a few seconds, his comment afterwards was, 'I thought that was my lot'; as Rawlins pointed out, another example of panic.

Thereafter followed, in quick succession, underwater escape trials using the French Etendard IV aircraft (which proved to be very similar to the Scimitar) and the Buccaneer aircraft and, finally, a series of aircrew training trials. Unfortunately, despite the success of the research programme, shortly afterwards a very experienced Buccaneer pilot and his navigator failed to escape when their aircraft stalled into the sea after carrier take-off, even though the pilot had been personally briefed on underwater escape procedures. Then a very similar incident occurred with a Sea Vixen, although here the crew did escape, just. In the case of the Sea Vixen, the great problem facing the crew had been that of releasing the restraint harness –

further evidence of the vital need for a fully automatic system. A significant advance had been made in this direction when the Walter Kidde Company successfully demonstrated at Farnborough a self-inflating dinghy, which Rawlins thought might be used to thrust a man out of his ejection seat subsequent to ejection. In January 1961 this idea was tested at Glen Fruin during the third phase of the Sea Vixen trial. It worked beautifully; the seat was fired, and automatic separation from the seat took place, followed by automatic deployment of the dinghy at the surface. To quote John Rawlins: 'It was clear that we had at last all the components of an underwater escape system which would demand not more than a single action on the part of the crew, and could easily be made fully automatic.'

Indeed, some time before the Walter Kidde demonstration at Farnborough, Martin-Baker had been approached on the problem of man-seat separation underwater, but little interest had been shown. Following the successful test at Glen Fruin, Rawlins was given formal permission to invite the Walter Kidde Company to develop an automatic seat-separation system for the Navy. This they proceeded to do and by April 1962 had produced a system that operated rapidly and reliably. It was, however, only semi-automatic inasmuch as the man still had to initiate ejection himself once underwater. Then, automatically, a cushion behind him inflated, the harness locks disconnected and, as he left the seat, both Mae West and dinghy inflated, taking the man to the surface. By this time, however, the Martin-Baker Company were taking an interest in the problem of man-seat separation underwater and had very quickly developed a fully automatic system which would initiate the ejection sequence without any action by the crew once a specific depth had been reached. In fact, the man-seat separation system the company adopted – automatically inflated air-cushions – was remarkably similar to that devised by the Walter Kidde Company. In June 1962 the Martin-Baker Automatic Underwater Escape System was put through its paces at HMS *Dolphin* using a Sea Hawk, with Sandy Davidson making the first live test with a successful through-canopy ejection. However, what was really needed was a through-canopy system for the Buccaneer, and so more trials were arranged for September of that year.

Problems arose immediately. In tests with dummies there was strong evidence of unacceptable neck flexion as the head went through the Buccaneer canopy, and the neck of one dummy was actually broken. Despite this, astoundingly, four live tests followed.

In three of these the subject failed to separate from the seat, sinking to the bottom jammed in the seat by expanded separation bags and unreleased harness. The fourth subject (Davidson) braced his head back deliberately to reduce risks of flexion, but later it was pointed out that an unconscious subject would not be able to do this. So John Rawlins agreed to eject with his neck relaxed. What happened is, once again, best described by the subject himself.

> In the test my head was forced violently onto my chest, the facepiece of my diving gear being fractured by hitting the canister of CO_2 absorbent. Both nose-clip and mouthpiece were displaced and there was, momentarily, a loss of vision which may have resulted from the sudden forced flexion of the neck. Separation failed and I started to sink, inhaling water through the broken facepiece. However, Davidson, clinging with one hand to the ladder, managed to support both me and the seat with my head above water until a line could be secured to the seat.

For Martin-Baker it was back to the drawing-board. On the advice of Davidson they modified their inflation system for the separation bags, adopting the method successfully employed in the Walter Kidde automatic separation system. Perhaps, more important, it became recognized by all that through-canopy ejection in the Buccaneer was just not on.

Although at this point Walter Kidde was ready to go into full production, Martin-Baker was to be awarded the final contract, despite the fact that the company had still not produced a satisfactory system, and the system it did have was largely that of the Walter Kidde Company. To be fair, Martin-Baker went on to produce a highly effective and safe underwater ejection seat, although this took rather longer than the five weeks initially anticipated.

The introduction of the Martin-Baker Mark 4 ejection seat, with its eighty feet per second ejection gun, produced another problem for the IAM team. There was concern – justifiable as it turned out – that the greater blast pressures generated might cause injury. Anaesthetized sheep were exposed to the shock waves in the mining-tank at HMS *Vernon* and did indeed suffer serious injury – damaged lungs and ruptured liver. The sheep were not actually exposed in an ejection seat, however, and it was argued by representatives of the Blackburn Aircraft Company, in whose

Buccaneer aircraft the new ejection gun was being introduced, that the shielding provided by the back of the Mark 4 seat would prevent any injury from occurring. So Rawlins gave it a try himself. He described the sensation as 'one of a fairly violent concussion, possibly accompanied by a momentary loss of consciousness, comparable with the effect of a sudden blow on the jaw'. According to an observer, Rawlins was lifted four inches in the seat by the explosion, and afterwards all the rivets holding the seat-back in position were found to be sheared. His symptoms afterwards were compatible with bruising of lungs and liver. Then it was discovered that the seat had not been located accurately with respect to the explosion, and, following correction, a sheep was once again exposed. It died. Some time later three more sheep were actually ejected. They too died. There was no more talk of using the eighty feet per second ejection gun in Navy aircraft where there was an underwater ejection requirement. Anyway, the advent, shortly afterwards, of Martin-Baker's prototype compressed-air system eliminated that particular problem.

To conclude this account of what was certainly one of the most dangerous research programmes ever undertaken under the auspices of the IAM, mention must be made of one final trial conducted jointly with the French in July 1962. It will be remembered that sink-rate had proved to be an important factor determining whether or not a successful escape could be made from a submerged aircraft. There was little doubt that the sink-rates measured at Glen Fruin were unrepresentative of what happened with intact aircraft. Information was needed on how long an aircraft would stay afloat, how sinking was affected by the aircraft attitude in the water, how fast the pressure built up across the canopy and at what pressure the canopy would collapse. And, ever since the Etendard IV escape trial in 1960, the French had also wanted answers to these questions. Despite French enthusiasm, the Ministry of Aviation was at first uninterested, but eventually they agreed to the trial, provided that it cost no more than £15,000.

The plan was to drop two aircraft, one French and one British into the sea off Toulon in various attitudes and at various weights and to record what happened by the use of appropriate sensors and underwater ciné photography. It was suggested by John Rawlins that the British should supply the cameras, and the French the remaining instrumentation. In fact, the photographic requirements were very exacting, and the British certainly had not got the easier half of the bargain. A photographic record had to be obtained of the track of the sinking aircraft, and of the collapse of the canopy. In addition, there was a need for a general record of all the test procedures. To Rawlins' consternation, it soon became apparent that there was no suitable underwater ciné camera available. Fortunately the RAE stepped in and agreed to design equipment specially for the trials team, on the understanding that there would be plenty of future use for the equipment. (As indeed there was; five years later Rawlins wanted to borrow the cameras from the RAE, only to find he had to join a long queue!)

The other problem was where to find an aircraft – and one was needed that could be 'written off' at the end of the trial – and then how to get it to Toulon. After all, the budget was only £15,000. Fortunately the cost of the underwater photographic equipment had been covered by the RAE as part of their financial allotment for research and development – just as well, since the sum involved represented two-thirds of the total budget. Then came another stroke of good fortune. Rawlins learned the whereabouts of an aged Scimitar with just a few hours flying-time left. It was his for the princely sum of £5. After flying it down to Toulon, it was completely out of hours and only good for dropping into the sea.

The trial was conducted outside Toulon harbour, the two aircraft – the French were using an old Etendard IV – being conveyed to the spot on a barge towed by a tug. A hundred-ton crane on another tug handled the aircraft for the drops and for the subsequent recovery from the sea-bed a hundred feet below. Six tests were carried out with the Etendard and five with the Scimitar. Retrieval of the aircraft was always tricky, particularly of the larger and heavier Scimitar. On one occasion the slings broke as the crane was lifting the aircraft clear of the water, and it plunged back down to the bottom – fortunately no divers were in the vicinity. Following a drop with the aircraft inclined 45° nose down, and after floating for nearly a minute, it sank so rapidly that the attending divers could not keep up, and it arrived at the bottom nose first. A team from Vickers had to rebuild the nose from scrap metal.

Overall, the trial was a great success. Sink rates were established, and it was proven that these were a function not of water density, as the Americans thought, but of the orientation of the aircraft in the water. The aircraft always sank nose-down or tail-down but never horizontally. Excellent pictures were obtained of the Scimitar canopy imploding at forty feet. In the final test the Scimitar was catapulted off the deck of HMS *Centaur* after it had been fitted with the Martin-Baker automatic escape system and a dummy pilot. Despite striking the sea with great violence, a perfect ejection was initiated, and the dummy came to the surface.

Yet, in one sense, all this research and tireless effort by John Rawlins and his colleagues came to nought. Even as the Toulon trial was taking place, rocket packs were being fitted to the Mark 4 and 5 ejection seats. The 'zero-zero' capability that rockets provided meant that pilots could now safely eject in the few seconds between ditching and sinking. There was no need for underwater ejection. There was, however, still plenty of need for further research into problems of ejection from aircraft. For, even after successfully ejecting, there are still hazards that have to be faced before the airman arrives safely on the ground. For example, there is what is known as wind-drag deceleration. When the man is ejected from his aircraft, he is still travelling at the speed of his aircraft. The air outside is not, however; in effect, it is stationary. So he hits a wall of air. The consequences are similar to striking a brick wall; there is a very rapid deceleration – a wind-drag deceleration. Clearly, the greater the aircraft speed, the more rapid the deceleration and, just as with the vertical acceleration of ejection itself, there is only a certain amount the human frame will withstand. Just how much this is, was determined in a now classic series of experiments in which an American, Colonel J.P. Stapp, had himself fired down a track in what was basically a high-powered version of the RAF rocket sled used by Bill Stewart and others from the IAM, for essentially similar purposes.[8] In the run which established what the maximum tolerable deceleration was likely to be, Stapp was propelled down the track at 647 m.p.h. The water braking-system, in bringing him to rest, decelerated the sled at a rate of 600g per second, producing a peak load of 35g! For several minutes after the experience, Stapp was in a severe state of shock, lapsing into periods of semi-consciousness. For a while he lost all vision, and when this returned, he was found to be suffering from small haemorrhages in and around his eyes and in the soft tissues of the face. He was in hospital for five days.

Windblast is itself hazardous to the man. In addition to being rapidly decelerated on hitting the 'wall' of air as he leaves the cockpit, there is also the pressure effect of striking that 'wall'. This pressure can be so great as to be irresistible, causing the limb flailing to which we have already referred. Totally uncontrollable as it often is, the flailing can easily lead to fractures or joint dislocations, which is why, during ejection, the limbs have to be held secure with restraints. Even more seriously, the windblast can also cause similar flailing of the head, leading to loss of consciousness and fatal brain damage. The problem is that, to design the most effective restraint system, you need to simulate the effects of windblast, and without a rocket track like Colonel Stapp's, or a wind tunnel, this is not easy. However, David Fryer of the IAM came up with a novel idea – use water.

To be fair, it was not entirely Fryer's idea. During the second underwater ejection trial at Glen Fruin in 1957, when subjects were being dragged across the lake clutching a trapeze, Ed Beckman had commented that the effect of the water pressure on the body was rather like windblast. The advantage of water is that, being about twenty-six times more dense than air, far lower velocities are needed to achieve the same effect. So in 1960 David Fryer, then a squadron leader, decided to try to put this idea into practice. But how would it be possible to attain the required velocities underwater, under conditions allowing scientific observation and measurement and adequate safety? The answer was by using the rotating beam channel at the Admiralty Research Laboratory. This was basically a fifty-five feet radius beam, from which could be suspended test vehicles to travel on or under the surface of water contained in an annular tank fifteen feet deep. A submersible support structure for a seat was built, a task undertaken by the RAE, and a restraint sytem devised for the legs, arms and head. Air was supplied to the subject through a hose from the surface, and a fail-safe communication system based on the 'dead-man's handle' concept was adopted; failure to keep two lightly spring-loaded buttons pressed resulted in the immediate termination of the experiment.

The object of the exercise was, basically, to evaluate the potential usefulness of this novel method of simulating wind blast. A system of strain-gauges provided measures of the loads imposed on various parts of the body and, in particular, of the forces tending to separate or flail the limbs. Some physiological measurements were made, including the pressures produced inside the subject using a water-filled balloon at the end of a tube which was swallowed. A total of fifty-nine experiments was carried out, involving just two subjects – David Fryer himself and a civilian, Mr Roy Needham. After being securely fastened into the seat, the subject would be rotated through the water at speeds which ranged from 3 to 22 m.p.h. At the higher speeds substantial pressures were exerted on the subject, and the

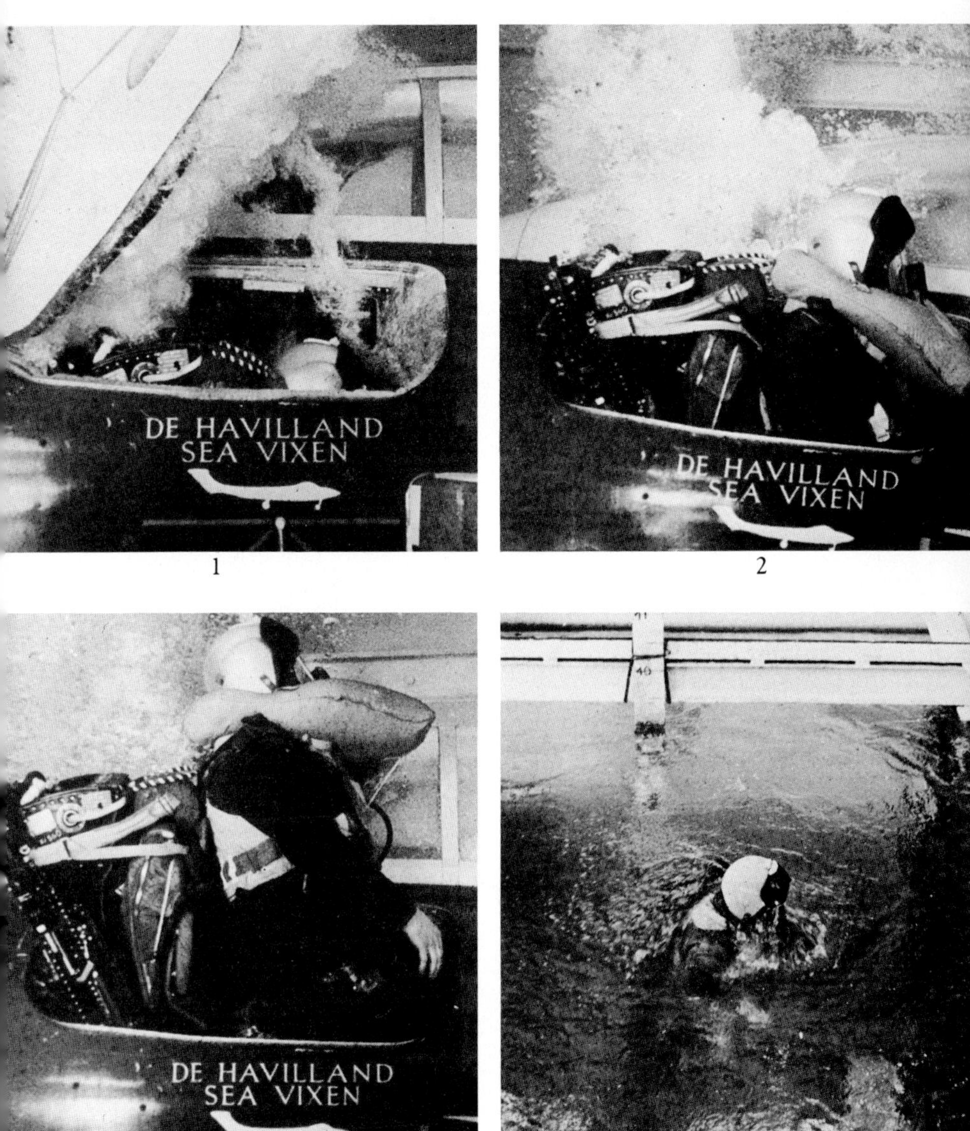

42 Underwater ejection from a Sea Vixen cockpit by Surgeon Lieutenant-Commander J.S.P. Rawlins, from canopy jettison to arrival at the surface

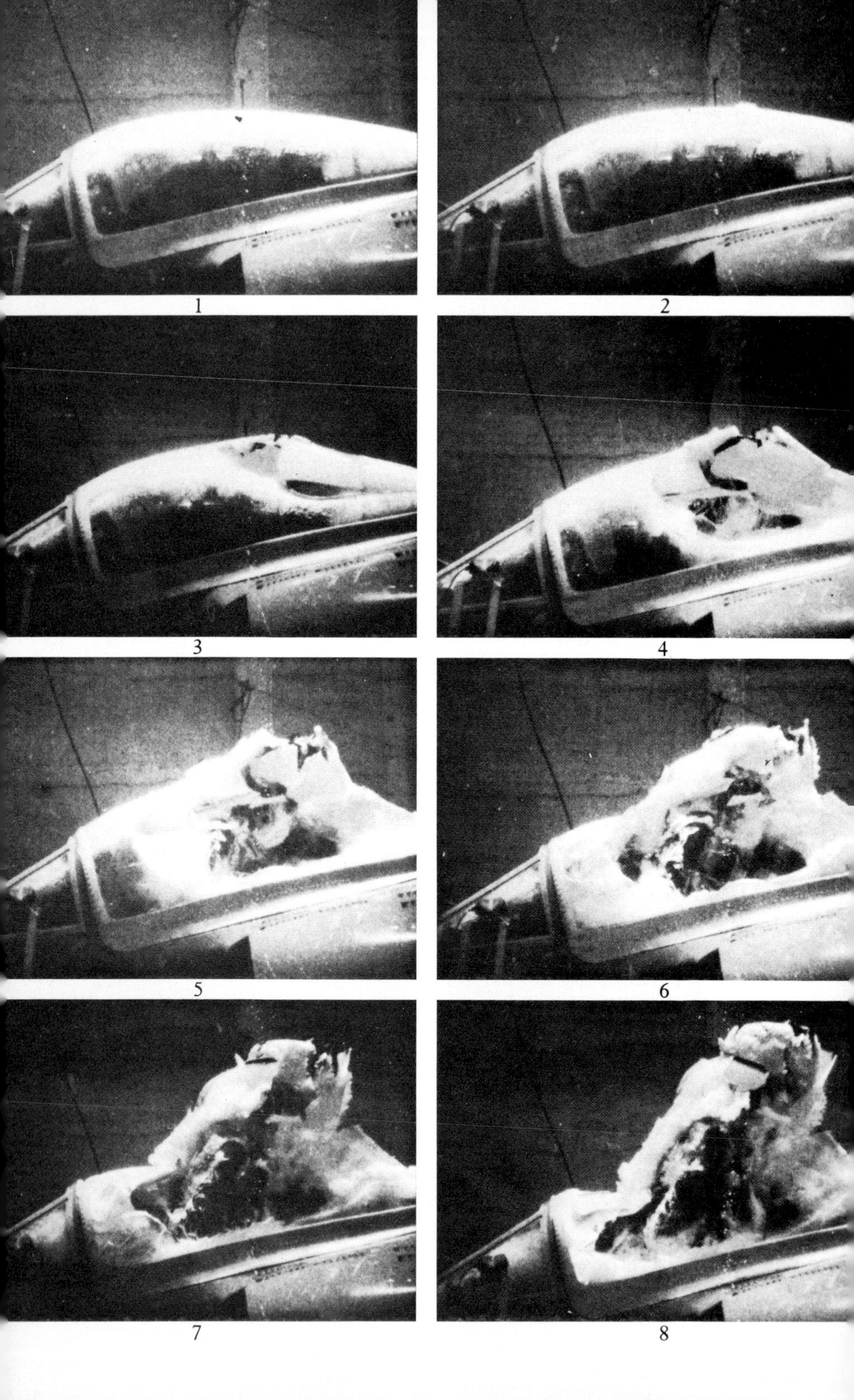
1
2
3
4
5
6
7
8

Left: Through-canopy ejection sequence

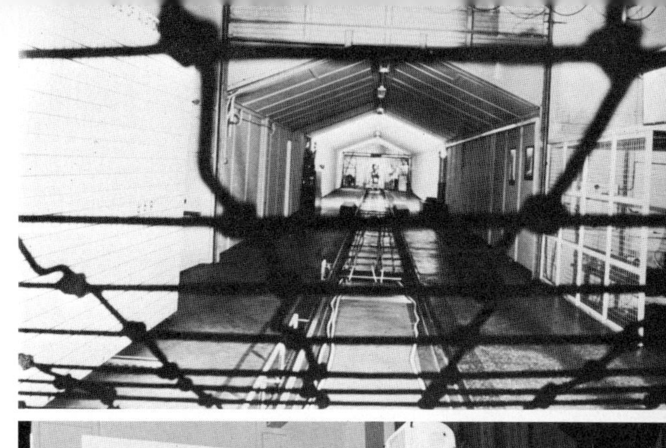

Right: The IAM decelerator track. The subject is Wing Commander David Reader

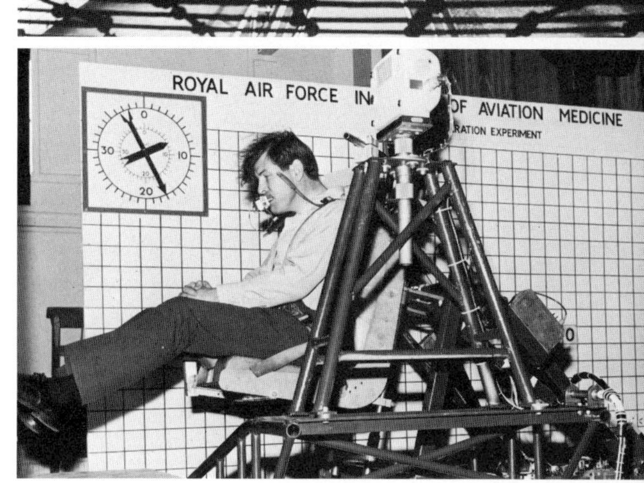

Group Captain A.J. Barwood OBE

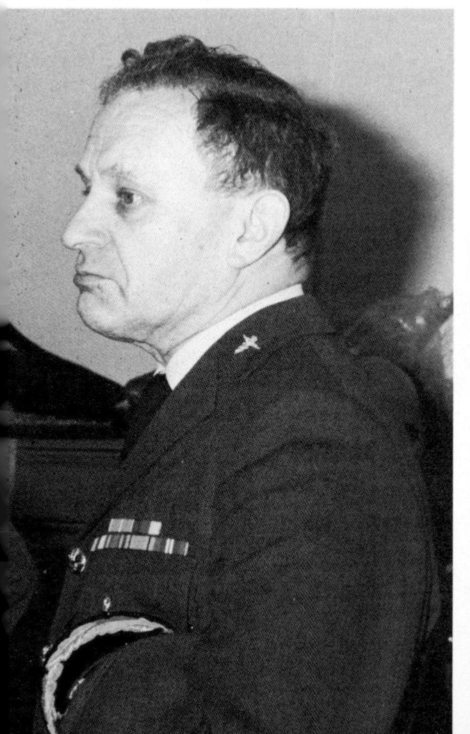

46 Professor E.A. Pask OBE

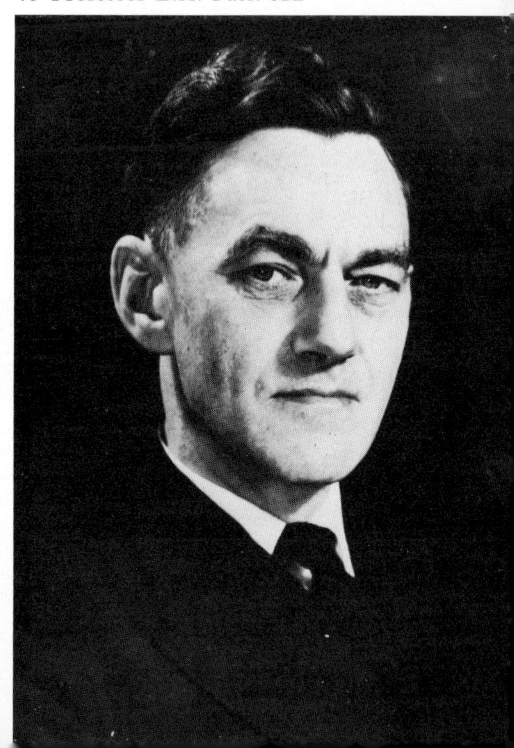

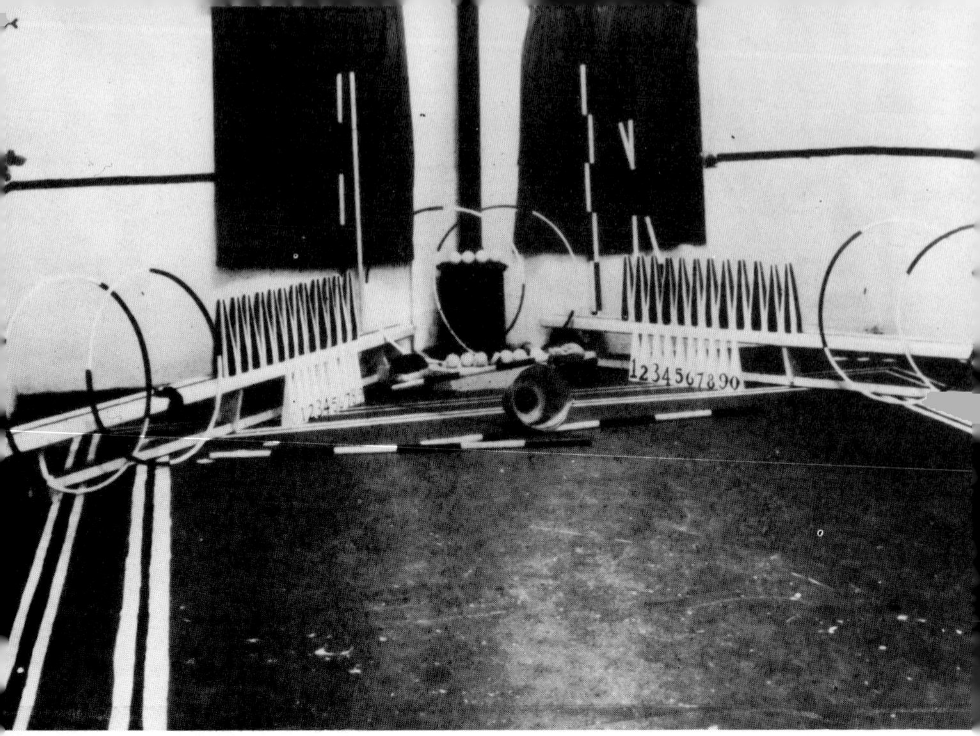

47 A night-vision gymnasium, containing apparatus to be used in very dim light

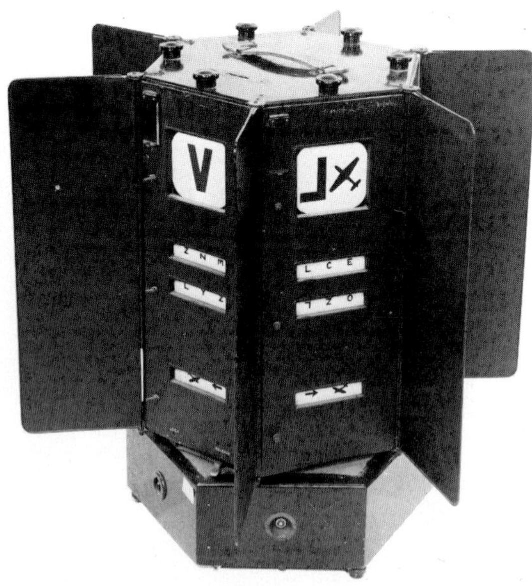

48 Livingston's rotating hexagon

49 A dual-visor helmet which has suffered a high-speed bird-strike in a high-performance aircraft, demonstrating the benefit of the clear, inner visor

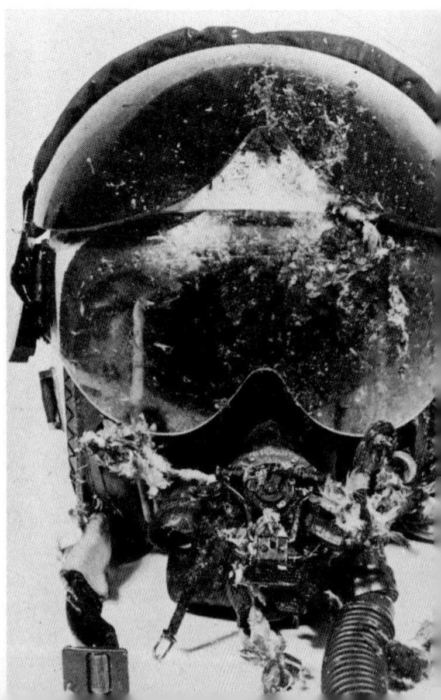

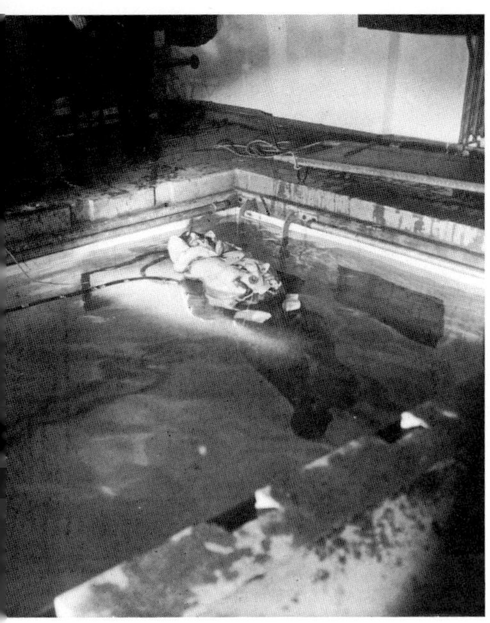

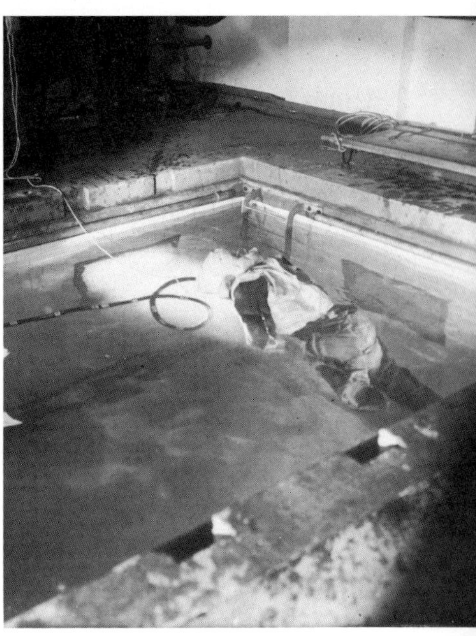

50 Pask's experiments to determine the floating posture of the unconscious body with different life-preservers; left, in the normal position; right, face-down, which leads to rapid drowning

51 The Air Ventilated Suit, Mark 1

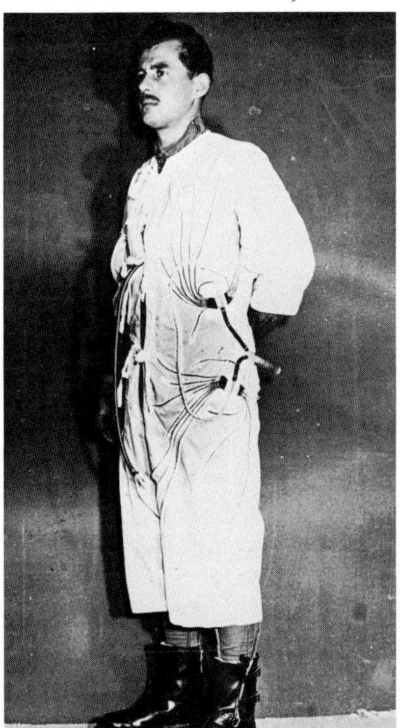

52 The Liquid Conditioned Suit

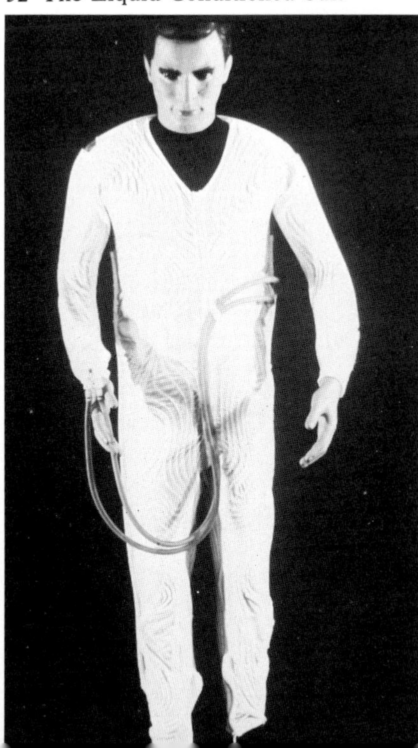

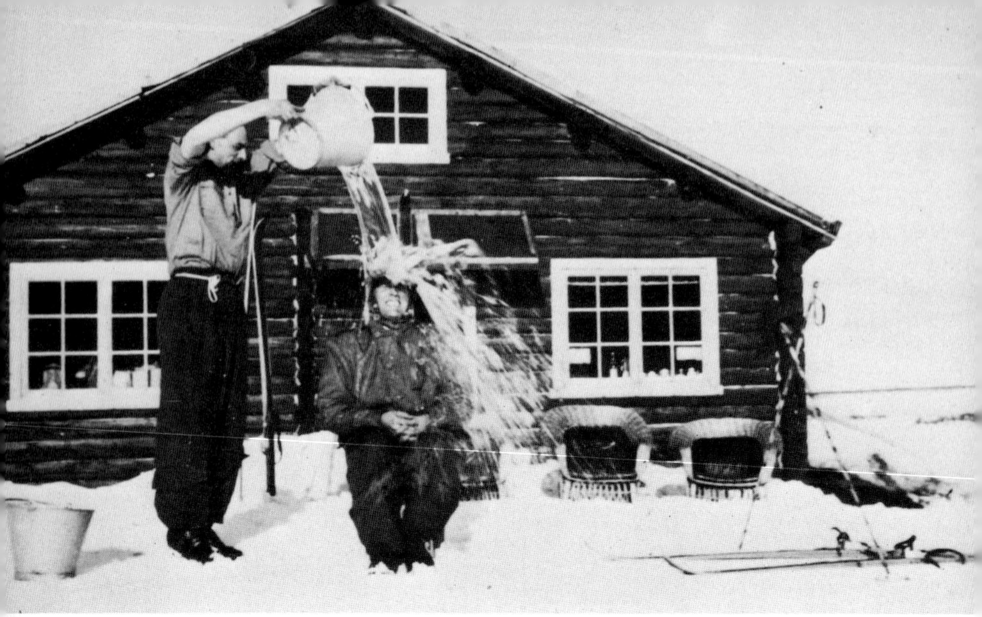

53 The application of science to the testing of flying clothing. Wing Commander Pat Ruffell-Smith (with the bucket) and Squadron Leader Peter Whittingham, Norway 1950

54 Flight Lieutenant John Billingham drinking snail juice and holding some of the snails in his hand

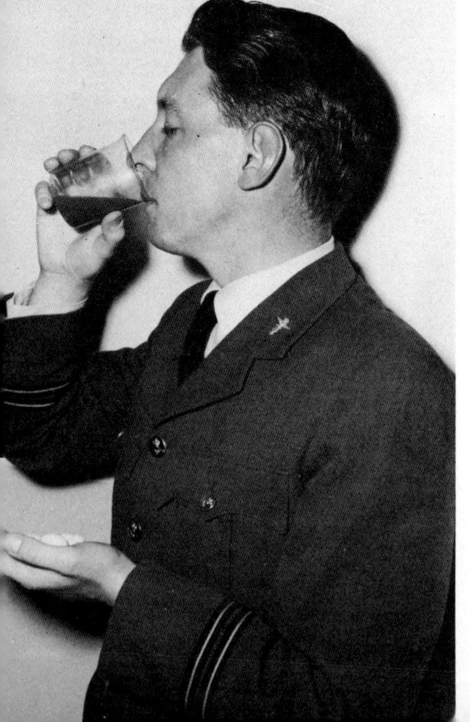

55 The Aircrew Respirator NBC No. 5

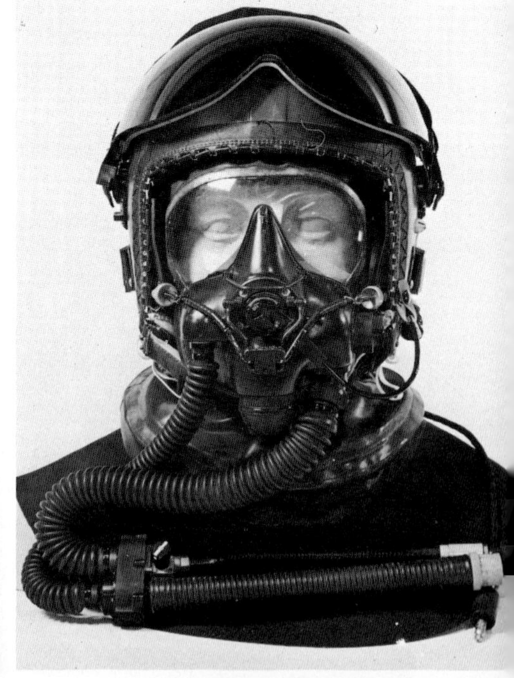

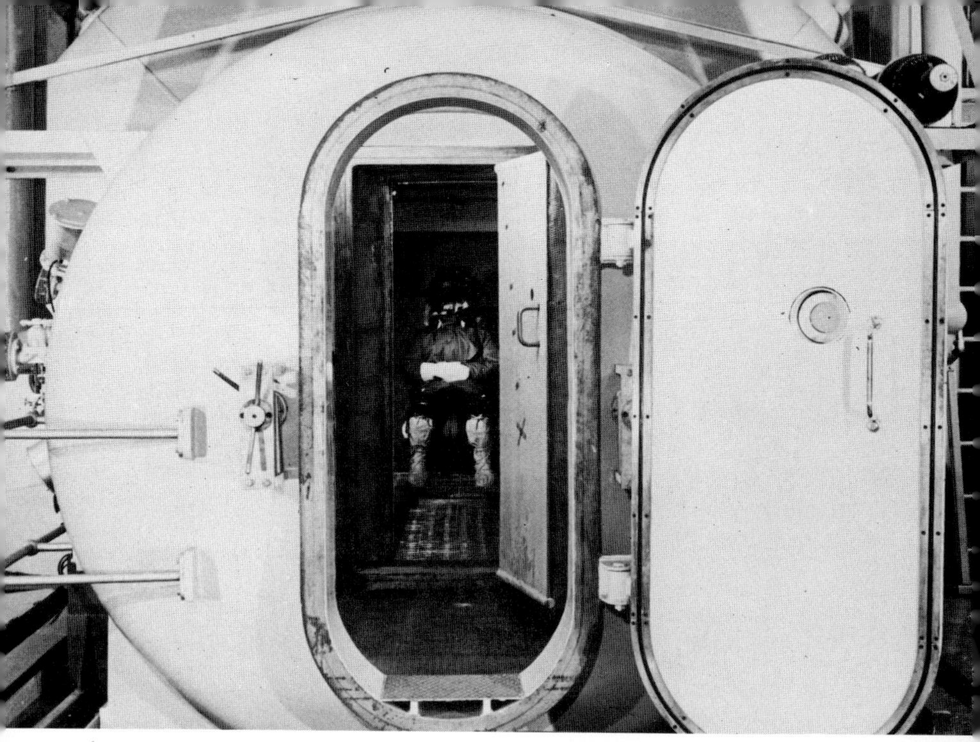

56 The IAM radiant heat chamber

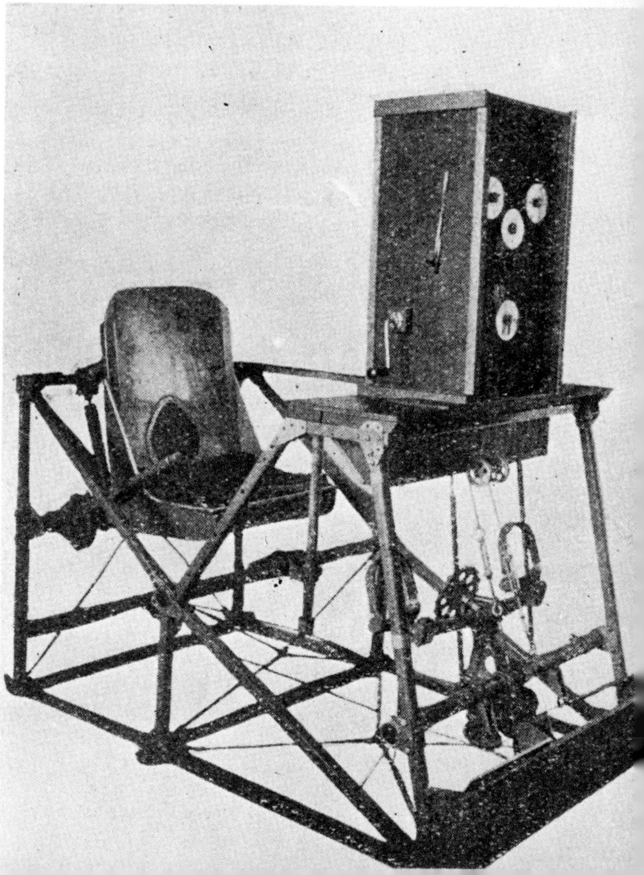

57 The Sensori-Motor Apparatus No. 3

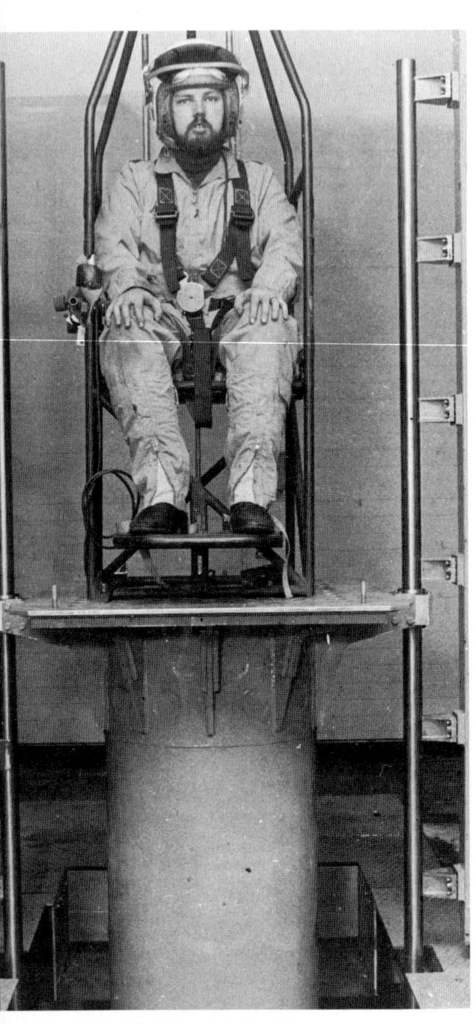

58 The IAM vibrator

59 The IAM oscillating table

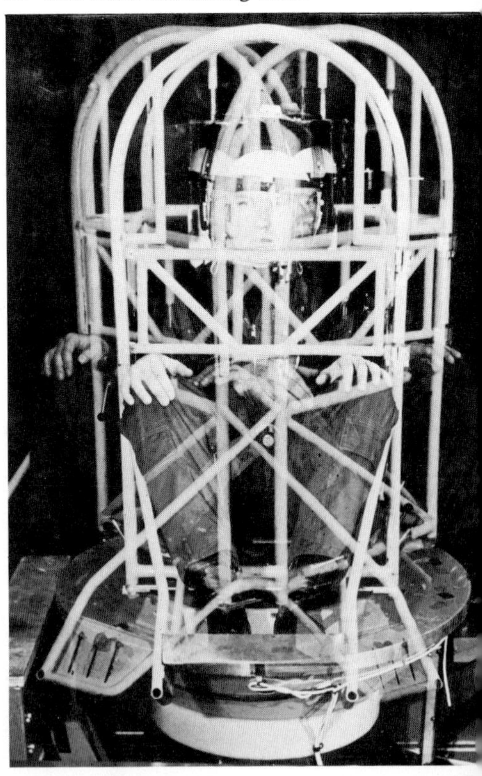

measurements of the separation loads on the limbs showed that these had been underestimated in the past. The limits of tolerance came at speeds of 20 to 22 m.p.h. (equivalent to an air speed of some 600 m.p.h.), with severe pain in the hips, thighs and spine being accompanied by numerous small haemorrhages on the upper arms. At these speeds the subject's impression of the run was blurred by what was described as 'sensory swamping'.[9] Indeed, vision began to be lost in a manner analogous to the grey-out of positive g, and the eyes suffered a similar but milder injury to that experienced by Stapp. No problems were encountered with head flailing, which was attributed to the very effective stabilization provided by Needham's especially designed head-cowl. All in all, these very successful experiments demonstrated the validity and practicability of underwater rotation as a means of simulating the effects of wind blast, and also provided valuable pointers to how the vexed questions of providing limb and head restraint might be resolved. However, the technique was never taken up again, and further studies of restraint systems at the IAM would have to await the construction of a decelerator track some years later. But at least Fryer could claim the world underwater speed record!

In all situations in which short duration accelerations are encountered, we have consistently emphasized the importance of the safety harness in preventing these accelerations from causing injury. It is not just a question of restraining the man in his seat; the design of the harness must be such that the forces generated during impact deceleration are optimally distributed over as large an area of the body as possible and are not localized at just a few points. Much theoretical work on this problem was carried out by Wing Commander Freddie Latham. Practical investigation, however, requires a linear decelerator, and consequently much of the early research at the IAM was carried out using the RAE rocket-propelled trolley. Thus it was Stewart's human deceleration experiments in 1944 that led to the development of a new RAF harness, the type Z. This replaced the Q-harness, which itself was only a modified version of the First World War vintage Sutton harness. In 1939 even Oliver Sutton would probably have been surprised to find his harness, still unchanged from World War I, installed in most fighter aircraft. Pilots of bomber aircraft were also provided with a Sutton harness, but it was generally not worn since it restricted movement. The remainder of the bomber crew were provided only with waist-belts, the inadequacy of which Stewart had demonstrated so effectively in the Battle aircraft. In truth, however, the Sutton harness really was not that much better. For a start, the harness would only withstand a decelerative force equal to 10g although, to be fair, this was no more than specified by the MAP. Yet the equivalent German harness could withstand 26g! Then, because of the absence of a restraint strap between the legs, the lower part of the body tended to slide forward off the aircraft seat. The harness was also uncomfortable to wear, difficult to adjust and put on and, when tightened as required, severely restricted mobility and, hence, the rearward field of vision. In some aircraft the straps were so close to the pilot's neck that they were reputed to have, on occasion, caused asphyxia and strangulation.[10] And all this was nearly twenty-five years after the harness had been introduced into service. Not that the war greatly stimulated development of a replacement. Although by late 1942 attempt were at last being made to improve the Sutton harness, it would be 1945 before the Q-harness entered service, and this was essentially just the old Sutton harness but with a lap-belt and a fixing-point for the straps which ensured that the harness was not incorrectly worn too high up.

Stewart's Z-harness was to remain the standard RAF safety harness for many years. Like the Q-harness, it had shoulder-straps joined to lap-belts at a central four-point quick-release box on the front of the abdomen. However, it used nylon webbing stressed to 35g, instead of the more bulky cotton, and it was provided with a mechanism for automatic separation from the aircraft seat after ejection. A disadvantage of all the early harnesses, however, including the Z, was that a separate parachute harness had to be worn beneath, and this led to a potentially confusing duplication of straps.

Throughout the fifties and sixties various combined harness systems were developed, these tending to be specific to particular aircraft. Some of the earliest combined harnesses were evaluated by Latham using the RAE track, in 1957. During these tests he took the opportunity of studying some aspects of human tolerance to linear deceleration, and he recorded very high intra-abdominal pressures at the moment of impact. He suggested that these pressures might be transmitted in the blood-filled veins to the head, there producing the local haemorrhaging in the soft, unsupported tissues of the face, and particularly the eyes, described by Stapp and experienced later by Fryer and Needham.

To test this hypothesis, Latham, with Peter Howard's support, set up a very strange experiment. Subjects lay on their back and, without warning, ten-pound sandbags were dropped six to twelve inches onto their unprotected abdomens. Intra-abdominal and venous pressures were measured – on one occasion, which included rapid inversion of the subject, from a needle in a jugular vein. Doubtless much to the satisfaction of the subjects, the hypothesis was at least proved inasmuch as the transmission of a pressure wave was demonstrated, although there was no evidence of capillary rupture and haemorrhaging.

Sandbags were all very well, and David Fryer's system for studying problems of limb restraint worked well enough too, although the rotating beam channel was thirty miles away at Teddington and in regular use; also it was difficult to imagine many people being very keen to act as experimental subjects. What was really needed was a decelerator. Indeed, so urgent was the need that in 1967 a low-cost, highly improvised device was constructed at the IAM. Cheap to build and simple to operate it may have been, but it would accelerate a sled to a velocity of sixty feet per second over a distance of fifty feet and produce smooth decelerations up to 40g. The sled was propelled not by rockets but by a number of less spectacular but far more reliable bungee rubber cords, which were stretched by a winch; the sled was brought to a halt by hydraulic energy absorbers which were adjustable to produce the required deceleration characteristics. Over a three-year period some eleven hundred test runs were completed, including many with human subjects. However, the short length of the track, and the fact that the bungee cords were not fully relaxed at the point of impact, meant that required deceleration profiles were not always reproducible and, more important, the sled was actually still accelerating at the moment of impact. This led, in 1970, to the construction of the present decelerator track, which is 150 feet long. Although the bungee propulsion system has been retained, the test vehicle is 'pushed' by an additional 'pusher' vehicle, which is arrested independently after eighty feet, allowing the test vehicle to coast (and cease accelerating) before it is decelerated, again by adjustable hydraulic energy absorbers.

Both tracks have been used for testing many different types of aircraft seat and restraint systems. Seats are studied for their ability to withstand crash impacts, and one of the earliest major discoveries was the very poor impact protection provided by helicopter seats. Tests are carried out with the seats mounted in different positions, to cover all crash possibilities, and at increasing g-levels, until damage is first noted. Strain gauges and high-speed ciné-photography provide a detailed record of events occurring at the moment of impact, this usually enabling the precise location of points of structural weakness to be identified. One type of study has been a comparison between the performance in an impact of forward-and rearward-facing airline passenger seats. This proved what everybody knows but nobody (except the RAF) does anything about – that you are far better off in a crash with your back to the direction of travel.

The Institute is little involved in the design of seats, although it can, and does, make strong recommendations and suggestions if a seat tested on the decelerator track is found wanting in terms of the impact protection it offers. On the other hand, the close relationship maintained with the Martin-Baker Company means that problems of this sort rarely rise with ejection seats. The Institute is, however, involved in the design of safety harnesses. One, a simplified combined parachute and restraint harness, designed by Wing Commander David Reader, recently entered service and is being used in most types of current fighter aircraft. An important consideration in modifying old or designing new restraint systems is the comfort of those who have to wear them. Thus, whilst dummies provide perfectly adequate subjects for seat testing, live subjects must be used at least during some stages of harness testing. Despite the risks involved, the Institute's safety record is impressive. Over the last thirteen years, human subjects have been used in many thousands of runs, with nothing worse being sustained than a few strained necks and sore limbs.

One of the most important functions of the decelerator track is the testing of aircraft seats and restraint systems that have been found to fail in accidents. Indeed, under the direction of Group Captain Tony Barwood (now retired but still very active in the field), post-crash investigation is an area of aviation medicine in which the Institute has built up on outstanding reputation over the years. Barwood is concerned mainly with aircrew personal equipment and why it sometimes fails, whilst Mr Roger Green, a psychologist, deals with human factor aspects – such as the thorny problem of whether pilot error may be a contributory factor in a particular accident. Perhaps Tony Barwood's most significant contribution to safety in the air was his pioneering work on the negative-g strap. This is a strap which comes up from the front of the seat between the legs to join the safety harness at the quick-release box and, as the name suggests, keeps the body firm in the seat during aircraft manoeuvres involving negative g. Without it the harness would ruck upwards, and the restraint provided is impaired. Another important aspect of Barwood's work was his uphill struggle to have the comfort of ejection seats improved, and further progress in this direction was made in the late 1960s and early 1970s with the work of Dr Jim Fitzgerald. With about fifteen per cent of the pilot population in the RAF suffering from back pain every time they flew, a superficially mundane medical problem was becoming, at this time, a serious handicap to operational efficiency. Fitzgerald's delightfully simple solution was cheap but individually contoured back supports, moulded and cast to match the curvature of the spine. These immediately relieved most, if not all, the symptoms of back pain.

It is over the last fifteen or so years, however, as an 'air crash detective', that Tony Barwood has made his own unique contribution to aviation medicine. He is an acknowledged world expert on ejection seats, using a lifetime's experience and knowledge to enable him to piece together the sequence of events leading to some crucial equipment malfunction. Having identified a fault or a potential weakness, he is able to suggest improvements to equipment and procedures. Not that it is always an easy job getting new ideas accepted. Battling against bureaucracy and obstinacy is an important part of the job, to which the Group Captain, with obvious relish, applies his own particular brand of fiery disdain for authority. If his characteristically blunt, forthright but always humorous approach to his job has not always endeared him to those in authority, it has most certainly made him a popular and respected figure amongst the aircrew whose cause he espouses; indeed, to many of them Barwood *is* the IAM. And the impression he has made is indelible in more ways than one. The upper surface of the personal survival pack, which forms the seat cushion of the ejection seat, has a contoured shape corresponding precisely, and by no coincidence, to that of the Barwood bum!

But to return to the decelerator track. A typical example of the type of post-crash investigation the Institute is asked to conduct is given by a Gannet aircraft which overshot the runway on landing and crashed into a building, causing fatal injuries to the pilot. A mock-up cockpit was built on the sled, and in the cockpit was mounted the appropriate type of aircraft seat, on which sat a dummy. By accelerating the sled to the known speed of the Gannet at the moment of impact, it was possible to reproduce the effects of the impact deceleration and so discover what injuries could be attributed specifically to movement – that is, to inadequate restraint – of the pilot. In another study it was discovered that injuries had been caused by seats shearing from their fixing-points. The IAM team went on to design and make new fixing-points, test them on the track and prove them much superior.

Some rather more basic research has also been carried out on the track. David Reader was interested in whether concussion caused by the type of head impact not uncommonly experienced during a crash landing might sufficiently impair judgement and performance to jeopardize the ability of a pilot to escape from his aircraft. The problem is not so much the actual bump on the head, since the helmet or bone-dome protects against impact, but more the fact that, if the skull inside the helmet is brought to an abrupt halt, the brain inside the skull keeps moving. It is this which can lead to concussion as a result of compression or even tearing of the soft and delicate brain tissues. So a number of subjects were fired off down the track, without any head restraint. Consequently their head was accelerated forward at impact, striking the chest vigorously. A simple task was carried out before and after the impact, and the results were compared. The subjects were found to have performed less effectively afterwards despite the fact that, for reasons of safety, only low levels of deceleration and, therefore, of impact had been used. Obviously at higher levels the effect would probably have been even more pronounced and longer lasting, with potentially serious implications in terms of reducing the ability of an airman to respond to the emergency.

9 To See or Not To See

Excellent night vision was an important attribute for many aircrew during the Second World War. Night interceptors needed to be able to pick up their targets before they themselves were spotted; bomb-aimers needed to be able to place their bombs accurately despite the attentions of searchlights and tracer; and pilots had to be capable of judging their landings correctly on darkened airfields. As Wing Commander Hugh Corner commented, 'Night flying brings out in intensified form the difficulties of day flying.'[1] In 1939 Wing Commander P.C. Livingston was well aware that this would be so, and he had impressed upon the FPRC the urgent need for research in this area, especially to try to find a way of enhancing night vision and to identify factors which impaired night vision.

Livingston was a recognized authority on problems of vision in aviation. He had obtained his pilot's brevet out in Iraq, where he had also carried out valuable work into problems of sun glare and on the effects of glare on night vision. When he came back to Britain, he continued with his vision research, especially after taking over from Clements at the CME. He started to relax the rigid and severe visual standards required of potential aircrew by Clements – later it was calculated that this change in policy released two thousand extra candidates for aircrew training during the Second World War.[2] Perhaps his most valuable work, however, was his design of a set of goggles for aircrew; these gave protection against air blast, dust and glare, whilst still giving a full field of vision. They remained fixed to the flying helmet at any speed and could be rapidly adjusted. Filters or corrective lenses could be changed easily, and the goggles could also be provided with a dark visor which could be tilted into position to enable the pilot to fly directly towards the sun with a minimum of discomfort. The goggles came into standard use in the RAF and, although the aircrew did complain that they were heavy, they were certainly the best available. Livingston also devised a rotating hexagon test which enabled visual tasks, representative of those actually carried out by night fighter pilots, to be simulated. The apparatus consisted of a revolving hexagonal drum, each face being similar and having a series of illuminated panels showing letters, figures and shapes, which could be presented under varying illuminations to simulate moonlight, starlight and dark sky. Six persons could be tested at a time. From an experimental series of eighteen thousand individuals, Livingston was able to set appropriate standards for those aircrew who were given night flying training. During the Second World War, the efficiency of the test was validated in terms of improved operational performance.[3]

Accepting Livingston's advice was one thing but getting the research underway was quite another. The ophthalmological department at the CME was too busy testing the vision of candidates for aircrew training to do any research, and the Physiological Laboratory was fully involved with oxygen systems and g-protection. It was not until February 1941, and the formation of the Night Vision Sub-Committee of the FPRC, that any research was carried out, mainly by three men – Livingston from the CME, Flight Lieutenant Goldie from the Lab and Dr K.J.W. Craik from the MRC Applied Psychology Unit at Cambridge. Together they conducted elegant and useful experiments across the whole field of vision research.

The Americans had reported that glucose greatly aided night vision. Craik, however, was unable to confirm this, and he even achieved the equivalent improvement in more than sixty per cent of his subjects by giving them the same amount of cold water as the Americans, but without the glucose! It was also known that drugs such as alcohol, benzedrine, caffeine, quinine, strychnine and moderate cigarette-smoking had no effect on night vision. Attempts were made to improve night vision by administering massive doses of Vitamin A, but this did not work. The Japanese tried a substance obtained from sharks, and after the war the IAM, checking a German claim, tried an extract from French marigolds. However, the only substance ever shown to improve night vision in normal people was oxygen. This had a marked beneficial effect at 17,000 feet and a slight effect at 9,000 feet. Subsequent work was to reveal a beneficial effect of oxygen at altitudes as low as 4,000 feet, and Bomber Command was advised that its aircrew should continue to use oxygen during a sortie right down to the ground if possible, to enhance their ability to pick up enemy fighters waiting for them to land. Finally night vision could be aided by special night binoculars, by concave lenses (to collect light from a wider area) or by eye movements controlled so as to have the best chance of spotting enemy aircraft from limited visual cues. There were six thousand pairs of night glasses available in the MAP, but the Commander-in-Chief Fighter Command had condemned them without a proper trial.[4]

The most urgent research required was into the exact conditions met on night-time operations – the dazzle from searchlights and guns, the glare from instrument lighting, and internal reflections on the aircraft windows. The flash from cannon and machine-guns was found not to affect night vision, although tracer did. The German searchlights were described as being intense, white or pale green, and very numerous. Searchlights impaired night vision, not only by their direct effect but also because the light was scattered by the aircraft windows and reflected from items inside the aircraft. For the bomb-aimer, it was not only searchlight glare that made life difficult. He also acted as the navigator and after making his way from the well-lit navigation desk to the dark bomb-aiming position, was effectively night blind for some time. Winfield described the frustration of the dark-adapted pilots who could see ground features that the hapless navigator could not. By the end of 1942 Bomber Command had made provision for an extra crew member specifically for bomb-aiming.[5]

Livingston and his colleagues conducted an experiment on a Wellington inside a darkened hangar and found that the ability to see a dim source of light, with glare from three simulated searchlight beams, was impaired by the perspex windows of the aircraft. The visual range through perspex was half that through glass, and this reduced to a quarter when the perspex was dirty. Also, plane glass surfaces were better than curved ones. However, the only short-term solution to the problem was the clear vision panel – a hole cut in the perspex window. Although these improved vision, they detracted somewhat from thermal comfort! Goldie built a useful device which he called a 'dirt-meter' and with which he travelled round Bomber Command to measure visibility through aircraft windows. He also took full advantage of the opportunity to indoctrinate aircrew on the importance of keeping the windows clean – although the impact of his message may have been lost when the aircrew saw Goldie's car, for its perspex windscreen had an opaque arc where the wiper had ground in the mud!

Another source of glare within the aircraft was from instrument lighting, a problem which had received some attention from Livingston and Clements in 1923. They had found that white or pale green light impaired dark-adaptation more than red-orange light, and the latter had subsequently been adopted. But in 1939 aircrew had decided that white floodlighting was an ideal way of lighting cockpits, and this, as well as highly luminous paint on the instruments, was introduced into service. Then in 1941 came a report from Canada which pointed out that red lighting of cockpit instruments allowed preservation of night vision and, in addition, that instruments could be read more accurately and with less fatigue than with luminous paint. However, at this time a system of using fluorescent paint illuminated by ultraviolet (UV) light was being developed at the RAE and looked very promising. Yet nothing was done for a year after that, even though the Vision Committee recommended that Commands should study the matter of instrument lighting as a matter of urgency. By August 1942, with Bomber Command still having taken no action, Air Marshal Whittingham sent Air Chief Marshal Sir Arthur ('Bomber') Harris, the C.-in-C. of Bomber Command, a copy of the Vision Committee's recommendations;[6] almost immediately the Bomber Command Development Unit at Boscombe Down started to study the problem. Thereafter most aircraft were fitted with red lighting until the UV system could be developed. Bomber Command were still carrying out trials on UV lighting in May 1943, and it was not until September 1944 that aircraft were coming off the production line equipped with the system.

Protection from glare could also be provided by goggles. These tended to be worn mainly in open-cockpit aircraft and by gunners in Bomber Command, and so they also had to protect against smoke, flame and foreign bodies such as splinters of glass. These requirements meant that either goggles had to have many layers of screen that could be swung into place as the occasion demanded, or they had to have interchangeable lenses. The design requirements were that the goggles should be optically perfect and as light as possible; because they had to be used by aircrew in battle, they also needed to be robust. Generally speaking, the flying-goggles worn throughout the war were considered unsatisfactory by the aircrew. The normal complaints were that they were too heavy, that the degree of tint was not optimal or that they misted up.

Goggles were also used for the pre-adaptation of aircrew to the dark. It was discovered first that dark-adaptation could be achieved by waiting in a darkened room before take-off, and then that the same result could be achieved by using dark goggles instead. Later the goggles were ruby tinted, which allowed the aircrew to continue with most of their normal activities whilst dark-adaptation was developing. Their benefit was demonstrated at Kirton-in-Lindsey aerodrome by Livingston when a gunner, with normal vision, could not see an aircraft forty yards away on a clear, moonlit night, five minutes after coming out of a brightly lit crew room, whereas another crew member with the same visual standards, who had been wearing pre-adaptation goggles for one hour, could clearly see aircraft parked 150 yards away.[7]

Training and experience also improved night vision. It was not the physiology of the airman that was being changed but the use to which he could put his eyes. Night-vision gymnasia were set up at various places throughout the country so that aircrew could practise various tasks in dim light and be trained in how to scan properly to make maximum use of the visual cues that were available. Some idea of the operational significance of night vision during the war is given by the fact that only a quarter of the submarines known to be on the surface in a given area were ever spotted. Livingston recommended the establishment of a visual training course at Felixstowe for special duty look-outs. The course consisted of lectures and indoor and outdoor training. The indoor exercises included the use of a silhouette room where model ships could be moved on a realistically lit background in such a way that they looked as they would do at sea when viewed from 2,500 feet altitude at a range of two miles.

Unlike the acceleration and oxygen research programmes, vision research during the Second World War did not, in general, produce definitive solutions to problems. This was mainly because the problems were so much more difficult to define and quantify. But this was not always the case. For example, Goldie and Gilson came up with a neat solution to a problem faced by some aircrew who had to keep watch by looking out of the aircraft window, focusing on infinity, and then had to switch to near vision when they looked at a cathode-ray screen; they often found that they could not adjust focus fast enough, and the screen would appear blurred. Goldie and Gilson devised a system that reflected the image from the cathode-ray screen onto the windscreen, focused at infinity, so that the crew member did not have to change his focus looking from the sky to the image. The system was tried in the Beaufighter – surely the very first head-up display, now so common a feature in modern military aircraft (Chapter 11).[8]

After the war, problems of vision became less urgent. The two main areas of research were concerned with effects of glare – from nuclear weapons as well as from the sun – and with laser safety. For more than twenty-five years all the Institute's vision research was spearheaded by one man, Tom Whiteside. Arriving as a Flight Lieutenant in 1949, he was to become Officer Commanding of the RAF's Aviation Medicine Training Centre at North Luffenham, and also Whittingham Professor of Aviation Medicine. Behind a façade of absent-mindedness (he would frequently 'lose' his car, only to find it again exactly where he had left it – at the local railway station), he concealed an acute scientific brain and an impressive linguistic skill. Since his departure from the Institute, the mantle of vision research has fallen upon Dr Derek Brennan, who maintains the high standards set by his predecessor.

In the immediate post-war period, glare was a particularly serious problem at high altitudes, when sunlight was reflected off the clouds beneath. The result was that the outside was so bright that goggles with anti-glare shields had to be used, but the inside of the cockpit, painted black to aid night vision, was so dark that the instruments could hardly be seen. At the same time, there was considerable dissatisfaction with the goggles then in service; the materials and workmanship were so poor that they frequently fell to pieces, and there was evidence that facial injuries during aircraft crashes had been caused by the rims of the goggles. Also, the flip-down filters were insufficiently dark to allow much to be seen out of the cockpit at high altitude but were still too dark to allow vision within the cockpit.[9] Flight Lieutenant Bazarnik suggested to the Vision Committee that a graded density filter was needed, dark at the top and paler towards the bottom, but it was discovered that this idea had been tried and rejected by the RAF in 1925. The best solution seemed to be a visor, attached to the flying-helmet, that could be easily positioned up or down as required. Visors had been assessed previously, but only before the war, when they had tended to blow off in the open cockpits.

Within six months Bazarnik had produced, with RAE help, a simple visor assembly which slid on a track attached from the centre of the back of the helmet to the front. The visor itself was of perspex, and it could easily be positioned up, down or half way. At the same time, an alternative visor, differing mainly in the raising and lowering mechanism, was being developed by Whiteside following a visit he had made to the medieval armour section of the British Museum! This differed from Bazarnik's by being hinged at the sides and being attached to the helmet by a band passing round the front and an elastic strap at the back. Whilst Whiteside's visor was more robust, less liable to accidental damage and easier to make than Bazarnik's, early versions tended to come off the head on sudden exposure to windblast. However, both types of visor were much superior to the goggles they were intended to replace, especially in terms of restriction of vision. By March 1951 both had been tested in flight. They remained in place during accelerations up to 6g, and remained on the face at speeds of up to 300 m.p.h. in an open cockpit – a speed at which the lenses of the goggles were pushed in.[10]

Apart from a misunderstanding with Coastal Command, when the aircrew used the visors all the time during visual search, rather than just to combat glare, the visor assemblies were universally liked and were incorporated on the new aircrew protective helmets. Bazarnik's, with the central track, went on the Mark 1 helmet and, in a more developed form, onto the early Mark 3 helmets, whilst Whiteside's, with an added mechanism that locked the visor down on exposure to the accelerations encountered during ejection (and which never actually worked quickly enough!), was incorporated onto the early Mark 2 helmet.

Since then, the only really significant development in visors has been the production of the double visor system. To protect aircrew from fragments of bird coming into the cockpit at high speed when the aircraft suffers a birdstrike, helmets now have two visors. Internal to the anti-glare visor is a clear visor of polycarbonate specifically for impact protection of the face. The IAM and particularly Derek Brennan, have been involved in checking that the visual characteristics of the visors are acceptable in aviation and that the shape of the visors is compatible with the oxygen mask. The latest version of the aircrew protective helmet, the Mark 4, will have independently operating dual visors so that either may be selected independently of the other, so reducing the number of layers of transparency that the pilot has to look through. Another clear visor that has involved a tremendous amount of work is that for the Aircrew NBC Respirator (Chapter 11). Not only does this visor have to be optically perfect but it also has, like the other polycarbonate visors, to retain that optical perfection after various protective coats have been applied.

With the introduction of atomic weapons into the armouries of the superpowers, it seemed that dazzle from these weapons might seriously impair airmen's eyesight, perhaps sufficiently to prevent them flying their aircraft. The explosion of an atomic bomb does, after all, produce a fireball which can be a hundred times brighter than the sun. There were really two problems: first, that of straightforward, temporary dazzle with the added complication at night of loss of dark-adaptation; and second, the possibility of retinal burns which could leave permanent damage. To study the glare problem, Whiteside had a small tower built on the roof of the IAM, and on this he had mounted a twelve-inch-diameter mirror. An assistant, directed by telephone, could aim the image of the sun to a viewing telescope, where a photographic shutter could control the exposure of a subject's eye to the unexpected flash. The recovery time was then measured. Sir Stewart Duke-Elder, the Civilian Consultant in Ophthalmology to the RAF, 'thought this suicidal' when Whiteside first related the experiments to the Vision Committee, but the Army adviser later described them as 'the only really relevant and reliable work on the human eye which has been done' in the field of nuclear flash.[11] Whiteside found that vision of the cockpit instruments could be regained within a few seconds as long as the instrument lighting was sufficiently intense, although some after-images remained for up to thirty-six hours. In addition, he felt that aircrew could be trained to prolong their initial involuntary blink and to keep their eyes shut for the rest of the duration of the flash; it was especially important to suppress the natural curiosity to look at the explosion. Air Marshal Sir George Mills, the Air Officer Commanding-in-Chief of Bomber Command, was stimulated to remind the Vision Committee that the simple precaution of closing the eyes to protect against atomic flash should not prevent other work going ahead on the project, for the time would come when 'atom bombs would be going off in fair numbers over a big target'. While Whiteside's experiments seemed to confirm that a potential problem existed, it was clearly important that detailed measurements should be made during an actual detonation of an atomic weapon. An opportunity arose in June 1956, when Air Commodore D.A. Wilson, the RAF Consultant in Radiology, was an observer for the test of a British bomb. He reported: 'The effect was almost identical with that produced by the experiments of Squadron Leader T.C.D. Whiteside at the Institute of Aviation Medicine in 1953.' But what could be done to protect the eyes? One possibility was an electromechanical shutter worn on the pilot's helmet, but it was initially thought that this would be unacceptable, and it was not known whether such a shutter could be made to react quickly enough. Nevertheless, this, together with suitable training, seemed to offer the best chance of success.

Technical design of a shutter was started by the RAE and also by the Atomic Warfare Research Establishment at Aldermaston, with the IAM, as the initiators of the project, keeping a close eye on developments. While the provision of a shutter that could successfully be worn by a pilot proved very difficult, and in this country well nigh impossible, Whiteside devised a system that he could use for experimental purposes and which he obtained permission to use during a nuclear test in the Pacific. The Vision Committee had pointed out that Whiteside's experiment was 'no more hazardous than those often used in eclipse observations of the sun', and it considered the risk a reasonable one to take, although the hazards could not be fully predicted. Unfortunately, when he went to Christmas Island, because 'the Air Ministry's position had not been sufficiently clarified as regards responsibility for retinal burns which the observer might sustain', clearance for attendance at the explosion did not reach the test site in time, so Whiteside came all the way home again without seeing an explosion. The minutes of the next FPRC meeting record tartly that the Committee 'could not see how a mechanical protective device could be tested otherwise than by the experiment proposed',[12] and Whiteside returned to Christmas Island. This time he was successful in viewing an explosion and in testing his device, which worked admirably. The after-image of the fireball lasted between two and three hours; apart from that, the only sensation was a prickling of the eye, similar to having dust in it, for five to six hours.

Unless a practicable shutter or some alternative protection could be developed for aircrew, the best chance of preserving vision was by training the aircrew not to look at the flash after the initial blink, although it was recognized that even this would not prevent retinal burns occurring. An aircrew training film was therefore made, with the script written by Whiteside. And that was how the situation remained until the Americans came up with PLZT (lead lanthanum zirconate titanate) anti-flash goggles, which were demonstrated to the FPRC in 1978. The UK requirement for PLZT is more stringent than the American specification, but development of a British version is under way.

Damage to the eyes can also be caused by lasers. Since the early 1960s these have been used increasingly by all three services, particularly for range finding. In April 1963 Air Commodore Stewart was approached for advice on the biological effects of lasers by three separate authorities, and this initiated a programme of research which continued until very recently. Attention has been focused on the threshold levels for retinal damage and on vision after exposure to lasers. The IAM also has tri-service responsibility for laser safety and for determining damage thresholds. This work, and collaborative work with the Institute of Ophthalmology, has been used in the formulation of safe codes of practice produced by the British Standards Institute, the International Electrotechnical Commission, the military authorities and other bodies.

The IAM has been interested in many other areas of vision research over the years. Examples include advising on the quality of the paper used in navigation tables, commenting on the effect of blink rate on the likelihood of mid-air collisions and doing experiments with the RAE on the Calvert airfield lighting system when it was first proposed. Much work has been carried out into the visibility of different colours and symbols for aircrew maps to be used under different lighting systems, and on the use of these maps in the cockpit. Following Dr Matthews' observation that, 'The old-fashioned unfolding of maps is quite out of the question at modern speeds', Wing Commander Ruffell-Smith invented a small track-keeping device which was worn strapped to the knee. All the pilot had to do was keep checking his course on the strip of map running through the box – indeed, an early version of today's moving map display. At about this time Mr Brownrigg, a retired squadron leader who was in charge of the IAM workshop, invented a map-cutting machine, which trimmed the aircrew map to a reasonable size and which saved folding and unfolding the map in flight. Unfortunately, during a demonstration to visiting dignitaries and brass hats, it went berserk, shredding the maps into confetti!

In 1952 Squadron Leader Peter Whittingham became involved in experiments to determine the most effective colour for survival equipment, especially dinghies. The standard colour for RAF dinghies was a shade of yellow known as 'air-sea rescue' yellow. However, the Americans and Australians had been using fluorescent paints on their dinghies in Korea, and there was an indication that they were being found sooner than RAF pilots. Whittingham's experiments proved that visual pick-up of a fluorescent orange dinghy was at three to four times the range of a yellow one. Unfortunately United States sources suggested that sitting all day in a fluorescent painted dinghy was extremely nauseating, and it required a further experiment from Whittingham to disprove this.

The MOS required some convincing, however, as they knew that fluorescent paint could not be applied to the dinghy material and that, even if it could, it would not stay there[13] – regardless of the fact that two of our allies were already doing it! They were eventually convinced, and all standard RAF survival dinghies and the stoles of life-preservers are now flame orange in colour.

The Institute has also been involved in setting standards for vision tests, in developing corrective spectacles, in assessing hard and soft contact lenses and in studying the effects of chemical-warfare agents on vision. Much of the work has been carried out in close co-operation with the RAF consultants in ophthalmology and with the Vision Committee of the FPRC. However, unlike during the war, the IAM's vision interests in the last thirty years have been intermittent and have not been characterized by the same intensive research effort which has been maintained in the fields of oxygen equipment and acceleration.

10 Dressed To Kill

Unpalatable and unfortunate though it may be, it is undeniably true that the military aviator's *raison d'être* is the destruction of the enemy. Since he is operating in an environment that is hostile in both a military and a physiological sense, his ability to survive to do his job depends on the degree of protection with which he is provided. And an important component of that protection is his clothing.

Although from 1917 onwards the concept of 'official issue' flying clothing became increasingly accepted, that clothing still represented what industry thought the RAF wanted rather than what the aircrew of the day actually wanted or needed. Until 1936 the Director of Equipment's department in the Air Ministry had to take on trust the bland assertions of commercial firms that the clothing they developed would do the job it was supposed to do. Consequently throughout the 1920s and 1930s – and, indeed, during the war itself – aircrews attempted to compensate for the inadequacies of their issue flying clothing by wearing various additional items of personal clothing, such as pullovers, extra socks or American flying jackets.

In 1936 it was at last appreciated that the Director of Equipment's organization was unsuitable for experimental work in connection with flying clothing.[1] Development of flying clothing became the responsibility of a Flying Clothing Committee which, from August 1940, was a sub-committee of the FPRC. At the Committee's inception, and until he became the DGMS in 1941, the Chairman was Air Commodore Whittingham. On this Committee sat those representatives from the Director of Equipment's Department who had previously been responsible for flying clothing, and representatives from the several Command Headquarters and from branches concerned with the inspection and distribution of clothing. In other words, the Committee represented an attempt to co-ordinate all the disparate groups within the MAP and the RAF who were in any way concerned with flying clothing. From 1939 onwards the

Flying Clothing Committee liaised closely with the FPRC, this being facilitated by the presence on both of Whittingham himself and Bryan Matthews from the Physiological Laboratory.

In 1936, however, the Committee was still faced with the same fundamental problem that had beset that Director of Equipment; that is, how to exercise some control over the design of flying clothing and, in particular, how to make sure that specifications agreed with commercial firms were actually met. Research into new fabrics and materials was conducted by private industry, with virtually no input from services until the Stores and Clothing Research and Development Establishment was created in 1967. For the clothing manufacturers, this meant that they had to rely on their own testing procedures, which, for flying clothing, needed to be highly specialized. In general, these firms did not have expensive environmental chambers capable of simulating the flight conditions their clothing was supposed to protect against, and even less were they able to flight-test prototype items of clothing. It should come as no surprise, therefore, to learn that the quality of flying clothing and associated personal equipment at the outbreak of war was woefully inadequate. To quote Air Vice-Marshal Harry Roxburgh, 'With some exceptions, the R.A.F. started the War with poor equipment which was quite incapable of protecting the aircrew under either routine or emergency conditions. Indeed, some of the emergency conditions were not catered for at all.' However, at least from August 1939 the RAF Physiological Laboratory was available for consultation. The usual way the Lab became involved in matters relating to flying clothing was by receiving an instruction from the Flying Clothing Committee transmitted either through the FPRC or, after mid 1942, by Whittingham himself at the meetings of the Flying Personnel Medical Officers (FPMOs) held at Farnborough every four weeks. In addition, there was the direct feedback from Winfield and the FPMOs themselves. The Physiological Laboratory was never to be responsible for actually making items of clothing, although Edgar Pask certainly carried out modifications and improvements to clothing he tested, and in 1943 the Laboratory acquired its own tailor. As Roxburgh recalls, if a clothing problem arose, then a meeting would be arranged to bring it to the attention of the manufacturer concerned. Either a new requirement would be established or some modification agreed. Prototypes would be produced by the firm and tested by the Physiological Laboratory. If unsatisfactory, more prototypes would be produced, and so on until a satisfactory result was achieved. Simple items such as gloves were assessed by operational squadrons or by the RAE test pilots in trials organized by the Laboratory. The same could apply to more complex clothing, like flying suits, although many tests were actually carried out using the cold decompression chamber at Synehurst Farm, an outstation of the RAE, with Winfield and Margaret Worthington often acting as subjects. In 1943 the Laboratory was provided with its own cold chamber which could be cooled to minus 40°C, decompressed and simulate wind to a speed of 25 knots.

Cold had remained one of the most serious problems facing airmen during the inter-war period. However, the solution was not to pile on more and more layers of clothing, since this unacceptably reduced mobility, but, as Winfield said in 1941, to provide adequate cockpit heating. Because it is far easier to heat a small cockpit than a large cabin, most of the complaints regarding cold and clothing during the Second World War came from the bomber crews. Huins described the 'special dodges' used to keep warm.[2] Silk pyjamas, cardigans and polo-neck sweaters, all personal clothing, would be worn beneath the flying suit. One officer wore Indian moose-hide moccasins and up to five pairs of loose stockings. However, it was the danger of frostbite which worried the bomber crews, rather than the cold itself. Those worst affected were the gunners, who often had to remain in their turrets for many hours. During 1941 and 1942 frostbite was a common occurrence and a major worry for Bomber Command. To prevent facial frostbite, crews would go without shaving and cover their faces with grease or oil. The real problem, however, was protecting the hands. When guns jammed, they had to be cleared, and if bare flesh inadvertently touched metal, the temperature of which could be well below zero, then the flesh froze instantly. The only protection was to wear silk gloves which both retained heat and allowed adequate finger movement.

In 1939 the basic item of flying clothing was still the Sidcot Suit. However, over the years this had changed considerably, and it was now very different from the suit introduced into the RFC in 1917. Fireproofing had been added early on, and by 1930 it had become a rubberized linen garment. However, the rubber made it too hot for comfort, and by the end of the decade a cotton material was being used instead, although the rubberized suit continued to be issued well into the war. The cotton permitted better ventilation and the relatively unimpeded evaporation of sweat from the skin surface. Also, during the 1930s, a kapok-quilted inner lining was introduced which was detachable and so could be worn with or without the Sidcot Suit. Yet, even when worn together, these failed to provide adequate protection against the bitter cold experienced at high altitudes. So in 1938 thermally insulated jackets were developed made of a flexible, reversed lamb-skin, with a dope treatment on the outer face. These jackets were the immediate predecessors of the Irvin Suits, soon to become the best-known item of World War II flying clothing.[3]

Beneath the flying suit were worn long underpants and a long-sleeved vest. Introduced originally with the Sidcot Suit, these had then been made of wool, which irritated the skin. Therefore in 1923 wool was replaced by cotton, which made them more comfortable but less warm. By 1939 the RAF had reverted to wool, the problem of skin irritation being overcome by plaiting one side of the woollen fabric with (artificial) silk. However, there was disinclination among pilots to wear wool; they preferred to be 'tough' and favoured the cheaper, and rather dingy, cotton underwear.

Footwear before 1930 had usually taken the form of leather ankle-boots, although knee-length boots were also available. Fug-boots had disappeared following the introduction of the Sidcot Suit. The disadvantages of the flying boots of the 1920s were that they were heavy, cumbersome and hardly waterproof. In 1930 a knee-length, sheepskin-lined suède boot was introduced, although in 1936 the suède was replaced by leather, and it was these which were in service at the outbreak of war.

Thus it can be seen that flying clothing at the start of World War II was, in some respects, barely distinguishable from flying clothing at the end of World War I. Neither did flying clothing seem to change much during the course of the war. Appearances can be deceptive, however, and during these six years considerable advances were made in clothing materials, design and fabrication. Attitudes changed too, with the realization that properly designed flying clothing could make a significant contribution to aircrew comfort and that increased comfort meant improved operational efficiency. As early as 1940 it is evident that the Flying Clothing Committee fully appreciated that the multiple-layer approach was the best for cold protection. It proposed that a hard-wearing cotton flying suit should be worn in normal (i.e. warm) conditions but that in the cold a separate kapok lining should be worn beneath. In the post-war period the cotton (later Nomex) flying coverall would become a basic item of the aircrew flying clothing assembly.

Incidentally, the idea for the now familiar pockets on the legs of the coverall originated with the clothing firm of Robinson and Cleaver, which had produced the first official issue flying suit in 1917 and was, in 1940, still submitting new designs for flying clothing.

Yet, throughout the war, manufacturers persisted with the single suit concept. The Irvin Suits were no longer issued from 1943, but, along with Sidcot Suits and American Shearling Suits, they were to remain in use for many more years. The suit that replaced the Irvin Suit was the Taylor Suit, in which thermal insulation was provided by a filling of kapok, and flotation pads of kapok were located in the breast pockets, in the collar and on the legs, so providing buoyancy in the event of a forced landing in the sea. There was also a separate electrically heated lining which was attached to the suit with buttons.

Electrically heated clothing was standard issue for aircrew during the war. Comprising a heated waistcoat, heated gloves and heated sole inserts for boots, the design was based upon the best of the various systems in use at the end of World War I. Be that as it may, experience showed that, overall, electrically heated clothing had not really advanced much since 1917. Examples of the type of problems regularly encountered were given by Roland Winfield: '... electric plugs are liable to pull out, short circuits develop causing complete failure, or hot spots occur and produce an insidious burn which is not noticed until after descent.'[4] The other serious problem was reliability; few electrically heated suits survived ten trips without causing trouble. Also, most wearers seemed to want some means of controlling the heat supply to the suit – a reasonable request one might think, and one easily satisfied by incorporating a rheostat. Yet the official attitude was that this would be '... wasteful as the excess heat would have to be absorbed in resistance'.[5] Incorporation of heat control was considered 'an unnecessary complication'.

Several alternatives to providing either layers of thermal insulation or electrical heating as a protection against cold were investigated during the early part of the war. One of the more exotic was to cover exposed areas of skin with a highly perfumed white ointment called Akrotherm. This was supposed to increase the resistance of the skin to cooling; in practice it was found admirable for dealing with chapped hands and sore skin but for little else – certainly not for cold protection. Another approach was to line the flying suit internally with aluminium. Essentially this was the space blanket concept of reflecting body heat back onto the body surface. That did not work either. A third and potentially more fruitful approach was to blow hot air through tubes fastened inside the flying suit. Unfortunately water tended to condense out of the hot air as it cooled, and not enough heat could be supplied to the hands and feet. By 1943 it had been accepted that the only solution to the cold problem was to provide better cockpit heating, and, indeed, thereafter references to cold are conspicuous by their absence from contemporary records. Another reason was that, even if the clothing itself did not improve much, at least the aircrew learned how to look after it properly. An education programme was begun which taught the importance of clean, loose-fitting clothing, of making sure that sweating was avoided and of adopting the layer principle. In truth, the cold problem in the RAF during World War II was resolved not by aviation medicine but by education and common sense. Problems of survival, on the other hand, were resolved by painful trial and error and by individual heroism and self-sacrifice.

With so much of the flying in World War II being over water, and often over very cold water, research into problems of survival at sea sustained a high priority throughout the war. For obvious reasons the Navy also had a keen interest in sea survival, and some problems were tackled and solved jointly by the RAF in conjunction with the Admiralty. The RAF Physiological Laboratory's most important contribution to flying clothing during World War II was undoubtedly the work on immersion suits and life-preservers conducted by Edgar 'Gar' Pask. Pask, on his arrival at the laboratory in 1941, had quickly acquired an interest in flying clothing, and particularly, in survival clothing.

His first major task was the development of an immersion suit for the pilots of the Merchant Ship Fighter Unit (MSFU). This unit had been formed to protect the convoys operating in the Atlantic and North Sea. One ship in each convoy would be equipped with a Hurricane aircraft which would, if the need arose, be catapult-launched into the air to engage enemy Condor aircraft. A Hurricane launched from a Catapult Armed Merchant (CAM) ship, could not, of course, land back on board, and so, if land was too far away, the pilot had to ditch in the water. For obvious reasons, therefore, a suit was needed which would enable the pilot to withstand a fairly prolonged immersion in very cold water. The suit had to be watertight and yet be comfortable enough to wear for prolonged periods whilst the pilot was on standby aboard ship. If this was to be achieved, three criteria needed to be met. First, the free circulation of water around the body had to be prevented. To accomplish this, all openings in the garments for the wrists, neck and feet had to be sealed to prevent entry of water. Second, a layer of heat-insulating material had to be preserved between the body and the sea. In practice this meant that the inside of the suit had to be kept dry, so retaining the insulating air. Third, the garment could not be completely impermeable, since then any sweat would not be able to evaporate and would instead condense and wet the internal fabric, lowering its insulation value. It was this last requirement of finding a material which was watertight but not air-(or vapour-) tight that presented the problems. So impossible did this seem at first that one physiologist suggested that the only solution was to use the skin and feathers of a sea bird.[6]

Two approaches were pursued. The first was to use leather, and the second was to develop a special cotton fabric. Leather possesses very small pores, and the problem of making it water-repellent was tackled by the British Leather Manufacturers Research Association. Eventually waterproofed, full chrome tanned leather garments were produced which were issued for trial in the CAM ships in 1942. Thermal insulation was provided by an interlining of Tropal, a material newly available during the war which was also used in life-jackets and flying suits. In addition to its insulation properties, Tropal was five times more buoyant than cork and could support thirty times its own weight. Before the 'flying coverall', as the immersion suit was known, was issued to the Hurricane pilots on the CAM ships, it received extensive laboratory and field testing, mostly by Pask himself. The effectiveness of the new suits was admirably illustrated one bitterly cold midwinter's day when Pask was testing one at Sullom Voe Loch, in Scotland. The test had to be discontinued because the observers in the accompanying launch became too cold to continue. Pask, who had been swimming vigorously, came ashore uncomfortably hot! Unfortunately, by the time the suits were ready to enter production, the need for CAM ships had ended. However, the Navy adopted the suits and continued with further development work.

The second approach was to produce cotton fabrics of small pore size and high water-repellency, a task taken up by the British Cotton Industry Research Association at the Shirley Institute. A special Oxford weave fabric was eventually produced which was both comfortable to wear and acceptably waterproof. The manufacturing and processing of garments from this material proved difficult, however, and required great skill from the weavers and seamsters.

Mr J. Silverstone, of Frankenstein Ltd, was responsible for solving many of the problems of tailoring the new fabric, and Frankenstein went on to produce the immersion suits, which were to be issued mainly to the Fleet Air Arm. They were not as waterproof as the leather flying overalls but were less bulky and heavy and therefore more popular. They were sufficiently waterproof to keep a ditched man dry long enough to inflate and board his survival dinghy. If some water did enter, then drain plugs were provided in the integral rubber boots. The immersion suits were used by the Air/Sea Rescue Service, as well as by the Fleet Air Arm, and by the crews of the high-speed motor launches which ran the blockade to bring vital equipment (for example, ball-bearings) from Sweden.

A third type of suit evolved from the immersion suit, and this was the exposure suit. Only half the weight of the immersion suit (i.e. about $2\frac{3}{4}$ lbs), it was inflatable and was intended to be donned either just before baling out or ditching or after entering the dinghy. It was made of two layers of impermeable balloon fabric and was quilted so that an insulating layer of air was maintained even at points of pressure. Again the idea for the suit was Pask's, although in this case the war was just about over before the exposure suit entered service.

Whilst the ideas may have been Pask's, the expert advice regarding which clothing fabrics were worth considering came from a civil servant within the MAP, Mr Harold Franks (who was no relation to the Canadian Wilbur Franks). With his keen interest in, and very considerable knowledge of, all matters relating to clothing materials and fabrics, he was to dominate flying clothing development over the next two decades. Also, with his abhorrence of red tape and bureaucracy, he was the ideal link between Farnborough and the Ministry. A close affiliation and mutual respect developed between Franks in London and Pask, Gilson and Roxburgh at Farnborough, which was the beginning of an essentially symbiotic relationship between the Ministry, industry and the Physiological Laboratory that has endured to this day.

The Lab tested several other types of immersion suit sent to them from elsewhere. The Americans and the Canadians in particular carried out extensive research into water-resistant fabrics, although it seems no suits comparable with the British ones were available during the war. Frankenstein Ltd appear to have co-operated with the Canadians, for on one occasion an employee of the company set out to take one of the firm's suits to Canada, presumably to demonstrate its effectiveness. He got no further than Liverpool, where, on Whittingham's instructions, the poor man was arrested. The immersion suit was taken from him, and then he was allowed to continue his journey. Matthews tells this story to illustrate the pathological obsession with secrecy that prevailed everywhere at that time. The absurdity of this attitude is reflected in the way in which the Canadians, and the Americans even before they entered the war, did everything possible to help Britain.

Squadron Leader Pask's other major contribution to the Laboratory's research effort into flying clothing was his pioneering work on life-jackets. These, like immersion suits, had received virtually no attention after the end of World War I, reliance being placed on the flotation properties of the kapok-lined flying suits. An inflatable life-jacket was actually produced during World War I, but, despite being comfortable and unobtrusive, the 'Perrin Arm Brace' never seems to have caught on. Traditionally, the RAF's first inflatable life-jacket is taken as being the 'Mae West', named after the 'resemblance' of the inflated jacket to the contours of the well-known film star of the period. In 1943 the primary concern was to determine whether the Mae West life-preserver was preventing unconscious survivors from drowning in the sea, and it was this problem to which Pask next directed his attention. It was quickly appreciated that a conscious man, however relaxed, could not imitate the inertness of an unconscious man. So, with Air Commodore R.R. Macintosh, then the RAF Consultant in Anaesthetics, a series of experiments was undertaken using an anaesthetized subject – and the subject was Pask himself.[7] Pask, however, was well qualified to perform this type of experiment and knew the risks involved, for he had been Macintosh's assistant from 1939 until he joined the RAF.

As a preliminary, it was decided to see what happened to an unconscious man unsupported by a life-jacket.[8] The result of the experiment was dramatic – Pask disappeared beneath the surface and came to rest at the bottom of the tank. Having thus conclusively demonstrated that a life-jacket was essential for an unconscious subject, the staff of the Physiological Laboratory proceeded with a full evaluation of the Mae West. To simulate entry into the water from a ditched aircraft, or entry by parachute, Pask would be literally thrown into the tank and then allowed to languish there whilst photographs were taken. By this means Macintosh and Pask were able to prove that the RAF life-jacket did provide a satisfactory floating position for the unconscious subject and that it had acceptable self-righting characteristics which prevented the subject from floating face down. The Taylor 'buoyancy' suit was shown to be highly unsatisfactory in this latter respect.

Some weeks later the procedure was repeated, again with Pask as subject.[9] This time the object was to test the efficiency of eight different types of life-saving equipment. One embarrassing discovery, at least for the Royal Navy, was that their tubular inflatable lifebelt repeatedly failed to turn the face-down Pask. Obviously any unconscious survivor unfortunate enough to fall face-down in the water would, if wearing the Navy belt, drown! And the Navy belt was not the only one unsatisfactory in this respect. Some lifebelts tended to maintain the subject in a near vertical position, where any vertical oscillations resulted in periodic immersion. Others failed to provide adequate support for the head, which consequently lolled from side to side, causing the nose and mouth to enter the water. But the most crucial revelation of all was that the Board of Trade life-jacket, which was manufactured in vast numbers and was widely used, also failed to keep the survivor's head out of the water. It was discovered that the optimum position for the body in the water was face-up at an angle of about 45 degrees. This stopped the tongue falling back into the throat and causing choking, and also minimized wave splash on the face. As a result of these discoveries, a new life-jacket was designed incorporating many improvements, notably providing increased buoyancy to lift the back further out of the water.

Pask's experiments are now, quite properly, regarded as classics, not just because of his outstanding bravery but also because his observations and findings have stood the test of time, providing the basic framework for all future research. Much of that subsequent work was done by Pask himself, but as a civilian and Professor of Anaesthetics at King's College, Durham, now the University of Newcastle-upon-Tyne. Realizing that his experimental technique was hardly likely to attract many volunteers, and presented with the need to conduct his experiments under the more realistic conditions of the sea, he proceeded to design a dummy which he could use instead. This would eventually have electronic equipment, devised by Pask himself, installed within it capable of recording the frequency and duration of the periods when the face of the dummy was immersed. Some experiments using the dummy were carried out in the late 1950s at the Institute.

Although nothing to do with survival clothing and equipment, it is appropriate to mention here another even more heroic experiment conducted by Pask. During the early part of the war there was little information available on the best means of resuscitating aircrew rescued from the sea. Pask, confronted with this question, thought an answer might be provided by a modification of his anaesthetized subject method. This time he not only had himself rendered unconscious but also had administered to himself the drug curare.[10] This, in the right dose, causes complete paralysis of the muscles used in respiration, and so the patient's life can then be sustained only by artificial ventilation. Preliminary conventional anaesthesia was necessary because curare affects mainly the muscles, leaving the brain 'awake' and functioning normally – a potentially terrifying state to be in. During the experiment the effects of alterations in the rate at which Pask's lungs were artificially ventilated on heart rate, blood-pressure and other physiological responses were examined.

Despite Matthews' restraining influence, there is no doubt that in this last experiment Pask did go too far; he was never quite the same afterwards, almost certainly as a result of having his lungs over-inflated. The question naturally arises as to whether the results of his experiments justified the permanent sacrifice of his previous good health. That the immersion suit work and the life-preserver work were eminently worthwhile cannot be doubted, for many lives were saved as a direct result of his efforts. This was very quickly recognized by the award of the OBE in the 1944 New Year's Honours List, and later some of his work would be portrayed in the film *In Which We Serve*. Whether the results of the resuscitation experiment can be similarly justified remains an open question. And, of course, Pask was not the only member of the Laboratory to suffer permanent injury – we have already referred to the damage to Bryan Matthews' vision caused by repeated episodes of decompression sickness. Under Matthews' leadership, morale and motivation were maintained at a high level at the Physiological Laboratory, and this, combined with the exigencies of war, perhaps resulted in some experimental work being pursued rather too enthusiastically. After all, this was long before ethical committees started telling medical researchers what they could and could not do. Pask, Matthews and Stewart were physiologists in the true Haldane spirit: 'You cannot be a good human physiologist unless you regard your own body, and that of your colleagues ... as something to be used, and, if need be, used up.'[11] Pask left the RAF in 1947 and took up an appointment as Reader in Anaesthetics at the University of Durham, where he was to remain until his death in 1966 at the early age of fifty-three. At first he wanted to return to aviation medicine, but the terms offered by the Treasury proved to be unacceptable to him. The FPRC tried to secure an improvement, and in early 1949 he was offered the position of Deputy Chief Scientific Officer at the IAM, with an annual salary of £500. However, by then the University had offered him a Chair, which he accepted, becoming only the second Professor of Anaesthetics in the British Isles.

Tom Macdonald remembers Pask as a modest man determined to do all he could to help the fighting airmen. And, as we have seen, Pask was also an incredibly brave man. Even the prolonged immersions he endured when working on the flying overall, and then the immersion suit – which seem fairly innocuous compared with the life-preserver experiments – were not without their own sacrifice, for Pask was particularly prone to sea-sickness. Yet, despite his unique contribution to aviation medicine, he remains something of an enigma. For example, his name appears only very rarely amongst the eminent scientists who contributed to the wartime publications of the FPRC, while his classical life-preserver work was not to appear in the open scientific literature until 1957. He was constantly providing advice on, and participating in, assessments of flying clothing. He attended virtually all of the FPMO meetings from the first in 1941 until he left the Air Force and, as the minutes show, regularly contributed first-class ideas, often in fields well outside his own particular expertise – something he would continue to do on his return to civilian life. He would be remembered after his death as a brilliant teacher and a man of stature in world medicine. The RAF Physiological Laboratory was indeed fortunate to have enjoyed the services of such a man.

Survival equipment apart, there were few developments in flying clothing during the war which led to any significant improvement in the comfort and well-being of aircrew. Compared with the achievements in hypoxia prevention or g-protection, those made in the field of flying clothing pale into insignificance. Nevertheless, some progress was made, most notably in terms in the new clothing fabrics and materials which were developed under the pressures of war. Largely, however, these were the products of the efforts of the clothing industry, and in the immediate post-war period considerable commercial benefits would accrue to the firms involved. What the RAF gained was an appreciation that flying clothing could not be regarded merely as a collection of individual items which could be put on and taken off at will; it had become a complicated assembly which, if it was to be effective, needed to be integrated with other personal equipment such as the parachute and harness-restraint systems, the communication system and the oxygen supply. Items like the anti-g suit and the Bazett pressure waistcoat provided just a foretaste of the ever-escalating complexity of flying clothing which has continued to the present day.

When clothing becomes highly specialized, there is an increasing need for that clothing to fit the individual properly if it is to operate effectively. The problem with aircrew is that they come in all shapes and sizes. Whilst there may be ample room on the flying suit of a tall individual to attach, say, an oxygen-supply hose, on a smaller individual that hose might foul on the restraint harness. The problem is far more serious when it comes to designing cockpits so that all instruments are accessible to pilots of any size. During the war very little information was available regarding the physical dimensions of the aircrew who wore the standard-issue clothing and who flew aeroplanes which often were an ergonomic nightmare. Almost certainly many of the flying clothing problems that did arise during the war simply reflected inadequate fit.

It was John Gilson and Harold Franks who first realized that a more scientific approach to the sizing of flying clothing was needed. The essential requirements was for details of the physical dimensions of the aircrew so that clothing covering an appropriate size range could be produced. In other words, what was needed was an anthropometric survey of aircrew, and to carry out such a survey the Physiological Laboratory acquired the services of the eminent anthropologist and statistician Dr G.M. Morant. Geoffrey Morant had established his scientific credentials during the late 1920s and early 1930s, with a series of elegant scientific papers. However, his most important anthropological works, certainly in terms of their practical and particularly political impact, came in 1939. Deeply disturbed by what he saw as Hitler's perversion of physical anthropology to 'prove' the Aryan purity of the German race, Morant responded with two powerfully argued expositions (the second of which was prefaced by J.B.S. Haldane) in which he ruthlessly but entirely scientifically destroyed the Nazi case and in fact demonstrated that the Germans were the most heterogeneous group in Europe!

Although it was 1944 before he actually became a member of the Laboratory's staff, he conducted a preliminary survey of 2,400 potential aircrew recruits in 1943. This revealed that the grading of sizes for flying clothing was highly unsatisfactory. But, more than this, garments purportedly of the same size proved to have widely varying dimensions. For example, a given waist size for trousers could vary by as much as ten inches between different manufacturers! From the measurements made, it was clear that specifications for new garments could be laid down far more effectively, for example, by reducing the number of different sizes available. For flying clothing these numbered seventeen, and for demobilization clothing forty. Until near the end of the war the size specification for RAF clothing was based on that laid down for the British Army in 1905, although many modifications had subsequently been made, on a trial-and-error basis, in response to criticisms of the stock-size garments. Unfortunately no statistics had been kept regarding the number of garments altered, and so a completely new range of sizes needed to be specified.

It was in response to this need that in 1944 Morant and Gilson carried out a detailed survey of body and clothing measurements on 550 RAF aircrew. The object was the acquisition of data for the specification of a size range for flying clothing. Morant and Gilson were able to provide Harold Franks with recommendations regarding an appropriate range of sizes for most items of flying clothing. The clothing was then manufactured in those size ranges and issued to the squadrons for an extensive fitting trial and general evaluation. As Roxburgh points out, anthropometric surveys are very time-consuming and produce mountains of figures. However, the work of Morant and Gilson brought order and science to the chaos and confusion surrounding the design and sizing of flying clothing, and their work has stood the test of time. If Pask's work represented the Physiological Laboratory's most significant contribution to flying clothing during World War II, then the work of Morant and Gilson must come a close second.

Application of the anthropometric approach has allowed the optimum use to be made of a limited size range of clothing. For most flying suits and coveralls, adequate fit can be obtained using only nine sizes, although to achieve perfect fit in the tailoring sense many more sizes than this would be needed. However, such an extensive size range would make neither economic nor logistic sense. What was also appreciated very early on was that aircrew clothing needed to be aircraft specific; so there is now a specific Aircrew Equipment Assembly (AEA) for each aircraft type.

In the 1950s and early 1960s flying clothing was categorized as high or low altitude and winter or summer. High-altitude winter was the most thermally insulating assembly, and low-altitude summer the least. A partial pressure-suit (for example, the combined pressure and anti-g suit) would be part of the high-altitude assembly, and an air-ventilated suit (described later) part of the low-altitude summer assembly. However, by the mid 1960s the high-altitude category had all but disappeared in the RAF, because of the realization that aircraft high up were very vulnerable to missile attack. The TSR2 was the last aircraft for which a full high-altitude AEA was planned. Since then Britain has operated a low-altitude air force; aircraft fly below the level of radar detection. So now there are just two categories of AEA – summer and winter.

The development of flying clothing over the last thirty years has tended to follow patterns and principles established, but not put into practice, during the war. The most important advances since the war have come from the new synthetic fibres developed by the chemical and textile industries, and this has had particularly important implications for the designs of cold-weather protective clothing and for immersion suits. It has also been especially important in developing fire-retardant clothing. For example, the lightweight flying coveralls in use during the latter part of the war, and for many years thereafter, were made of windproof gabardine. However, in 1966 the Mark 11 coverall was introduced, and this was made of a Flax/Terylene fabric which offered better fire-protection. Since then many more fire-resistant fabrics have been developed, of which two, Nomex and Teklan, are currently in use. Although both are rather expensive, Nomex is some two to three times more resistant to abrasion, tear and tension than Flax/Terylene and so is more durable.

Pressure and anti-g suits apart, three themes have dominated flying clothing since World War II: protection against cold, against heat and against the chemical agents which could be used in any European war. It may seem surprising that cold was still a problem, despite the realization during the war that cabin heating was the only really effective way of keeping aircrew warm. The trouble was that, whilst cabin heating is fine in theory, in practice it needs heavy conditioning plant if it is to be an adequate solution to the problem. This immediately incurs a penalty in terms of reduced payload or restricted operating range. So there has to be compromise. But this compromise resulted in totally ineffective heating systems being installed in aircraft like the Shackleton Mark 1 and several Marks of Canberra. Some light training aircraft have no heating at all, and some fighter and bomber aircraft have heating only after the engine has been started, making any prolonged stand-by in wintry conditions a chilly business.

Cold is, of course, particularly associated with altitude. Consequently, the problem did tend to diminish in importance once the RAF started operating mainly at low altitudes. Also, because so little flying is now done at high altitude, there is no longer the serious concern expressed during the 1950s of the intense cold that would be experienced following failure of the pressure cabin. Nevertheless, severe cold can still be experienced flying at low altitudes in the European winter; helicopters, flying in the search and rescue role and the anti-submarine role, do so with doors open or even removed. Then there is still the problem with which Edgar Pask was so concerned – how to protect against the cold of immersion in the sea. Hence, in the post-war period there has remained a need to protect aircrew from cold in the air, in water and, indeed, on land too. Most of the time this has been possible only by providing appropriate flying clothing and equipment.

Although the thick, bulky Sidcot, Irwin, Shearling and Taylor flying suits continued to be used for several years after the war, the basic philosophy behind environmental protection was based on the use of multi-layer clothing, so that a single clothing assembly could be applied to the wide range of environmental conditions encountered by aircrew. Thus, with one or two exceptions, flying clothing was no longer designed exclusively for protecting against specific adverse climatic conditions but rather for integration and co-ordination with other items.

This concept is well illustrated by the first of the post-war cold-weather overalls, which evolved as a result of the experiences of, amongst others, Squadron Leader Tony Barwood from the IAM, who participated in survival exercises in the Canadian Arctic and in Norway in the late 1940s. The Overall Mark 1 was a two-piece garment which could be worn under all conditions in which the RAF were likely to operate. For ground survival, the jacket and trousers could be separated to allow ventilation – one of the greatest problems of physical exercise in a dry, cold environment is not so much keeping warm but keeping cool! With all the clothing insulation, the body temperature rises quickly, leading to sweating. Sweat, if it condenses on the clothing, not only causes the clothing to feel cold and clammy, but more importantly, reduces the insulation of the clothing. A cardinal rule in cold climates, therefore, is 'don't sweat'. The multi-layer principle allows this rule to be followed, as clothing can be easily and quickly stripped off – and put back on – as required.

The cold-weather overall was also intended to form part of the high-altitude flying clothing assembly. However, it was soon discovered that, for the level of temperature likely to be experienced – minus 40°C to minus 85°C – it was unrealistic to rely on insulation alone. The only solution seemed to be some sort of personal heating. Air was tried first, but all that was achieved by blowing hot air through the RAF's personal cooling garment, the air-ventilated suit, was an unlikely combination of second-degree burns and frostbite![12] Electrical heating was tried next.

Electrically heated gloves and socks, as well as complete electrically heated suits, had remained available, usually as ex-wartime stock, throughout the 1950s. The two-piece suits were, however, very uncomfortable, and so the late Dr John Nelms, a national serviceman who stayed to become a civilian at the Institute and later Director of the Army's equivalent of the IAM, the Army Personnel Research Establishment, developed a one-piece garment for wear next to the skin. Wire and terylene yarn were knitted together, giving a close-fitting but elastic and comfortable suit. All the signs were that this would have been a very successful and worthwhile item of flying clothing, with every chance that it would have been far more reliable and durable than earlier electrically heated suits. Unfortunately two things happened. First, there was the shift from predominantly high-altitude to predominantly low-altitude flying; second, the two-piece acrilan-pile coverall, or 'Bunny Suit', appeared. All development work at the Institute on electrically heated suits stopped, and it has never restarted.

Acrilan pile was a product of advances made in artificial-fibre technology. The disadvantage of natural fleeces and piles is that they are bulky and heavy. They are also expensive, and they tend to aggregate and flatten with wear, which adversely affects the insulation they provide. Synthetic materials, on the other hand, are relatively cheap, and they launder and wear well without deterioration of the insulation. The Bunny Suit is now the first line of defence in protecting against the cold, with further layers of insulating clothing being added according to the severity of the conditions.

Opportunities to evaluate the effectiveness of cold-weather flying clothing assemblies arise each year during the winter training exercises held in northern Norway. The IAM has, on several occasions, sent staff as observers – or sometimes even as participants. These exercises have shown that the clothing available is generally adequate; if there are complaints, they are usually about cold hands, about which little can be done. Because today's aircraft do have better cockpit heating systems than the aircraft of two or three decades ago, cold is no longer the severe, routine problem for aircrew that it once was. On the other hand, the strategic importance of NATO's vulnerable northern flank means that the RAF must remain prepared and able to conduct military operations under Arctic conditions. Indeed, as the 1982 South Atlantic campaign demonstrated, it must also be prepared to operate under near Antarctic conditions. The military conflict over the Falkland Islands does, in fact, admirably illustrate the single most difficult cold protection problem that the RAF (and the Royal Navy) has to face, routinely; that is, protecting its people from the sea.

Immersion in the sea represents the ultimate in cold-survival. Like the South Atlantic, the open sea around the UK is cold even in summer, and the size of the British Isles, coupled with the restricted and overcrowded airspace, means that some flying over the sea is virtually obligatory. Consequently the aircrew of today are just as much in need of protection from cold-water immersion as were the Hurricane pilots operating from the CAM ships. As then, the need is for a completely waterproof outer cover, but also one which will allow the outward passage from the skin of evaporated sweat. The search for the perfect fabric is still being pursued just as vigorously today as it was by Edgar Pask at the Physiological Laboratory during the war.

From Pask's leather 'flying overall' to the present Mark 10 immersion coverall, all have had one overwhelming disadvantage: they have always been designed to be worn over the top of all other flying clothing, the idea being, of course, that everything underneath is kept dry and therefore keeps the wearer warm. The trouble is that the immersion suit then blocks access to the pockets of the flying coverall. The importance of these pockets to aircrew must not be underestimated. On the latest coverall there are eight of them, and all are usually bulging with maps, pens, briefing notes, checklists and manuals to which the airman needs ready access. There are other disadvantages of an external immersion suit. For example, being worn over the other clothing means that it is susceptible to damage. Even small tears or punctures, such as might easily occur during ejection or even climbing into or out of an aircraft, could mean the difference between death and survival in the sea. What is needed is an immersion suit that can be worn underneath the aircrew coverall, but, at least until recently, this has not been possible because of the suit's bulk and inherent inflexibility. However, research conducted at the Shirley Institute and by industry has resulted in a much improved cotton ventile cloth, and so now it seems likely that an internal immersion coverall will be feasible. If so, then it will be the most important step forward in the development of flying clothing for a very long time.

Looking back over the years since the war, there have, in fact, been remarkably few new developments in flying clothing. Until the 1970s the only new items to have appeared have been those designed to protect against the heat. Flying in hot climates presents its own special problems with regard to flying clothing. Aircrew tend to suffer severely from the heat whilst on the ground and waiting to take off, and then, as they climb to altitude, a rapidly falling air temperature combines with clothing wet with sweat to produce the reverse problem – cold. Between the wars the standard tropical flying kit was shorts and short-sleeved shirt, and this had not changed much by the time of the Middle East Campaigns of 1941, although lightweight khaki flying overalls were available. It was only after the war that the problems of flying in hot climates received any real attention. The urgent need for some form of protection was emphasized by the FPMO of Fighter Command after the war, Wing Commander Cellars, who, during a visit to units of the Middle East Air Force, saw for himself 'the drenching sweats which accompany flight in the Vampire at speed at low level', which 'reduce the blackout threshold and aid the onset of fatigue'.[13] Even though the RAF has now withdrawn from areas where severe environmental heat is regularly encountered, heat stress, perhaps even more than cold stress, remains a potentially serious operational hazard. One reason for this is that, whilst the effects of cold can be countered to a certain extent by piling on extra layers of clothing, there is a limit to how much flying clothing can be left off. Increasingly since the last war, formerly optional items of flying clothing have become essential. For example, the anti-g suit, which contributes significantly to the heat load, is an integral part of the modern AEA. Of even greater significance has been the more recent introduction of nuclear, biological and chemical (NBC) protective clothing, which adds an extra layer over the entire body surface. Not only does this represent an increase in the total clothing insulation, but also NBC clothing is less permeable to water vapour than conventional flying clothing. This means that body sweat is less able to evaporate and so is less effective in cooling the skin. Another reason is that, coinciding with the progressive withdrawal of British forces from these regions, there was the shift in emphasis from high- to low-altitude flying. At low altitudes the air is denser, and so the frictional or aerodynamic heating of the aircraft becomes greater. So flying at low altitude tends to be considerably hotter than flying at the same speed and air temperature at high altitudes. To make matters still worse, the engineers have, over the years, been putting more and more electronic equipment into aircraft, all of which produces heat. Consequently aircrew of fast jet aircraft still need to be protected against the heat.

At first sight a cockpit air-conditioning system might seem the obvious solution. However, just as with cockpit heating systems, there is a penalty to be paid in terms of reduced aircraft load-carrying capacity or operating range. The conditioning air has to be bled from the engines, which means less thrust. It has to be cooled, which means carrying the additional weight of heat exchangers. And, if the air-conditioning is to be at all effective, a high throughput of air is necessary, which creates noise that interferes with communication systems. Consequently, although all fast jet aircraft do have cockpit conditioning, this is often barely adequate, and, even under the generally temperate summer conditions of Germany and the UK, flying can be a hot, sticky and therefore very uncomfortable business.

A more economical way of providing air-conditioning is to supply the cooling air not to the entire cockpit but just to the aircrew. The originator of this idea seems to have been Wing Commander Tom Macdonald. During a visit to the Middle East Command in the winter of 1940-41, he had suggested that one solution to the heat-stress problem might be to circulate cold air through the flying suits on the ground and at low altitudes, and then warm air at high altitudes. Nothing was to come of the idea, however, until it was 'resurrected' by Tony Barwood nearly ten years later. By then the RAF, as Cellars had found, were encountering really serious problems with heat stress in pilots flying from bases in the desert and Tropics. High-altitude flights were the norm, and so the aircrew were having to wear thermally insulating clothing, even through a significant proportion of sortie time was spent on the ground, at readiness, waiting for take-off. Consequently the heat load was severe – so severe as to represent a threat to operational efficiency. Squadron Leader Barwood's solution was the air-ventilated suit (AVS). In its earliest form this was a nylon garment with a ventilating harness of narrow-bore, polyvinyl chloride tubing through which cooled air was passed. At that time there was no climatic chamber at the Institute, and so this prototype AVS had to be evaluated in the 'hot' room – a room heated simply by the large number of boiler and central-heating pipes that converged there. Nevertheless, a temperature of 40°C could be attained, and the test certainly showed that air personal conditioning seemed to work. But to prove the point beyond doubt and to justify continuing to put more time, effort and money into the project, it needed to work in an aircraft in a hot climate. So a flight trial was arranged in Khartoum. This took place in May 1950 and involved, besides Barwood, Wing Commander Ruffell-Smith, Squadron Leader Howitt and Flight Lieutenant Latham. The equipment was ferried out by Dakota, whilst Howitt flew the Institute's Vampire aircraft, in which the trial was conducted, over from Farnborough. To increase the severity of the thermal stress, some high-speed low-level flights were flown in which cockpit temperatures reached 56°C. Despite some problems with the air-supply and cooling systems, the AVS most definitely reduced the strain induced by these very high temperatures. Air-ventilated suits had arrived.

Over the next two years development of the AVS continued under Tony Barwood at the Institute, and by 1954 it was in service with Canberra and Venom aircraft. In its final form, the suit covered only the trunk and thighs and was made of a lightweight nylon fabric with the air tubes stitched to the outer surface. This partial body coverage was, however, a serious disadvantage from a physiological point of view. Cooling was provided by the ventilating air evaporating sweat as it was produced – and sweat is produced over all of the body. Presumably, if aircrew considered that so much benefit could be obtained from such a suit, then surely even more benefit would accrue from a suit which covered all of the body. Also, with the experience gained with the Mark 1, it became obvious that the air-distribution system could be made much more effective. Between 1954 and 1957 the RAE, in conjunction with the IAM, worked on the problem. The result was a suit, the Mark 2, which covered the whole body. As before, a nylon fabric supported a network of branching PVC tubes; however, there were many more of these than in the Mark 1, and so the ventilating air could be distributed evenly over the body surface, increasing the effectiveness of heat exchange. The Mark 2 remained in service with the RAF into the 1970s. Widely used when first introduced in 1958, demand for personal conditioning gradually became less during the 1960s, until only Vulcan squadrons operating from Cyprus were using the AVS in the early 1970s. Although it was never very popular, nobody questioned that those flying in very hot conditions were much better off with it than without it. One reason for its unpopularity was the unusual way it was put on – rather like a surgeon's operating-gown, with ties at the back. Another was that the nylon material of the suit made the AVS unnecessarily hot when unventilated – a cotton-based material would have been far more sensible.

Research into air personal conditioning systems continued at the Institute throughout the 1960s and into the 1970s, although, as it turned out, to little avail. A serious disadvantage of both the Marks 1 and 2 was that they cooled by evaporating sweat. This meant that the wearer had to be producing sweat, and therefore be already hot, before the suit started to work. Flight Lieutenant John Billingham, later to become Director of Life Sciences for NASA, was the first to show that a suit which removed heat by convection was just as good, if not better, than one which removed heat by evaporation. That was in 1960, and over the next few years it was the convective, as opposed to the evaporative, AVS which dominated personal conditioning research. An important feature of this research effort was that design principles for convective personal conditioning were no longer just empirically based but were established in addition by theoretical considerations of the many factors influencing heat exchange. This approach was, of course, hardly new to the engineers of the RAE, who had contributed to the design of the Mark 2 evaporative AVS. It was new, however, to many physiologists, who tended to forget that the laws of physics apply to human beings just as to everything else. The biophysical approach to physiological heat-exchange mechanisms was fostered at the Institute by Dr David Kerslake. Kerslake, like John Nelms, was an ex-national serviceman who stayed on afterwards as civilian. His application of mathematical and engineering principles not just to the optimization of designs for personal and cabin air-conditioning systems but also to the study of physiological temperature regulation, earned him international recognition.

Although much of the credit for the work on air personal conditioning systems must go to John Billingham, it is not for this that he is best remembered by his colleagues. The IAM is always being asked for advice on matters relating to survival, whether in the Arctic or desert, jungle or sea, and in 1961 Billingham was consulted on a problem of desert survival. Would the millions of white snails found in the Libyan Desert not provide a valuable source of water? There was only one way to find out.

An initial sample of a thousand snails was obtained, and a variety of tests carried out to check that the liquid they contained was safe for human consumption. Having established that it was, a further ten thousand live specimens were flown from North Africa, and smashed to obtain some twenty litres of liquid. During an experiment in which Billingham himself was exposed for six hours a day for four days to a simulated desert environment in the Institute's climatic chamber, he drank the snail juice, half a pint at a time, at a rate which satisfied his thirst. Apart from some nausea at the end of the first day, allayed by adding flavouring, the liquid had no adverse effect, and it was concluded that these snails could provide a valuable source of water to desert survivors. But the two undying memories of those who assisted with the experiment are of escaping snails crawling everywhere, leaving their slimy trails over doors, walls and windows – even in the kitchen – and of John Billingham's breath, which smelled so awful that nobody would approach within two yards of him!

By 1970 experiments had shown that not only did the convective AVS provide much more cooling than the evaporative AVS but that it was almost as good as what was generally regarded at that time as the ideal personal conditioning system – water cooling. The basic principle of water cooling is the same as air cooling – the circulation through a suit of fluid which removes heat from the skin surface. An important difference, however, is that, having a far greater thermal capacity than air, much less water is required to extract the same amount of heat. In fact, whilst air flows of up to seven hundred litres per minute are necessary for some AVSs, water needs to flow through a suit at only one litre per minute.

Cooling by circulating liquid through pipes in a suit was regarded as something of a novelty until the Apollo space programme proved the concept to be sound in practice as well as in principle. Sound it may be, but liquid-cooled suits are not being used by the RAF or by any other air force. Yet the concept, which dates back to 1959, is British in origin, and the first prototype garment was produced at the RAE in 1962, by Mr Des Burton, in collaboration with John

Billingham from the IAM.[14]

A number of experiments were performed in which the suit was used not just for cooling subjects exposed to hot environments but also for heating subjects exposed to cold environments. And so impressive were the results that shortly afterwards NASA requested a demonstration of the RAE suit. A second prototype was quickly prepared for the demonstration, which took place at Houston, Texas, late in 1963. The subject wore the garment beneath a full pressure suit, and with considerable additional clothing insulation, whilst carrying out light exercise in a 37°C environment. Without cooling he could work for no longer than forty-five minutes and sweated profusely; with cooling sweating gradually diminished, and the subject was able to continue working in comparative comfort. Clearly the liquid-cooled suit (LCS) provided extremely good protection against the heat. The Americans therefore undertook a development programme of their own for the liquid-conditioned suit, which was to culminate, in the late 1960s, in the Apollo suit.

It was not until some twenty months after the first experiments with the prototype suit, and eight months after the demonstration to NASA, that the RAF expressed any interest in the concept of liquid cooling. It was decided that a formal programme of research should be undertaken, with a view to providing liquid-conditioned suits to aircrew whose operational role required them to wear pressure clothing, and to aircrew employed on low-level operations in hot climates. By early 1965 the Frankenstein Group Ltd had accepted a contract to manufacture LCSs for the RAF, and over the next two years several different types of garment were produced, and evaluated jointly, by Frankenstein Ltd, the RAE and the Institute. To begin with, problems were encountered with over-cooling of the skin, and these were solved by enclosing the tubes in fabric tunnels and doubling the length of the tubing from 60 to 120 metres. Some of the very earliest suits were evaluated in Libya, and the results were encouraging; they were considered comfortable, the cooling adequate and acceptable, and the profuse sweating seen in aircrew not wearing the LCS was completely absent. Certainly by 1966 the future for the LCS looked promising. However, then came two flight trials, both in Lightning aircraft, in which the LCS proved totally unreliable, providing insufficient cooling, leaking and tearing at the wrists and ankles. Although the inadequate cooling was the fault of the too small refrigeration unit used to cool the liquid circulating through the suit, rather than of the suit itself, the official report was damning. Indeed, the LCS was regarded by one pilot as being sufficiently uncomfortable to 'constitute a flight safety hazard'.[15] The consequences were dramatic; all research was halted for eighteen months. It was only in mid 1968, with an official request for a 'proper trial of reasonable proportions – to determine the future of the LCS for the British Services',[16] that work resumed. That trial took place in Cyprus in 1972, and, although no physiological measurements were taken, an assessment of Vulcan aircrew reactions to the LCS based on questionnaires, showed that they much preferred it to the evaporative AVS they habitually wore.

By this time chemical defence was becoming a recognized part of the UK defence strategy. It had been originally intended that the RAF's new multi-role combat aircraft, the Tornado, should be provided with the convective AVS personal conditioning system, but it would clearly be the height of folly to use such a system in a chemically contaminated environment. To begin with, it was thought that the air could be filtered first, but this so reduced the flow that the cooling provided was totally inadequate. With the evidence that aircrew liked the LCS, there was only only solution – adopt liquid conditioning for the Tornado. So what killed the convective AVS saved the LCS. But this was only a temporary reprieve. Despite impressive evidence from further laboratory evaluations at the Institute regarding the suit's potential – it could keep subjects comfortably warm over four hours at minus 26°C, and comfortably cool over four hours at 50°C, both potentially lethal environmental conditions – the entire liquid-conditioning research programme was halted following the 1978 Defence Review. It might be thought that the financial saving resulting from not producing liquid-conditioned suits for Tornado aircrew would be almost negligible compared with other items of military expenditure by the RAF. In point of fact, the problem lay not with the suits but with the system needed to supply the suits with cool liquid. To provide liquid at a suitably low temperature in a hot environment and pump it through the suit had needed a fairly substantial refrigeration and pumping plant. This presented no problem in the laboratory nor in the aircraft trials in which transports and bomber aircraft had been used. It did present a problem in the small fighter aircraft where space was at a premium.

By 1973 a possible solution had emerged. Mr Douglas Bewley, an engineer in the Experimental Physics department of the RAE, put forward the idea of a 'one-man conditioning pack'. The plan was for a cockpit-mounted heating and refrigeration unit capable of supplying one LCS. From the start, extremely severe size limitations were imposed – too severe as it turned out. The overall size was to be about that of an ordinary house brick – hence the name by which the unit became more familiarly known, the 'Bewley Brick'. Development work proceeded for a few years, but then the project ran into difficulties, the most important of which was that the system was proving very expensive – it was going to cost upward of £3 million just to equip Tornado aircrew with liquid personal conditioning. Taken with the fact that there was no evidence that there would be a heat problem in the Tornado, the decision to abandon the programme was hardly surprising. However, even had the programme continued, it is doubtful whether the design specification for the 'Bewley Brick' could have been met within the size limitations imposed, at least in the short term. Miniaturization of refrigeration equipment had not, in 1978, proceeded quite far enough. So nearly twenty years of research and development had apparently come to nought.

The story of the development of liquid personal conditioning systems in the UK is a long and unhappy one. Unfortunately, as we have seen before, neither is it atypical. On the other hand, given the right stimulus, the gestation period for an item of clothing or equipment can be drastically reduced. An excellent example of this came recently during the Falklands crisis. For many years the RAF has used a stretcher restraint harness that is heavy, complicated and expensive. Faced with the need to replace many which had reached the end of their useful life, the Ministry of Defence asked the Institute to suggest a new design. This it did, and a new harness was being constructed, and tested successfully on the decelerator track, at the time Argentina invaded the Falkland Islands. The RAF had to prepare for the possibility that large numbers of casualties would need to be evacuated by air, so the Ministry decided that a thousand of the new harnesses should be made. Within five weeks of that decision, all thousand harnesses had been made and delivered to the RAF Aeromedical Evacuation Squadron, although, in the event, they were not needed.

However, as far as protection against the heat is concerned, for aircrew there is, at present, none! The important question is whether this really matters. To answer it, information is needed on how hot aircrew become when flying fast-jet aircraft. Over the last ten years considerable effort has been made to obtain this information using automatic thermal data-recording (ATDR) equipment especially designed and built at the Institute. This equipment has allowed the measurement not just of how hot and humid the cockpit of a fighter aircraft becomes during operational sorties but also of how hot the pilot becomes and what happens to his heart rate. These measurements have shown that some aircraft cockpits become very uncomfortable places, even on relatively cool days. Until the development of the ATDR, laboratory simulations of in-flight thermal conditions were largely a matter of guesswork. There was no real evidence that the temperatures used were representative of those actually experienced in an aircraft. Yet laboratory simulations are the only economical and safe way of determining whether, for example, some new item of flying clothing significantly increased thermal discomfort or whether an air- or liquid-conditioned coverall provides adequate protection against a particular level of environmental temperature. This was precisely why the Institute had acquired a climatic chamber in 1952. The chamber comprises a heavily insulated tunnel, roughly oval shaped, around which air is circulated by a large axial-flow fan. An elaborate heating, ventilating and air-conditioning plant permits control of air movement, temperature and humidity over a wide range and within very close limits, so that virtually any type of climate, apart from severe cold, can be reproduced. Furthermore, the effects of sun and rain can also be simulated. Over the last few years the chamber has been extensively used for investigating the increased heat stress imposed by NBC clothing.

In the mid 1960s it became apparent that there was a possibility of chemical weapons being used if there were another war. It was obvious, therefore, that aircrew would need to be protected from chemical agents, and since then the Human Engineering Division of the RAE, together with the IAM and the Chemical Defence Establishment (CDE) at Porton Down have played a leading part in the design of clothing and equipment to protect aircrew in chemically contaminated conditions. Below the neck, protection is provided by coveralls impregnated with activated charcoal to absorb and neutralize chemical agents. Ground personnel wear chemical protective overgarments, but this is unsatisfactory for aircrew, since all their specialist equipment would be inaccessible underneath, and the various hoses which would pass through the overgarments would be a contamination hazard. In the early 1970s Mr R.E. Simpson of the RAE suggested that the chemical protective layer should be moved underneath the other layers of clothing. Thus items such as the life-preserver, the g-suit and the flying coverall would be allowed to become contaminated and would be re-used in a contaminated condition. Bob Simpson, in conjunction with Wing Commander Derek Beeton of the IAM (now unfortunately deceased) and the CDE, came up with the NBC aircrew under coverall.

Above the neck, the eyes, lungs and skin also had to be adequately protected against chemical agents. The problem was to devise a respirator which could be used with the existing protective helmet, oxygen mask and communication system. For several years the solution was thought to be a form of overhood, but the total head assembly proved so large that head mobility was unacceptably restricted and the big domed visor found to be incompatible with the many optical systems the modern pilot is expected to use. Then in 1976 Simpson suggested a respirator worn under the protective helmet, and it is this concept which has been adopted. Basically the respirator comprises a rubber cowl which encloses the head and is sealed at the neck. Blown, filtered air is supplied to the inside of the respirator, thus maintaining a positive pressure which prevents the entry of chemical agents. It is, perhaps, difficult to imagine such a device actually providing adequate protection, whilst at the same time being safe for flying and acceptable to aircrew. That the Aircrew Respirator (AR) NBC No 5 is safe for flight, has achieved a high degree of acceptability and has been processed from concept to production in just three years (when ten years is a good average for items of new equipment), reflects the greatest credit to the Farnborough research establishments, particularly Group Captain John Ernsting and Mr Arnold Cresswell of the IAM and Mr Bob Simpson of the RAE.

The AR 5 is to be worn beneath the RAF's latest protective helmet, the Mark 4. Rather surprisingly perhaps, we only have to go back to 1951 to find the very first of the 'bone-domes', the Mark 1 Protective Helmet. Before that, helmets – flying helmets as they were then called – were all of the cloth or chrome leather variety, which offered little by way of impact protection. The very first of these had, as we have seen, entered service during the final months of World War I, and it remained the RAF's only flying helmet until 1930. It was then replaced by the Type B, which accommodated the latest developments in radio-communication. With the similar cork Type A, intended for wear in hot climates, it saw service until 1942. It was never very satisfactory, however, being too tight and too hot. By the time a replacement was being considered, responsibility for helmet design had been transferred from the Director of Equipment's organization to the Physiological Laboratory and the RAE. At the Lab, John Gilson was involved in the design of the new helmet, the Type C, which besides being comfortable, could be used with the Types E and G oxygen masks. Variants of the C made of khaki, aertex and cloth were also produced, and all remained in service for several years after the war.

That the RAF acquired a protective helmet at all was largely due to the Navy – in 1951 the Admiralty had raised a requirement for a protective helmet for Naval aircrew.[17] Three years before, the Air Staff had actually stated that there was no requirement for a crash-helmet for pilots of high-speed aircraft. Because the helmet was ostensibly being produced for the Navy, much of the early development work was carried out by the Navy. However, the man tasked with the job was none other than Surgeon Lieutenant John Rawlins, who at that time was just beginning what was to be a very long tour of duty at the IAM.

The helmet he designed and built became known as the RAF Mark 1. Made of laminated nylon, it was designed as an over-helmet to be worn on top of the cloth Type G flying helmet, a lineal descendant of the Type C. Having to wear two helmets caused problems, not least of which was the tendency of the protective helmet to blow off during ejection. In 1960, therefore, it was decided to develop a Mark 2 protective helmet which would be an integral assembly. Dr J.E. Gabb was responsible for much of the preliminary design and development work, and he also devised testing procedures for determining the degree of impact protection afforded by helmets. Subsequently, under the guidance of David Glaister, the Institute would become an internationally recognized authority on standards for helmet design, making important contributions not just in the military sphere but also in the provision, for example, of head protection for motor-cyclists and climbers. Aircrew helmets damaged in accidents are also sent to the Institute, where tests and examination provide valuable information on causes of structural failure, and aid in future design.

The Mark 2 is still in service with the RAF, although in 1966 it was joined by the Mark 3. Although successful, the Mark 2 was generally regarded as being too bulky, and very little saving in weight had been achieved compared with the Mark 1. Weight is always a problem with protective helmets. The early British reservations regarding the very first protective helmet introduced by the

Americans in 1950, the Lombard helmet, were based on the assumption that during high-g manoeuvres too great a load would be imposed on the neck. Ironically British helmets have subsequently always been heavier than their American counterparts. This is because the British consider impact protection to be the most important consideration, whilst the Americans regard protection against buffeting during ejection as of paramount importance.

The Mark 3 helmet is basically the same as the 2, the only difference being in the mechanism for operating the visors. So the criticism regarding weight and bulk still remained. One or more visors which protect against glare, wind blast to the face, and the havoc that can be created by a bird striking the cockpit canopy, have been a feature of all recent protective helmets.

An attempt to reduce the weight of the helmet has been made with the Mark 4. Indeed, the basic shell is lighter, largely as a result of cutting away the sides near the face, and the back. However, this achievement has been largely nullified by the greater weight of the latest visor system which is incorporated into the helmet. Not everything has been lost, however, as the cut-away sides of the helmet have resulted in a significant increase in visual field – a vitally important factor in air combat. In contrast to the Marks 1 and 2, no single person can be credited with the design of the Mark 4. It has very much been a team effort, involving staff from both the IAM and the RAE. However, like all previous helmets it is manufactured by the firm of 'Helmets Limited', and it will shortly enter service, eventually replacing all other designs.

11 'Coffins or Crackers'

The expression 'coffin or crackers' was coined by the bomber crews in World War II who,[1] at one stage, had about a one-in-ten chance of surviving a full tour of thirty sorties; roughly translated, if the Hun didn't get you, the 'Funny Farm' would! Neurosis induced by the pressure of wartime flying was taken very seriously by the RAF Medical Branch, and an intensive research programme was mounted to identify and alleviate what Martin Flack had first described as 'flying stress'.[2] It is now recognized that flying stress has many causes, ranging from physical factors such as noise, vibration, heat and cold, which simply make flying uncomfortable, to the physiological consequences of those physical factors if the airman is not adequately protected, and to psychological factors such as anxiety, depression, fear of death and general problems of morale.

The precursor to neurosis is often fatigue, and fatigue itself is a serious condition because it can lead to accidents – or at least that is what James Birley thought in World War I[3] and what Air Commodore Whittingham thought in June 1939, when he proposed to the FPRC that suitable tests for measuring fatigue should be devised and that recommendations should be submitted to the Air Ministry regarding how fatigue could be avoided.[4] Because the issues involved in flying fatigue were psychological rather than physiological, and because the Professor of Psychology at Cambridge University, F.C. Bartlett, was a member of the Committee, it was logical that the necessary researches should be carried out in his department. Another advantage of Cambridge was that nearby was an RAF Initial Training School, which could provide a research team with an ideal supply of experimental subjects. So for a while the Psychological Laboratory at Cambridge became the psychological equivalent of the Physiological Laboratory at Farnborough. And the man who was given the job of devising a test for measuring flying fatigue was Kenneth Craik.

We have already referred to Craik's work on dark adaptation and cockpit illumination for the Physiological Laboratory. A brilliant scientist, in 1944, aged only thirty, he became the first Director of a new Unit for Research in Applied Psychology at Cambridge, only to die, tragically, just two years later in a cycle accident. In 1940, however, he designed the piece of equipment for which the Psychological Laboratory was to become most famous, the Cambridge Cockpit.

The Cambridge Cockpit was actually a Spitfire cockpit donated by Farnborough. It had intact controls and was fitted with an instrument panel very similar to the 'real thing'. All instruments on the panel could be mechanically operated by the experimenter. Their appearance was almost the same as those of an aircraft in flight, and they responded in a realistic manner to the actions of the pilot, whose timing and accuracy were objectively recorded. Thus the pilot could be 'sent out' on a simulated flight of any duration, and throughout all his movements would be recorded and then analysed afterwards. The hypothesis that Bartlett set out to test was that fatigue was a major factor causing pilot error and that consequently, as fatigue increased towards the end of a long sortie, so errors would become more frequent. As he pointed out to the FPRC, 'Without exception every serious and prolonged investigation of flying accidents that has ever been made has come to the conclusion that a very large number of such accidents are due to mistakes made by the pilots or some other member of the aircrew.'[5] Bartlett went on to put the fraction of accidents attributable to human error at 'about seventy per cent'. Writing after the war, Air Marshal Whittingham put the figure even higher, at eighty per cent.[6] To lose highly trained aircrew because of enemy action was one thing; to lose aircrew because of mistakes was entirely another. For the RAF this was a tragic, unacceptable waste of men and machines. However, after more than three years of careful experimentation involving several hundreds of subjects, the hypothesis, if not actually proven false, was certainly not proved true. Certainly pilots made mistakes, and the total number of mistakes tended to increase during the first part of the test, but only for a half hour or so, after which they declined. Some types of error, for example, allowing the aircraft to drift off course or failing to take an instrument reading, did tend to occur more often towards the end of a 'flight', but these could not be satisfactorily explained in terms of fatigue. The difficulties then, as now, were the enormous between-subject variability and the intermittency of error responses.

What the experiments did show was that temperamental factors were of great importance in determining the safety of an individual as a pilot. Errors depended upon stability of skill under stress, and in some pilots skill was affected adversely not just by stress but also by the anticipatory tension of stress.

This failure to ascribe a specific role to fatigue in the causation of flying accidents was supported by no less than four quite separate investigations. In the first of these Professor Bradford Hill, the eminent statistician and FPRC member, with Wing Commander G.O. Williams, investigated the rates of landing accidents at the end of operational sorties of different lengths. In sorties of between two and ten hours (the most common sortie duration), there was no increase in accident rate with sortie time, and therefore no evidence that fatigue caused accidents that did occur.[7] The accident rate was higher in sorties less than two hours, probably due to aircraft being recalled because of some special difficulty, and also in sorties of longer than ten hours – and here fatigue may have been a contributory factor.

In 1943 a series of experiments was conducted on behalf of the FPRC at the RAF Station at Harrogate.[8] The aim was to discover what qualities were associated with various forms of inefficiency in bomber pilots. Tests of the type employed in personnel selection and interviews were used, and about one-third of the one thousand or so pilots investigated were also given a cockpit test. An important finding was that a small proportion of pilots had significantly more accidents than others; in other words, some were accident-prone. Furthermore, it seemed that these accident-prone pilots could be identified by psychiatric assessment, although the end of the war supervened before this could be confirmed.

Finally Squadron Leader D.D. Reid carried out two surveys of errors made by the crews of bomber aircraft flying sorties over enemy-occupied territory.[9] In both, the error rate was greatest at times when emotional stress was at a peak – for example, as when crossing well-defended areas. There was no increase towards the end of flights as would have been expected had fatigue been an important factor.

Until the Cambridge Cockpit experiments were carried out, it had been assumed that flying fatigue was the major, if not the only, cause of 'human error' and that, consequently, if fatigue could be eliminated, then the accident rate would diminish. In one sense, therefore, the experiments dispelled a myth – a myth that fatigue caused accidents. However, both the Cambridge Cockpit and the Harrogate experiments had indicated that some pilots were really not that good at their job and that perhaps, therefore, the selection procedure for aircrew was not sufficiently rigorous. Indeed, it had been obvious for some years that there was something wrong with the RAF's method of selecting pilots. In 1939, of the many hundreds who were accepted for pilot training, only forty-one per cent reached a stage when they could fly operationally. Nearly thirty per cent of candidates failed even to make it through preliminary training. Despite the fact that this wastage was costing the RAF some £120 MILLION EACH YEAR,[10] virtually no steps had been taken between the wars to improve selection procedures, which is truly astounding when considered in terms of how much money might have been saved. As early as 1925 Whittingham had appreciated the importance of 'weeding-out' inefficient aviators, and he had written a paper suggesting various tests, later adopted, which might be of some help.[11] The only other advance during the inter-war period had been the development by Squadron Leader Williams and Dr E.J. Shuster of the Sensori-Motor Apparatus No.3, or SMA 3. This apparatus required candidates to carry out co-ordinated movements of one arm and both legs, whilst being distracted by visual or auditory stimuli which had to be cancelled using the other arm. William and Shuster found that their new apparatus provided a good indication of flying ability, just as the Reid Reaction Tester had done many years before. Williams had also modified two other tests used by industrial psychologists for studying causes of accidents, and Professor Bartlett considered that these, with the SMA 3, 'should at once become a part of the routine examination at entry ... and that failure in them should be made a basis for immediate rejection'.[12] However, his recommendation was not accepted by the Air Ministry, probably for two reasons. First, whilst Williams' tests certainly eliminated many of those unlikely to pass successfully through the course of flying training, they also eliminated a few who almost certainly would have been successful. It is clear that Bartlett knew, and that the entire Cambridge team knew, that a perfect 'psychological filter' was an impossible dream;[13] the Air Ministry, however, did not know it. Second, the Air Staff wanted to distinguish between potential fighter pilots and potential bomber pilots; the former were assumed to be individuals who 'get into their stride at once' and who 'do best when they work in short, intense, spurts', whilst the latter required 'a longer "warming-up" period' and were 'better when they have longer periods of concentration'.[14] For reasons which were not made clear even to Professor Bartlett, the Air Ministry refused to evaluate the tests further despite the fact that the SMA 3 had already demonstrated its clear superiority to all other forms of test then available. What the Ministry demanded was a new set of tests developed 'mainly with a view to attempting to use techniques which might bring out fighter qualities more clearly'.

So at the beginning of the war there were NO tests in use for aircrew selection. There was just a board of serving officers 'who were afforded no more definite briefing than to find the right types'.[15] By implication, therefore, there were 'right' and 'wrong' types for aircrew duties, and officers were best at identifying 'the best type'. One can be forgiven for thinking that little had changed since the outbreak of the previous war. It had not, but it was about to. By early 1940, as part of the general assessment of the Aviation Candidate Selection Board, medicals and interviews were accompanied by verbal intelligence tests, an elementary mathematical test and a written (fifty-word!) essay test. Professor Bartlett was instrumental in devising these tests, and consequently they became known as the 'Bartlett Tests'. The Cambridge Psychological Laboratory also had a battery of twelve aptitude tests for evaluation, which were designed to try to discriminate between fighter and bomber pilots. These tests, which became known as 'Pre-selection Tests', took into account variation in physical, intellectual and temperamental qualities. One of them was the Cockpit Test. Over the next few months they were evaluated both at the Cambridge Laboratory and at the Initial Training Wings (where candidates for flying were sent for preliminary training before proceeding to a Flying Training School), and by the end of the year they had been reduced from twelve to five. By then the Air Ministry had decided to use the SMA 3 on all candidates who had passed the medical examination for flying – a welcome reversal of its earlier attitude towards Williams' apparatus.

At first there seems to have been strong support for the tests devised by the Cambridge psychologists, and four pre-selection units were actually established. However, by mid-1941 scepticism was being expressed by the Director of Flying Training, Air Commodore the Hon. R.A. Cochrane, regarding their value. He pointed out that the results obtained from the tests were no better than those obtained from service assessments. These were standard tests at prescribed intervals during a twelve-hour period of initial flying training, conducted by RAF staff. Although, as Professor Bartlett pointed out, the pre-selection tests discovered in hours what the service took months to do, the fate of the Cambridge battery of selection tests was sealed by a damning report from Professor Bradford Hill, who considered that the opinion of the pre-selection teams seriously biased the assessment.[16] This ended the involvement of the Psychology Laboratory in the development of pre-selection tests, which thereafter became the responsibility of Professor E.A. Bott, a Canadian from Toronto University, who centralized all work on selection and training under one authority. What eventually emerged in 1944 was a two-day testing programme that involved a battery of aircrew aptitude tests designed to yield aptitude measures for all categories of aircrew. Many of the tests were American in origin. Only two were from the Cambridge Psychological Laboratory, and one of these was the SMA 3. Whether the 'Air Ministry approved' test battery was any better or was any more successful than the original twelve tests proposed by Professor Bartlett and his team would have been is impossible to say, as there was never any comparison. Indeed, by the time the 'Aircrew Aptitude Test Battery' became generally available to the selection boards, the war was just about over!

Improving selection procedures to 'get the right type' was a very indirect way of trying to reduce flying stress. What needed to be done was to eliminate the causes of that stress. Unfortunately, as Bomber Command knew to its cost, there did not seem to be much that could be done, at least in the short term, about the most serious cause of flying stress – poor morale. It had always been anticipated that anxiety and depression would be a common problem, but only in those who had been fatigued by long periods of operational duty. What actually happened in Bomber Command was that, once heavy losses started to be sustained with the inception of daylight bombing operations, morale plummeted and neurotic breakdowns multiplied, reaching a peak in the winter of 1942–43, even though by then daylight bombing had long been replaced by night attacks. In Fighter Command the problem was much less acute, although Training Command suffered the same high incidence.[17]

Why was morale so low in Bomber Command? The reasons were pretty clear, mainly as a result of reports received from the field medical officers and from Flying Personnel Medical Officers such as Corner and Huins, whose task it was to visit operational squadrons and investigate all aspects of aircrew morale. For example, the bomber captain, certainly early in the war, operated alone; at night navigation was difficult, and the weather often awful; night fighter attacks became increasingly effective as the war progressed; physical discomfort was acute during the first two years of the war, mainly, as we have already seen, due to cold; and there was the widely held (and correct) belief that the bombing was achieving little of military significance. As is now accepted, in the early years only about one third of all bombs actually fell within a five-mile radius of the target. To do any good, the bombs had to hit the target; if they did this, it was largely by chance. Often it was impossible to find the target because of cloud or industrial haze.[18]

One way of reducing the stress to which each man was subjected, and so reducing the chances of breakdown, was to restrict the amount of operational flying he was required to undertake. This became increasingly obvious as the war progressed, and when Whittingham became the DGMS, he arranged for some studies to be carried out. In 1942 Air Commodore Charles P. Symonds, the RAF Consultant in Neuro-psychiatry, with Wing Commander Denis J. Williams, a specialist in the same field, was tasked to investigate the factors that increased the risk of neurotic illness. Their findings[19] confirmed much that was already known or becoming known: i.e., that certain types of individual were more susceptible to breakdown than others; that emotional tension was the most important element of stress; and that existing methods of psychiatric assessment were capable of identifying a predisposition towards psychological disorders. Unfortunately these assessments identified the predisposition only *after* personnel had exhibited some psychological disorder, and consequently the RAF psychiatrists were unable to reduce the high incidence of breakdowns occurring after candidates had been through the selection procedures. The other finding of note from the study was 'that the 30 sortie limit was within the boundary of endurance for those who survived the first stage of an operational career'.[20] It is fair to conclude, therefore, that whilst important advances were made during the war in understanding psychological disorders in flying personnel and in appreciating the causes of poor morale, these were of little immediate benefit to the aircrew themselves except, perhaps, after they had become candidates for the 'Funny Farm'.

The other way of reducing flying stress was to make aircraft more comfortable to fly, and in trying to do just this the Cambridge Psychology Laboratory made some of its most important contributions to aviation during the war, whilst at the same time giving birth to a new science – ergonomics. Ergonomics is the study of work in relation to the environment in which it is performed and the personnel who perform it. The Laboratory pioneered the then (and perhaps still!) radical notion of considering the design of machines in terms of the needs of the human operators and applied this principle, in particular, to the design and positioning of aircraft controls. It was shown that correct design could eliminate errors of manipulation and reduce fatigue. Inappropriately located aircraft controls could lead to disaster, as demonstrated by the many accidents in the Mosquito aircraft which could be directly attributed to the asymmetric controls. Recommendations regarding principles of design, control and display were circulated to aircraft designers for consideration in connection with future aircraft types. Attempts were also made to improve instrument panel displays, which in many aircraft were haphazardly arranged, badly marked and poorly illuminated.

After the war, the ergonomics of cockpit design was to receive regular attention, although at Farnborough rather than at Cambridge, following the transfer of the RAF's psychology research programme to the Institute. To begin with, it was Ruffell-Smith who maintained the momentum of the Cambridge work, but during the 1950s the Institute's psychology research effort generally was boosted by the recruitment of several newly graduated psychologists. As far as the designers of aircraft cockpits were concerned, the problem was how to cram even more instruments into an extremely restricted workspace. The IAM's psychologists made recommendations concerning how the instruments should be arranged in terms of their relative importance and how sudden deviations from 'normal' readings might best be brought to the attention of the aircrew – for example, by using auditory or visual warning systems. Another consequence of the escalating complexity and sophistication of fast-jet aircraft is the greatly increased workload imposed on the aircrew, especially in the single-seat fighter, and this too has been subject of much investigation. The Institute has also studied, on behalf of British Airways and the Civil Aviation Authority, the workload imposed upon pilots during routine flights, with attention being focused on take-off and landing, which are both the most stressful and the most dangerous phases of flight.

Another aspect of the psychological research conducted at Farnborough has been the study of the effects of physical factors, such as vibration, noise and mild hypoxia, on performance. Even today flying military aircraft can be an uncomfortable business. It is obviously less so than it was during the First World War and probably less so than it was during the Second. Yet from the earliest days of flying it has been unusual to hear complaints. When complaints are made, it is safe to assume that something is seriously wrong. To airmen discomfort is simply part of the job; in time of peace it is an acceptable penalty for being allowed to indulge in what has recently been described as 'the sport of kings'[21]; in times of war it fades into insignificance besides more fundamental problems, like surviving. In other words, motivation overrides considerations which, in any other circumstances, might be expected to make the job intolerable. This is the major reason why it is difficult to show, in a laboratory environment, whether physical factors which might be expected to impair performance actually do so in the air. Particularly since the end of the last war, developments in protective flying clothing have done much to alleviate the worst effects of, for example, hypoxia, acceleration and cold, whilst advances in aircraft design and engineering have reduced, if not eliminated, some of the worst 'mechanical' sources of stress – vibration and noise being the most notorious examples. Vibration remains a serious problem in aircraft, especially helicopters, because at certain frequencies instruments become so blurred that they are impossible to read. However, it has been found that characteristics of instrument displays, such as luminance contrast and the amount of information presented, can have a profound effect on the intelligibility of a vibrating instrument. This, of course, has important implications for the design and layout of instrumentation and for how information is presented to the pilot.

Early in the war it had been assumed that the high level of noise prevailing in the cockpits of the bomber and fighter aircraft would have an adverse influence of flying efficiency. Rather surprisingly, however, a large number of laboratory experiments carried out using the Cambridge Cockpit failed to reveal any definite adverse effect of noise. On the other hand, the incessant roar of the engine during flight was certainly a strain on the aircrew, a strain which was aggravated by the poor communication system then in service.

Here again was the old familiar story. The end of World War I had seen the introduction of the Mark 1 flying helmet with mounted microphone and side pockets for earphones, which permitted ground-to-air and air-to-air communication. However, this very great advance in communications was neither improved nor exploited by the RAF, and it was to be the late 1930s before radio communication became widely adopted. Even then the system was highly unsatisfactory, great difficulties being experienced in receiving and interpreting signals transmitted from one aircraft to another. Professor Bartlett suggested that the whole problem be submitted for investigation to Dr A.F. Rawdon-Smith and Dr R.A. Sturdy, experts in electronics and psychology at Cambridge University. This suggestion was accepted, and over the next few months Rawdon-Smith and Sturdy proceeded to carry out a comparative evaluation of the existing RAF communication system, a new RAF set which was being developed by the RAE for the MAP, and a set of their own. The tests showed the Cambridge system to be considerably superior to both the RAF system, and Dr Rawdon-Smith very magnanimously put forward several constructive suggestions as to how the new RAF equipment, referred to as the A 1134, might be improved. It was eventually agreed that contracts be placed for the production for service trials of both communication systems. Unfortunately thereafter a series of misunderstandings regarding what had actually been agreed, and regarding the placing of contracts, led to increasingly acrimonious exchanges between those responsible for developing the two systems. In essence, the RAE maintained that, after making the suggested improvements in the A 1134 system, it was now just as good as the Cambridge system. A year later neither system had been introduced, comparative trials were still being conducted and the Rawdon-Smith set was still the better. In the absence of the necessary authority from the Air Ministry for the British manufacturer of this set, Pye Ltd of Cambridge, to proceed with full production, Air Marshal Whittingham, perhaps in exasperation, suggested that they might be made in the USA and fitted to aircraft supplied from there.[22] But it was not to be; the Rawdon-Smith communication set was never introduced, whilst the A 1134 was; aircrew had to suffer a second-rate system throughout the war. If there were extenuating circumstances which justified this appallingly negative official attitude towards a serious operational problem, then they are hard to find.

Neither is this the only example of an incomprehensible official attitude in the field of communications. Incredible though it may seem, the communication system used in training-aircraft at the outbreak of the war was based on Gosport tubes – even though electrical communication systems had been available for twenty years. In 1940 Professor Bartlett pointed out that a number of accidents in training aircraft could be attributed directly to this poor communication system.[23] Although improvements were supposedly being 'rapidly effected' early in 1940, Gosport tubes were still being used two years later, and it was September 1942 before a comprehensive programme of re-equipping training aircraft with an electrical intercommunication system was underway. Undoubtedly this reflected the delays in taking a decision about which communication system to adopt.

The ultimate aim of the IAM's psychology research programme is to try to reduce the potential for human error; hence the emphasis on information display, warning systems and workload. Laboratory evaluation of alternative systems is greatly facilitated by the Institute's research flight simulator, which can be programmed to reproduce the characteristics of various RAF aircraft. It is often used for workload studies, since one way of reducing the chance of human error is to give the human less to do. This is being made possible by the introduction of automatic navigational and weapon-guiding systems and by Head-Up Displays which give the pilots access to key information without his having to look down at his instruments. A reflecting panel directs the image from certain instruments to a point outside the cockpit canopy, so that the information displayed is superimposed upon the external world. As we have seen, this idea goes back to the days of Gilson and Pask. The problem in recent years has been deciding what symbology to use for presenting the necessary information, and it is in this area that the Institute's psychologists, notably Joe Huddleston, have led the field. Head-Up Displays are also one of the great success stories of British aviation technology, and they are to be found in many of the latest jet fighters.

It is not just in the air that there is potential for human error. Today air defence has become a highly complex operation, and the man on the ground is just as important as the man flying the aeroplane. Studies of the 'human factor' in the overall air-defence system began at Cambridge during World War II, then lapsed, but were picked up again by the IAM in 1956. Bill Stewart himself was the driving force behind this work. Possibly as a result of Bartlett's influence, he had become aware that psychology was just as important a part of aviation medicine as physiology and that consideration of human factor problems had, apart from Ruffell-Smith's work, been largely ignored. This point was certainly reinforced during a sabbatical leave he spent at McGill University, where he worked with the eminent Canadian psychologist Hebb. On his return, studies began of problems of tracking and control of guided weapons, and of human performance at following radar displays. And closely allied to the work on human factors in air-defence systems has been that on human factors in air-traffic control. Essentially the problems are the same – the integration of a large number of operators into a single functioning system. In 1964, following preliminary trials of various air-traffic control systems, the Institute participated in talks with various interested authorities on the desirable impact of human factors on air-traffic control, and since then there has been continuous participation by IAM psychologists in air-traffic control evaluation. From 1974 this work has been formally supported by the Civil Aviation Authority, which also provides the necessary funding.

Another problem with which the RAF has always had to contend is airsickness, although it was only in 1940, with the vast increase in the number of aircrew trainees, that its operational significance came to be appreciated; for then airsickness became a major cause of drop-out from flying training, whilst at the same time becoming a recurrent, albeit minor problem on operational squadrons. Roland Winfield carried out a thorough investigation of the problem for the FPRC which revealed, hardly surprisingly, that the most common cause of airsickness was 'bumpy' weather. This was the main reason why Coastal Command was worst afflicted; the average height of a patrol was one thousand feet, where bumpy conditions were more likely to be met than at higher altitudes. However, noise, cold and vibration were also contributory factors. Another problem was the food eaten by the aircrew during the long patrols, which could last up to twelve hours. A high carbohydrate diet was recommended, but in practice crew had to make do with what rations could be acquired from the mess beforehand. These usually took the form of tinned food and meals that had to be cooked on board; and the only convenient means of cooking was by frying. So not only did the sickly smell of frying meat waft around the cabin, but also the crews were served with greasy, fatty foods, hardly ideal for a queasy stomach.[24]

Some personnel did suffer severely from airsickness – those air-lifted in the big troop-carrying aircraft, for example, and also those unlucky enough to be carried by glider. According to Roland Winfield, even pilots who had never been airsick in their lives would be sick within minutes in a glider. Since air-lifted troops are often required to be fully operational on landing, particularly in wartime, this was a serious problem. For the same reason airsickness amongst paratroopers was always a cause for concern, and both Roland Winfield and his brother were involved in medical aspects of paratroop selection and training programmes. It was clear, therefore, that something had to be done to try to reduce the debilitating effects of airsickness in such personnel. Winfield had helped to identify the cause; what about the cure?

The short answer is that none was found. Of the many drugs tried, hyoscine ('Quells') was the only really effective one, as it still is. Attempts have been made, periodically, to predict predisposition to airsickness, but these have not met with any success. The only real advance in the treatment of airsickness has been the desensitization programme for aircrew initiated by Group Captain Tom Dobie (now retired) in the mid 1960s. The basis of his treatment was to expose the subject to repeated provocative stimuli, as similar as possible to those actually experienced in flight but graded in duration and intensity so that adverse symptoms were kept to a minimum. This could best be accomplished on the ground, and Dobie used a turntable on which the subject could be tilted to induce symptoms of motion-sickness. Over a period of days the severity of the stimuli would be increased by appropriately altering the speed of the turntable and increasing the number of tilts during any one run. In successful cases, about two to three weeks were necessary before a satisfactory degree of 'acclimatization' was achieved, and the subject then went on to a course of rehabilitation flying. Over the next few years Group Captain Dobie returned thirty-eight pilots, all of whom were regarded as suffering from intractable airsickness, to full, unrestricted flying.

From the beginning Dobie maintained a close liaison with the IAM and especially with Dr Alan Benson, who for many years has been responsible for all the Institute's work on problems of balance and disorientation with which airsickness is associated. Since 1976 the desensitization programme has gradually been transferred to the Institute from the RAF College at Cranwell. Now the subject sits in a box on a stable turntable and, under instruction, moves his head forwards or sideways as he is rotated – a very effective way of inducing nausea! The rehabilitation flying programme is also conducted at Farnborough using the Institute's Hunter aircraft. So far a dozen or more pilots have been treated annually at the Institute, and of these potential losses to the Air Force, about seventy per cent have been sent back to full operational duties. Not only is the cost of the desensitization programme itself covered several-fold, but the financial gain to the RAF represents a substantial fraction of the Institute's total research budget.

The treatment of airsickness forms only part of a dedicated research effort aimed at identifying the causes and nature of disorientation. Disorientation has always been regarded as a potential cause in many fatal accidents not attributable primarily to mechanical failure. Yet, surprisingly, until the mid 1950s the only research conducted in this important area, at least in the UK was that of Sir Henry Head at the close of World War I. What prompted the renewed interest was the realization that the greater angular and linear accelerations of which the second-generation jet aircraft were capable might produce serious disorientation. Then Squadron Leader Melvill Jones from the IAM on visiting operational squadrons, discovered that most aircrew considered disorientation a problem even in the slower, first-generation jet aircraft. As a direct result, he initiated a programme of research which continues to this day, the main aim of which is to determine how the eyes and the vestibular apparatus of the inner ear appear in certain situations to act in conflict, producing symptoms of nausea and disorientation. Studies have been made, using a specially constructed rotating chair, to discover how factors like rotation and oscillation influence a pilot's perception of his orientation in flight. This research contrasts in one important respect with that carried out into the physiological effects of hypoxia, acceleration, heat and cold; against these some protection can be provided, whilst against disorientation it cannot. The only action that can be taken is to establish by experiment where the human limits lie and then to persuade the engineers not to design systems which require these limits to be exceeded.

It is also important that the aircrew themselves appreciate where their limits lie. If they could be made aware, at a very early stage, of the causes and effects of disorientation and then learn strategies for coping with these effects, perhaps incidents and accidents caused by disorientation would be reduced. With this notion in mind, the Institute has designed and built a Spatial Disorientation Familiarization Device (SDFD) which has been installed at the Royal Air Force Aviation Medicine Training Centre at RAF North Luffenham for the specific purpose of demonstrating to aircrew the 'fallibility of their senses'. This device, which is basically a cab containing various displays mounted on a turntable, permits the demonstration of a number of the most common vestibular illusions and visual disturbances encountered during flight. Since its introduction in October 1974, the device has received wide acceptance not just from students but also from experienced aircrew. Indeed, so successful has the 'illusion familiarization' programme been that a second SDFD was installed at North Luffenham in 1978.

Of course, it is always possible to try to extend human limits artificially – with drugs. During the last war there was great interest in drugs for reducing fatigue, and as early as 1940 the FPRC were offered a wonder drug, Bioglan, which would reduce nervous strain, induce tranquillity and a spirit of calm confidence, maximize concentration and mental alertness, allay emotional instability, confer a capacity for instantaneous decision and provide practical immunity from infection.[25] And all this could be achieved by two injections per week for six weeks, at a cost of just £5.10s. The Committee was not impressed. Neither was it impressed by a suggestion that aircrew fatigue might be reduced by either 'supercharging the tissues of the body with oxygen' – by direct injection – or by exposing aircrew to UV radiation.

On the other hand the Committee was interested in any artificial means by which the effect of fatigue might be delayed or prevented. To begin with, it was thought that sleep would be a major problem, since the noise from air attack and ground defence would be so great that aircrews would be unable to sleep. A search was therefore begun for suitable 'British drugs which would give sound sleep without deleterious after-effects'.[26] Forty years on, that search is still continuing. However, early in the war emphasis quickly shifted to methods of reducing fatigue, and the archives of the FPRC are replete with investigations into, and claims for, the supposedly beneficial effects of vitamins, food supplements, minerals and even extracts of body tissues known to be concerned with resistance to stress, such as the adrenal cortex. Consideration of the latter was initiated following a report that the Germans had shifted fifty tons of adrenal glands to Germany from South America! The conclusion was always the same – no demonstrable effect in normal, healthy subjects. The only agent that was ever officially sanctioned for use in preventing fatigue was the stimulant drug benzedrine. It had become known early in the war that this was being used by the Germans, and so Roland Winfield arranged for trials of the drug to be conducted using crews from Coastal and Bomber Commands. The outcome of the trials was generally favourable, although some subjects found it difficult to sleep for many hours after taking benzedrine. Consequently the drug was never widely used, tending to be issued by squadron medical officers only for specific missions when fatigue was likely to be a problem.

In more recent years the Institute has become very actively involved in the study of drugs which may help aircrew perform their duties more effectively. The major problem facing the RAF is that, in times of tension or war, its personnel, particularly the aircrew, will be obliged to work under extremely disturbed and irregular conditions of rest and activity. A rather similar problem routinely affects civil aircrew operating on transmeridian, long-haul routes, when disturbance of the normal twenty-four-hour body rhythms disrupts normal sleep patterns. In both cases the results are increased fatigue and reduced operational effectiveness. Under Group Captain Tony Nicholson, the man who carried out the anti-g suit work in the early 1960s, the Institute has become recognized internationally as a centre for research into the effects of drugs both on performance and on sleep and wakefulness. In essence, the problem is to find a drug which will put a pilot to sleep and yet have little after-effect when he wakes up. As all drugs have some after-effects, this is by no means an easy task.

By using a battery of performance tests, confirmed with recordings of the electrical activity of the brain and heart, a number of drugs have been identified which do not disturb sleep patterns and which are without any significant adverse effect on awakening. The use of changes in the brain's electrical activity for determining whether sleep is impaired by a drug is a technique which has been pioneered by the Institute. As these changes may be fairly small and there can be literally hundreds of yards of either paper or magnetic tape with data for analysis, the problem has been how to reduce all the information to manageable proportions. Dr Mick Byford, for many years the IAM's 'computer king', has developed a technique for the automatic analysis of the electrical records, and so now brain activity can be used, routinely, as an indicator not just of the effects of drugs but of stress and fatigue. For example, it has been used in the aircrew workload studies conducted for the Civil Aviation Authority.

The IAM's drug-research programme is not restricted just to sleep-inducing drugs. Since the RAF requires a twenty-four-hour operational capability, the search is still on for the ideal stimulant. Certainly better drugs than benzedrine are now available. Other drugs being evaluated are those which may be prescribed for therapeutic purposes, such as the anti-allergy drugs, and drugs which lower blood-pressure. In general, aircrew undergoing a course of treatment with drugs are 'grounded'. However, if specific therapeutic agents could be shown to have no adverse side effects – for example, an anti-hayfever drug which did not cause drowsiness – then a change in policy might be possible.

12 The Achievement

The RAF Institute of Aviation Medicine's *raison d'être* is neatly encapsulated by its motto: *Ut secure volent* – 'That they may fly safely'. A measure of the Institute's achievement is provided by the success with which the ideals implicit in the motto have been realized – at least it is if some criteria on which to judge 'success' can be agreed. In fact, there are in science well-recognized indices of excellence, of individuals, departments and institutions. Quality of scientific achievement is measured by papers in prestigious journals, by invitations to present lectures to learned societies, by requests for advice and assistance and by the respect which only original contributions to science can earn. On all of these counts the RAF Institute of Aviation Medicine has been judged and has not been found wanting.

But is this enough? After all, it is essentially just a judgement, albeit a peer judgement, of scientists by scientists. Whilst there may be no argument that those qualified in science are best able to assess the quality of science, are they necessarily also best qualified to assess its value? And if not, who is? Perhaps it is the historian. As Friedrich von Schiller wrote, '... history is the world's court of judgement'.[1] If the British achievement in aviation medicine is to be properly judged in that court, then the evidence must first be submitted, and it must be submitted in a manner comprehensible to a jury not all members of which will be familiar with the language and idiosyncrasies of the scientist. Chapters 1 to 11 represent our submission to Schiller's court.

In departing from orthodox scientific objectivity, especially when trying to determine the value of a nation's contributions to and achievements in a particular scientific discipline, there is a very real danger of appearing chauvinistic. Also, since the British were such late arrivals on the aviation medicine scene, there is a certain risk of being accused of arrogance. After all, apart from the brief but productive flowering at the end of World War I, the British achieved very little until 1939. The world's very first School of Aviation Medicine was American, founded in 1918 – although it had virtually 'died' only seven years later. Today several countries besides Britain and America pursue research programmes in aviation medicine. Hopefully our history will be seen to have avoided the Scylla of chauvinism and the Charybdis of arrogance and yet to have demonstrated that British aviation medicine has realized the ambition expressed in '*Ut secure volent*'.

These twin dangers apart, there is another difficulty – our story is recent history. As Peter Howard succinctly points out, 'Data and opinion from the remote past may be difficult to amass, but they are comparatively easy to describe because, despite the ancient tag, it is permissible to be sharply critical of the dead.' Our task might have been made easier had longevity not been such a dominant characteristic of many of the key practitioners of aviation medicine in Britain! On the other hand, data and opinion from the remote past make for sterile history; human anecdote and experience make for living history. The personal records of men like Whittingham, Matthews, Gilson, Macdonald, Rawlins, Roxburgh, Ruffell-Smith and Barwood have, we believe, added colour and vitality to the story of how Britain has helped man fly in safety.

In judging the achievement, it is perhaps worth asking how it compares with the achievements of others – of the Americans, for example. Is the British contribution to aviation medicine unique? How the Americans themselves regarded British aviation medicine during the last war is demonstrated by reference to a memorial lecture given by Major General Harry G. Armstrong in honour of Air Vice-Marshal Stewart, in 1969.[2] Speaking of the co-operation between the two nations in aviation medicine, he said that, 'There can be no question that this program was an important factor in the winning of the air war and the ultimate Allied victory.' He went on to point out that the joint research effort 'greatly reduced the wound and death rate of the airmen involved'. What is so remarkable about the British achievement is that until August 1939 there was virtually no aviation medicine research being conducted in Britain, and yet just a few years later Britain led the world. This was, of course, an achievement born out of dire necessity. Without Matthews' Oxygen Economizer and without Stewart's raised rudder pedals, physiological limitations would have seriously compromised the British airman's fighting potential. Beyond any doubt, finely poised as the war in the air was in 1940, the help provided by the RAF Physiological Laboratory was crucial. If the solutions to the problems of protecting against hypoxia and acceleration were, as later developments would show, not ideal, they did work, and in 1940 that was all that mattered.

After the war, whilst maintaining a close association, the Americans and British have tended to go their own ways. The Americans have their own anti-g suits, their own oxygen masks and regulators and their own flying clothing assemblies – as do many other nations. In most cases, however, there is a basic similarity indicative of a common ancestry, an ancestry the origin of which lies with the wartime researches not just of the British and Americans but of the Germans too. Occasionally one nation will steal a march on the others. The Americans, learning from the Germans, were the first to develop the modern demand oxygen regulator, for example. More recently it has been the British who have taken the lead in the development of the NBC clothing – to the benefit not just of NATO but of the trade balance too! Strangely, however, achievements in aviation medicine are not usually measured in terms of one nation outdoing another. As Harry Armstrong observed, 'There is in aviation medicine a remarkable spirit of co-operation at the international level which is seemingly much greater than for any of the other sciences.'

Whilst the spirit of the Institute's motto may transcend national boundaries, it is only proper that some positive benefit should accrue to the nation that pays for the research. To put it crudely, what does the British taxpayer get for his money? In fact, as we have pointed out (Chapter 11), the Institute contributes significantly towards its own running costs, and so the burden on the taxpayer can hardly be described as onerous – unless, that is, the RAF itself is regarded as a needless expense, and this, we suspect, would be a minority view. Nevertheless, financial considerations are not the only ones that matter. Have there been any other benefits?

To some it may seem unfortunate that aviation medicine in general, and our history in particular, has such a strong military bias – to which one response might be that it is unfortunate that so much of scientific research has a strong military bias; witness the recent furore over the 'peaceful exploitation' of space, which both the Americans and Russians are attempting to fill with military hardware. However, aviation medicine does have a non-military aspect. Civil aviation medicine was born out of military aviation medicine, and most of its early practitioners were (and some still are) ex-RAF and Royal Navy doctors more familiar with combat aircraft and combat flying than with the mundane, unspectacular problems of commercial aviation – problems such as aircrew selection, route planning, aircraft design and disease control. Mundane and unspectacular though they may be, these problems are not so dissimilar from those faced by the RAF. As we have seen, co-operation between the civil airlines, represented by the CAA and the RAF, represented by the IAM, is close, and this co-operation has led to important advances being made which have contributed significantly towards much greater flight safety. A classic example of this was the investigation into the cause of the Comet disasters in the early 1950s, which was conducted jointly by representatives of the airline concerned, the CAA, the RAE and the IAM. Whilst the loss of the two aircraft was a crushing blow to the British aviation industry, the application of the lessons learned about metal fatigue undoubtedly saved thousands of lives later.

Then there are benefits of a more medical kind. David Glaister's work on the relationship between the structure of the human lung and its function has, as we have seen (Chapter 7), yielded new insights into how the lungs work which have direct application to understanding the aetiology of certain lung diseases. Alan Benson's work on disorientation and motion-sickness has considerable diagnostic implications, whilst the widespread general application of Tony Nicholson's research into sleep-inducing drugs, and into stimulants which are neither addictive nor have adverse side-effects, is obvious.

The Institute itself is a national asset from another point of view. It is unique within Europe not just in possessing all the capital research facilities so necessary for conducting co-ordinated research programmes in aviation medicine but also in having all these facilities together in one place. This results in greater economy of time, effort and money. Industry too avails itself of the remarkable hardware the Institute possesses, and so do the other two services and the universities – which is why it is such a tragedy that economic cuts are now threatening the very existence of what has become an important and respected part of Britain's scientific heritage. Ever since the early 1970s the Institute, along with many other national laboratories, has suffered savage cuts of its complement of scientists. Bans on recruitment, freezing of posts and the complete elimination of posts, have brought a halt to many research programmes, some of which could have led to developments of considerable economic benefit to the country, and others which would have contributed significantly to the greater understanding and better treatment of a number of medical conditions. The programmes which disappear are those which are considered to be of least short-term benefit, and this always means basic research. Yet, as history shows time and time again, it is from the discoveries which emerge, often accidentally, from basic researches that new technologies grow. Failure to recognize this fundamental fact of life in our scientific age is surely a significant factor contributing to the decline of what used to be justifiably and proudly referred to as 'Great' Britain.

The futility of short-term political and economic expedience is not the only lesson history teaches. As in many other success stories, the international respect and prestige that have come to Britain as a result of its contributions to aviation medicine are largely a result of the individual efforts of men like Whittingham, Stewart and Matthews. But they are the giants of aviation medicine not merely because they were innovative and academically brilliant men who achieved great things but more because they knew how to inspire others to give of their best too. They earned honour and respect because they were, above all else, capable of leading other men of science and medicine. Such leadership demands perspicacity and sagacity tempered with humanity. All too often, under the pressures of leadership, a capacity for profundity of thought becomes an excuse for intellectual arrogance. Brilliant men only rarely make brilliant leaders, and in Whittingham, Matthews and Stewart, Britain had three in one field of expertise at the same time. All three are remembered not just with respect but with affection too, probably because they always showed interest in and concern for the men and women they led; they knew when to call for order, but they knew too how to encourage with praise, appreciation and honesty. They also had the advantage of living and working through a period when first the RAF Physiological Laboratory and then the Institute of Aviation Medicine could be seen by all to be serving the airman who was living, and sometimes dying, 'at the sharp end'. This must have added both spice and excitement to those endless battles with pettifogging bureaucrats who, even in wartime, seemed more concerned with the maintenance of the *status quo* and with directing countless memoranda up and down endless channels than with the urgent needs of the men doing the fighting. As we have seen, there were many occasions when common sense did not prevail and when indecision meant that the poor airmen ended up both with second-rate equipment, and with equipment delivered long after the need for it had passed. Today there are still some criticisms about delays and inadequate personal equipment, and increasingly these criticisms are being directed not at the bureaucrats in London but at the IAM. This is because the Institute is becoming increasingly removed, through little fault of its own, from direct contact with the aircrew whom it exists to serve. If the spirit is still willing, the body is weak. Let us hope a proud tradition and glorious era are not to end in a sea of neglect.

We began by saying that the problems in aviation medicine have largely remained the same from the earliest days of aviation to the present; only the solutions have changed. Some hundred thousand words further on, this can be seen as not being quite true. Yes, the problems are the same, but so too are some of the solutions. It is just that the same solution is 'rediscovered' at regular intervals – sometimes intervals as little as ten years. The reason became obvious as we delved deeper and deeper into those filing cabinets bulging with reports of all shapes and sizes; nobody knew they were there, nobody knew what was in them, and few cared. So little of the material had been made generally available, and so transient was the 'passing through' the Institute of many of the reports' authors that, to quote William Cowper,

> Where once we dwelt our name is heard no more …
> 'Tis now become a history little known …[3]

We have brought some of these names and some of their achievements out of scientific obscurity and onto the world's stage. Those who for the sake of others regarded their own bodies 'as something to be used, and, if need be, used up' deserve no less.

References

Note: All FPRC documents were listed consecutively as they appeared. References to selected FPRC papers, minutes and reports therefore give only the serial number and date; the complete FPRC archives are now held by the RAF Institute of Aviation of Medicine.

1. *First Awakenings*

1. Frankland, N., *A Short History of the Royal Air Force*, Air Ministry Pamphlet 348, 1956, page 2.
2. Ibid., page 3.
3. Ibid., page 6.
4. Wells, H.V., *Journal of the R.N. Medical Service*, 1915(i): 55-60 and 1916(ii): 65-71.
5. Anderson, H.G. See Bibliography.
6. Heald, C.B., 'Genesis of Aviation Medicine in the Royal Flying Corps and Royal Air Force', Cabinet Office Historical Section, 1965.
7. Ibid., page 12.
8. Frankland, N., op.cit.

2. *All You Need is 'Hands'*

1. Rippon, T.S. and Manuel, E.G., *The Lancet*, 28 September 1918, pages 411-15.
2. James, A.W.H., *R.A.F. Quarterly*, 1930, 1: 534-8.
3. Medical Research Council Special Report No.53, 1920, *The Medical Problems of Flying*. This work details the experiments of Bazett, Briscoe, Cheatle, Corbett, Flack, Head and others.
4. Heald, C.B., op.cit., page 21.
5. Birley, J.L., *Bulletin of the Information Section, Air Service, A.E.F.*, 6 June 1918, Vol IV, no.182, page 3.
6. Dudley, S.F., *J.R.N. Medical Service*, 1918, 4: 131-40.
7. Birley, J.L., Goulstonian Lectures, published in *The Lancet* on 29 May, 5 and 12 June 1920.
8. Greer, L. and Harold, A. See Bibliography. The account of First World War flying clothing is based on this book.
9. Lucas, J., *The Big Umbrella* (1973), Chapter 6. See Bibliography.
10. Scott, S., Report of the Air Medical Investigation Committee, 1919, no. 37.
11. Reid, G.H. and Burton, H.L., *Proc. Roy. Soc. Med* (War Section), 1924, 17: 43-53.

3. *Ever Higher, Ever Faster*

1. Marshall, G.S., *J. Roy. Aero. Soc.*, 1933, 37: 389-410.
2. Marshall, G.S., unpublished paper to DMS (RAF), 24 June 1932.
3. Jacques, C.N., 24 June 1934, letter reference 256429/33/RD Inst 2/J.
4. Haldane, J.S. and Priestley, J.G. See Bibliography.
5. Davis, R.H. See Bibliography.
6. Marshall, G.S., 1933, op.cit.
7. Ibid.
8. Ibid.
9. Ibid.
10. FPRC 13, March 1939.

4. *Birth of 'The Lab'*

1. Livingston, P.C. See Bibliography.
2. Minutes of meeting held on file AF/A3328/64 Part 1.
3. FPRC 1, January 1939; FPRC 2, 9 February 1939; FPRC 13, 8 March 1939.
4. FPRC 37, 7 June 1939.
5. Ibid.
6. Macdonald, T.C. Personal communication.
7. Matthews, Sir Bryan. Personal communication, and FPRC 267, 27 March 1941.
8. FPRC 61a, September 1939.
9. FPRC 76, December 1939.
10. FPRC 186, 11 September 1940.
11. The accounts of Winfield's work during the war are partly taken from his book (see Bibliography) but are mainly based on his unpublished notes.
12. Roxburgh, H.L. Unpublished papers.
13. Ibid.
14. Macdonald, T.C. Personal communication.
15. FPRC 108, 17 March 1940.
16. Barwood, A.J. Personal communication.
17. Macdonald, T.C. Personal communication.
18. Matthews, Sir Bryan. Personal communication.
19. Farren, W.S., in letter P/DRAE/32 to DGMS dated 11 September 1942.
20. Goldie, E.A.G., *J.Sci.Inst.*, 1942, 19(2): 23-5.
21. FPRC 513, 23 February 1943.

5. *Growing in Stature*

1. FPRC 564, 25 January 1944.
2. FPRC 423(x), 12 September 1945.
3. FPRC 748, 13 October 1950.
4. FPRC 887, 21 July 1954.
5. FPRC 1040, 27 February 1958.
6. A.314847/58 dated 5 December 1958. Minutes of FPRC Working Party on future policy for the IAM.
7. ME Department Admin. Notice 1/61 dated 8 May 1961.
8. FPRC 1160, 3 August 1961.
9. Total calculated from the flight authorization books held by the IAM.
10. Ruffell-Smith, H.P. Personal communication.

11. Recounted in an expurgated form by Maycock (see Bibliography). The unexpurgated version was told to us by Group Captain Ruffell-Smith.

6. *Too Little Oxygen ...*

1. Cited by Ernsting, J. and Stewart, W.K., in *A Textbook of Aviation Physiology* edited by J.A. Gillies (see Bibliography), Chapter 11, page 212.
2. FPRC 511, January 1943.
3. FPRC 366, 15 October 1941.
4. FPRC 374, November 1941.
5. RAE Departmental Note No.H333, April 1939; SB1382/RD Inst 3, November 1943.
6. FPRC 111, March 1940.
7. FPRC 137, 8 May 1940.
8. Matthews, B.H.C. and Roxburgh, H.L., 29 January 1942. Enclosure 2 on RAF Physiological Laboratory file PL/24/13/2.
9. DGMS/5/23 dated 2 March 1944. The modifications did increase the output at altitude, where it was needed.
10. FPRC 70a, December 1939.
11. B.99635/40/RD Inst 2/A dated 20 September 1940. (Files with 'RD Inst.' in the title are MAP files, but the letters were sent to the RAF. Physiological Laboratory and are therefore held on Lab files.)
12. FPRC 232b, 25 January 1941.
13. Letter DAD/RD Inst., dated 13 May 1941.
14. RAE Technical Note No. Inst.743, February 1943.
15. Matthews, Sir Bryan. Personal communication.
16. Ernsting, J. Personal communication.
17. IAM Report No.R126, August 1959.
18. Glaister, D.H., PhD Thesis, University of London, 1966.
19. B.153842/40/RD Inst/A dated 28 March 1941.
20. B.153842/40/RD Inst 3/A dated 10 October 1941.
21. B.153842/40/RD Inst 3/A dated 4 December 1943.
22. Res.Inst.4223/RD Inst 3/EFA dated 12 March 1945.
23. PL/AJB dated 16 July 1946.
24. FC/S 41762/Ops Req dated 21 October 1952.
25. FE/15058/1/Med dated 12 May 1953.
26. IAM/1024/8/7 dated 11 June 1954.
27. Marshall, G.S. *Proc.Roy.Soc.*, 1937, 30: 995-1006.
28. CME/BM/38, dated 31 October 1939.
29. FPRC 267, 27 March 1941.
30. Unreferenced, undated (but probably 1942) report to FPRC on file PL/12/2.
31. CTP/G/1/73, dated 6 December 1943.
32. Cited by Brown, H.H.S. in *A Textbook of Aviation Physiology*, Chapter 9, pages 153-4. See Bibliography.
33. FPRC 437, March 1942.
34. C.39912/49 dated 31 May 1950.
35. This was not so much a pressure suit as a personal pressure compartment, containing a seat. It looked like a suit of armour, metal and articulated, and was made by Normalair Ltd. It is now in the Fleet Air Arm Museum.
36. IAM Report No. R320, April 1965.

37. Greene, R., in *The Lancet*, 17 November 1934, 1122-3.

7. ... *And Too Much Acceleration*
1. FPRC 13, 8 March 1939.
2. Armstrong, H.G. & Heim, J.W., *J. Aviat. Med.* 1938, 9: 199-214.
3. FPRC 233, January 1941.
4. Surprisingly little information concerning the early investigations at the Physiological Laboratory into blacking out is available from the records of the FPRC. The account here is based largely on Stewart's unpublished notes and on his paper, 'Some observations on the effect of centrifugal force in man', published in the *Journal of Neurology, Neurosurgery and Psychiatry, 1945, 8, 24-33.*
5. Ibid.
6. Gorham, W.G., 'Anti "G" Suits. The development and production of equipment which has enabled our fighters to outfly the enemy', published in the *Dunlop Digest* by the Dunlop Rubber Company, September 1945.
7. Interview with Dr W.R. Franks published in the *Newsletter* of the Canadian Society of Aviation Medicine, 1980.
8. Ibid.
9. Greig, D'Arcy A., 'Report on practical flying tests carried out with "Special Flying Suit" (designed by Dr Franks) between June 1st and June 5th, 1940 in Spitfire L.1090.'
10. FPMO Meeting Minutes, November 1943.
11. FPRC 584 and 584a, July 1944.
12. FPRC 407, January 1942.
13. Piper, R.K. Personal communication on behalf of the Australian Department of Defence, Historical Studies.
14. FPRC 599, October 1944.
15. Stewart, W.K., op.cit.
16. Mayer, M. *Air Surgeon's Bulletin*, August 1945, Vol.2, No.8.
17. PL/WKS 7/Inventions/5629 dated 19 November 1948.
18. Allen, G.R. Personal communication.
19. FPRC 500. November 1942.
20. FPRC 758a, May 1951.
21. Ruffell-Smith, H.P. Personal communication.
22. FPRC 943, November 1955.
23. FPRC 212, December 1940.

8. *Down to Earth*
1. Winfield, B.J.O. In FPMO Meeting Minutes, January 1946.
2. *History and Development of Martin-Baker Ejection Systems* (Martin-Baker Aircraft Company Ltd, Higher Denham, Middlesex, 1968).
3. Wragg, D.W., *A Dictionary of Aviation* (Osprey Publishers, Reading, 1973).
4. Jewell, J., *Engineering for Life*, (Martin-Baker Aircraft Company Ltd, 1979). The account of the ejection-seat work is based on this book and the publication at reference 2 above.
5. Howard, P., *Air Clues*, June 1962.
6. IAM Report No. R131, July 1959.

7. Rawlins, J.S.P., 'A summary of research carried out at the Royal Air Force Institute of Aviation Medicine, Farnborough, during the period January 1958 to December 1963.' The account of the underwater ejection research programme is based entirely upon this unpublished report.
8. Stapp, J.P., *J.Aviat.Med.*, 1955, 26: 268-88.
9. FPRC 1167, July 1961.
10. FPRC 274a, April 1941.

9. *To See or Not To See*
1. FPRC 75, December 1939.
2. Livingston, P.C., op.cit., p.187.
3. Reid, D.D. *Brit.J.Psych.* (Statistical Section), 1950, 3(3): 141-9.
4. FPRC 290, 21 March 1941.
5. FPMO Meeting Minutes, 1 November 1942.
6. FPMO Meeting Minutes, 2 August 1942.
7. FPRC 297, April 1941.
8. FPRC 315, 20 June 1941.
9. FPRC 706, 5 November 1948.
10. FPRC 756, 13 March 1951.
11. FPRC 957, 17 February 1956.
12. FPRC 1054, 17 July 1958.
13. FPRC 826, 31 March 1953.

10. *Dressed To Kill*
1. FPRC 231, January 1941.
2. FPRC 107c, April 1940.
3. Greer, L. and Harold, A. See Bibliography.
4. FPRC 389, December 1941.
5. FPRC 138, April 1940.
6. Pask, E.A., 'British Immersion Suits' in *The Maker-Up*, May 1946, 225-8. The account of the development of the RAF immersion suit is taken from this article.
7. FPRC 550, August 1943, and *Doctors in the Air* by R. Maycock. See Bibliography.
8. Smith, F.E., *Survival at Sea*, pp. 36-7. Royal Naval Personnel Committee report No. SS 1/74, December 1974.
9. FPRC 550a, February 1944.
10. Maycock, R., op.cit.
11. Clark, R., *The Life and Work of J.B.S. Haldane* (Hodder and Stoughton Ltd, London, 1968), p.61.
12. FPRC 1026, May 1958.
13. FPMO Meeting Minutes, July 1949.
14. RAE Technical Note No. M.E.400, 1964.
15. Aeroplane and Armament Experimental Establishment Technical Report No.343, Parts 1 and 2, 1967.
16. Quotation from a letter from OR26a (RAF) dated 3 July 1968.
17. FPRC 847, August 1953.

11. *'Coffins or Crackers'*
1. Reid, D.D., 'The historical background of War-time research in psychology and

psychiatry in the Royal Air Force', FPRC committee paper no.1696b, July 1976.
2. Flack, M., 'Flying Stress' MRC Air Medical Investigation Report, 1918.
3. Birley, J.L., First Goulstonian Lecture, *The Lancet*, 29 May 1920.
4. FPRC 44, June 1939.
5. FPRC 447, April 1942.
6. Whittingham, Sir Harold, *Brit.Med.J.*, 13 July 1946, pp. 39-42.
7. FPRC 423m, July 1943.
8. FPRC 529m, April 1944.
9. Russell-Davis, D., 'A lecture on fatigue in flying', University of Cambridge Applied Psychology Unit Report no.95/49, 1949.
10. FPRC 13e, February 1939.
11. Whittingham, H.E., *Journal of State Medicine*, 1925, Vol.33, pp.511-20.
12. FPRC 13e, op.cit.
13. FPRC 118, March 1940.
14. FPRC 13e, op.cit.
15. Vernon, P.E. and Parry, J.B. See Bibliography.
16. FPRC 404, January 1942.
17. Rexford-Welch, S.C., *The Royal Air Force Medical Services*, Vol.II, HMSO, 1955.
18. Frankland, N., *The Bombing Offensive Against Germany* (Faber and Faber, London, 1965).
19. Symonds, C.P. and Williams, D.J., *Psychological disorders in flying personnel of the Royal Air Force*, Air Publication 3139, HMSO, 1947.
20. Reid, D.D., op.cit.
21. *Fighter Pilot*, British Broadcasting Corporation documentary film, 1981.
22. FPRC 273, April 1941.
23. FPRC 226, December 1940.
24. FPRC 220a, December 1940.
25. FPRC 98, February 1940.
26. FPRC 46, July 1939.

12. *The Achievement*

1. Schiller, F. von., 'Resignation'.
2. Armstrong, H.G., *Aerospace Medicine*, 1969, 40 1169-75.
3. Cowper, W., 'On the receipt of my mother's picture'.

Bibliography

Anderson, H.G., *The Medical and Surgical Aspects of Aviation* (Oxford University Press, 1919). The first book on the subject. Contains many fascinating photographs.

Chant, C., *Aviation. An Illustrated History* (Orbis Publishing, London, 1978). A useful general history of aviation.

Davis, R.H., *Breathing in Irrespirable Atmospheres* (Siebe Gorman & Co Ltd; published privately). An interesting account of one firm's contributions. Well illustrated.

Dhenin, G.H. (editor), *A Textbook of Aviation Medicine*, two volumes (Tri-Med, London, 1978). A general account of aviation medicine principles.

Gillies, J.A. (editor), *Textbook of Aviation Physiology* (Pergamon, Oxford, 1964). A detailed account of aviation physiology. Now out of print.

Greer, L. and Harold, A., *Flying Clothing. The Story of its Development* (Airlife, England, 1979). Contains many interesting photographs. Text inaccurate in places.

Haldane, J.S. and Priestley, J.G., *Respiration* (Oxford University Press, 1920). An account of some of the early work on oxygen systems.

Jewell, J., *Engineering for Life* (Martin-Baker Aircraft Company Ltd, Denham; published privately, 1979). A history of the Martin-Baker Aircraft Company and Sir James Martin.

Livingston, P.C., *Fringe of the Clouds* (Johnson, London, 1962). Autobiography of a man who pioneered vision research in the RAF and who became DGMS.

Lucas, J., *The Big Umbrella* (Hamish Hamilton, London, 1973). A history of the parachute.

Maycock, R., *Doctors in the Air* (Geo. Allen & Unwin, London, 1957). An inaccurate, coy but well-known book about selected aspects of the IAM.

Penrose, H., *British Aviation. The Pioneer Years, 1903-14* (Cassell, London, 1967). An immensely detailed, well-illustrated and readable book.

Robinson, D.H., *The Dangerous Sky* (G.T. Foulis & Co. Ltd, Henley, Oxfordshire 1973). Aviation medicine history from the American viewpoint. Well readable.

Vernon, P.E. and Parry, J.B., *Personnel Selection in the British Forces* (University of London Press, 1949). Details of selection of aircrew during the Second World War.

Winfield, R.H., *The Sky Belongs to Them* (Kimber, London, 1976). Posthumously published autobiography. Concentrates on his exploits away from the IAM.

Index

Illustration numbers appear in italics